Caring for people with chronic conditions

A health system perspective

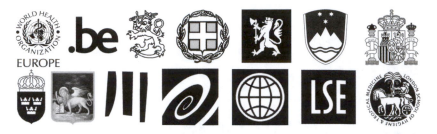

The European Observatory on Health Systems and Policies is a partnership between the World Health Organization Regional Office for Europe, the Governments of Belgium, Finland, Greece, Norway, Slovenia, Spain and Sweden, the Veneto Region, the European Investment Bank, the Open Society Institute, the World Bank, the London School of Economics and Political Science, and the London School of Hygiene & Tropical Medicine.

Caring for people with chronic conditions

A health system perspective

Edited by

Ellen Nolte and Martin McKee

Open University Press

Open University Press

Open University Press
McGraw-Hill Education
McGraw-Hill House
Shoppenhangers Road
Maidenhead
Berkshire
England
SL6 2QL
email: enquiries@openup.co.uk
world wide web: www.openup.co.uk
and Two Penn Plaza, New York, NY 10121–2289, USA

First published 2008

A catalogue record of this book is available from the British Library
ISBN 978 0 335 23370 0 (pb)
ISBN 978 0 335 23369 4 (hb)

Library of Congress Cataloging-in-Publication Data
CIP data applied for

Typset by RefineCatch Limited, Bungay, Suffolk
Printed in the UK by Bell and Bain Ltd., Glasgow

The McGraw·Hill Companies

European Observatory on Health Systems and Policies Series

The European Observatory on Health Systems and Policies is a unique project that builds on the commitment of all its partners to improving health care systems:

- World Health Organization Regional Office for Europe
- Government of Belgium
- Government of Finland
- Government of Greece
- Government of Norway
- Government of Slovenia
- Government of Spain
- Government of Sweden
- Veneto Region
- European Investment Bank
- Open Society Institute
- World Bank
- London School of Economics and Political Science
- London School of Hygiene and Tropical Medicine

The series

The volumes in this series focus on key issues for health policy-making in Europe. Each study explores the conceptual background, outcomes and lessons learned about the development of more equitable, more efficient and more effective health systems in Europe. With this focus, the series seeks to contribute to the evolution of a more evidence-based approach to policy formulation in the health sector.

These studies will be important to all those involved in formulating or evaluating national health care policies and, in particular, will be of use to health policy-makers and advisers, who are under increasing pressure to rationalize the structure and funding of their health system. Academics and students in the field of health policy will also find this series valuable in seeking to understand better the complex choices that confront the health systems of Europe.

The Observatory supports and promotes evidence-based health policy-making through comprehensive and rigorous analysis of the dynamics of health care systems in Europe.

Series Editors

Josep Figueras is Head of the Secretariat and Director of the European Observatory on Health Systems and Policies, and Head of the European Centre for Health Policy, World Health Organization Regional Office for Europe.

Martin McKee is Head of Research Policy of the European Observatory on Health Systems and Policies and Professor of European Public Health at the London School of Hygiene and Tropical Medicine as well as a co-director of the School's European Centre on Health of Societies in Transition.

Elias Mossialos is Co-Director of the European Observatory on Health Systems and Policies, and Brian Abel-Smith Reader in Health Policy, Department of Social Policy, London School of Economics and Political Science and co-director of LSE Health and Social Care.

Richard B. Saltman is Associate Head of Research Policy of the European Observatory on Health Systems and Policies, and Professor of Health Policy and Management at the Rollins School of Public Health, Emory University in Atlanta, Georgia.

European Observatory on Health Systems and Policies Series

Series Editors: Josep Figueras, Martin McKee, Elias Mossialos and Richard B. Saltman

Published titles

Primary care in the driver's seat
Richard B. Saltman, Ana Rico and Wienke Boerma (eds)

Human resources for health in Europe
Carl-Ardy Dubois, Martin McKee and Ellen Nolte (eds)

Health policy and European Union enlargement
Martin McKee, Laura MacLehose and Ellen Nolte (eds)

Regulating entrepreneurial behaviour in European health care systems
Richard B. Saltman, Reinhard Busse and Elias Mossialos (eds)

Social health insurance systems in western Europe
Richard B. Saltman, Reinhard Busse and Josep Figueras (eds)

Health care in Central Asia
Martin McKee, Judith Healy and Jane Falkingham (eds)

Hospitals in a changing Europe
Martin McKee and Judith Healy (eds)

Funding health care: options for Europe
Elias Mossialos, Anna Dixon, Josep Figueras and Joe Kutzin (eds)

Regulating pharmaceuticals in Europe: striving for efficiency, equity and quality
Elias Mossialos, Monique Mrazek and Tom Walley (eds)

Purchasing to improve health systems performance
Joseph Figueras, Ray Robinson and Elke Jakubowski (eds)

Decentralization in health care
Richard B. Saltman, Vaida Bankauskaite and Karsten Vrangbæk (eds)

Health systems and the challenge of communicable diseases
Richard Coker, Rifat Atun and Martin McKee (eds)

Contents

List of figures   ix
List of tables   xi
List of boxes   xiii
List of contributors   xiv
Forewords   xvi
Acknowledgements   xx

one   **Caring for people with chronic conditions: an
         introduction**   1
         Ellen Nolte and Martin McKee

two   **The burden of chronic disease in Europe**   15
         Joceline Pomerleau, Cécile Knai and Ellen Nolte

three   **Economic aspects of chronic disease and chronic
         disease management**   43
         Marc Suhrcke, Daragh K. Fahey and Martin McKee

four   **Integration and chronic care: a review**   64
         Ellen Nolte and Martin McKee

five   **Preventing chronic disease: everybody's business**   92
         Thomas E. Novotny

six   **Supporting self-management**   **116**
              Mieke Rijken, Martyn Jones, Monique Heijmans
              and Anna Dixon

seven   **The human resource challenge in chronic care**   **143**
              Carl-Ardy Dubois, Debbie Singh and Izzat Jiwani

eight   **Decision support**   **172**
              Nicholas Glasgow, Isabelle Durand-Zaleski, Elisabeth
              Chan and Dhigna Rubiano

nine   **Paying for chronic disease care**   **195**
              Reinhard Busse and Nicholas Mays

ten   **Making it happen**   **222**
              Ellen Nolte and Martin McKee

              Index   245

This volume has been produced with the generous support of the United
Kingdom Department of Health

List of figures

1.1 Health system activities covered in this book. 7
2.1 Burden of death and disease attributable to stroke in selected
countries in the World Health Organization European Region, 2002. 20
2.2 Estimated and projected prevalence of diabetes mellitus in 2003 and
2025 in selected countries in Europe. 23
2.3 Burden of death and disease attributable to diabetes in selected
countries in the World Health Organization European Region, 2002. 24
2.4 Burden of death and disease attributable to chronic obstructive
pulmonary disease (COPD) in selected countries in the World
Health Organization European Region, 2002. 26
2.5 Prevalence of clinical asthma in selected countries in Europe. 27
2.6 Burden of death and disease attributable to asthma in selected
countries in the World Health Organization European Region, 2002. 29
2.7 Burden of disease attributable to unipolar depressive disorder in
selected countries in the World Health Organization European
Region, 2002. 31
2.8 Frequency of multiple conditions in Germany, 2002. 33
4.1 Levels of integration and user need. 73
4.2 Population management levels of care. 74
4.3 The Chronic Care Model. 75
5.1 Overview of the burden of disease framework. 93
5.2 Age-standardized annual mortality from all cardiovascular diseases
in men and women aged 35 to 64 years in Finland, 1969–1982. 96

5.3 Cumulative risk of lung cancer mortality men in the United
Kingdom, based on 1990 smoking rates.   97
5.4 Overweight and obesity in the European region.   98
5.5 Proportion of diabetes attributable to weight gain by region for
adults aged over 30 years.   99
8.1 Conceptualizing clinical decision tools.   176
8.2 Summary of applying clinical decision support (CDS) to improve
outcomes in healthcare organizations.   180
9.1 Financial flows related to paying for chronic care.   195
10.1 Experience of patients with chronic conditions in seven countries.   223

List of tables

3.1 Examples of direct, indirect and intangible costs 45
3.2 Healthcare costs for cardiovascular disease by EU country, 2003 46
3.3 Selected cost-of-illness studies in which cost is expressed as percentage of national health expenditure 47
3.4 Costs and benefits of chronic disease management 54
4.1 Summary of evidence on effectiveness of the components of the Chronic Care Model 79
5.1 Deaths and burden of disease attributable to common risk factors, 2001 94
5.2 Population goals for nutrients and features of lifestyle consistent with the prevention of major public health problems in Europe 101
5.3 Cost per quality-adjusted-life-year saved by interventions to reduce or prevent obesity 102
5.4 Key elements for prevention of chronic diseases in clinical settings 110
6.1 Self-care, self-management and self-management support for chronic conditions: key characteristics 118
6.2 Overview of behavioural theories and related self-management support interventions 122
6.3 Level of inactivity among patients with at least one chronic disease by level of physical disability and income, 2005 132
6.4 Knowledge about medication use in 440 patients with chronic obstructive pulmonary disease by educational level, 2006 134

8.1   Factors relevant to decision support system design for
      different health system actors   175
8.2   Clinical decision support intervention types   178
8.3   Evidence for the effectiveness of computerized clinical
      decision support systems   185
8.4   Evidence of effectiveness of telehealth and interactive health
      communication applications   188
9.1   Purpose of financial incentives and regulation for chronic
      disease care   204
9.2   Examples of financial incentives for chronic disease care in
      selected high-income countries   206
9.3   Examples of indicators, targets and point values for chronic
      disease management in the United Kingdom NHS general
      practitioner contract   209

List of boxes

2.1   Congestive heart failure   17
2.2   Dementia   30
4.1   "Alternative" care concepts   70
4.2   International adaptations of the Chronic Care Model   76
4.3   Case management in England   82
4.4   Nurse-led clinics in Sweden   84
6.1   Examples of self-management support programmes   126
7.1   Developing integrated organizations   146
7.2   Changes to provide a person-centred service   148
7.3   The development of new roles for chronic disease management   150
7.4   Primary care networks in Canada   155
7.5   Redefinition of the role of nurses in Sweden   156
7.6   Different payment models   163
8.1   Electronic decision support for Australia's health sector   179
9.1   Definitions of key terms   195
9.2   The Quality and Outcomes Framework (QOF) in the United Kingdom NHS general practitioner contract   208
10.1   Transmural care in the Netherlands   226
10.2   Evaluating the Australian Asthma 3+ Visit Plan   237
10.3   Auditing health networks in France   238

Contributors

Reinhard Busse is Professor of Health Care Management at the Berlin University of Technology as well as Associate Head of Research Policy and Head of the Berlin hub of the European Observatory on Health Systems and Policies.

Elisabeth Chan is resident in Public Health at Paris hospitals, France.

Anna Dixon is Director of Policy at the King's Fund, London, UK.

Carl-Ardy Dubois is Associate Professor in the Faculty of Nursing Sciences at the University of Montreal.

Isabelle Durand-Zaleski is Professor of Medicine at the University of Paris and head of the Public Health department at Henri Mondor hospital, Paris, France.

Daragh K Fahey is a public health consultant and medical director working for Croydon Primary Care Trust (London) and Health Dialog UK (Cambridge).

Nicholas Glasgow was the Foundation Director of the Australian Primary Health Care Research Institute and is Dean of the College of Medicine and Health Sciences at the Australian National University.

Monique Heijmans is a Senior Researcher with the research programme 'Health Care Demands of the Chronically Ill and Disabled' at NIVEL (Netherlands Institute of Health Services Research), Utrecht, The Netherlands.

Izzat Jiwani is a research associate to the Chair of Governance and Transformation of Health Organizations at the University of Montreal, and has an independent practice as a health policy and health systems analyst, with a primary focus on chronic disease prevention and management systems.

Martyn Jones is a Reader in the School of Nursing and Midwifery, University of Dundee and Associate Director of the Social Dimensions of Health Institute in the Universities of Dundee and St Andrews.

Cécile Knai is a Research Fellow at the London School of Hygiene & Tropical Medicine.

Nicholas Mays is Professor of Health Policy in the Health Services Research Unit, Department of Public Health and Policy, London School of Hygiene & Tropical Medicine.

Martin McKee is Head of Research Policy of the European Observatory on Health Systems and Policies and Professor of European Public Health at the London School of Hygiene & Tropical Medicine.

Ellen Nolte is a Senior Lecturer at the London School of Hygiene & Tropical Medicine and Honorary Senior Research Fellow at the European Observatory on Health Systems and Policies.

Thomas E Novotny is a Professor of Epidemiology and Biostatistics at the University of California, San Francisco, School of Medicine. He is Associate Director for Global Tobacco Control in the UCSF Center for Tobacco Control Research and Education.

Joceline Pomerleau is Lecturer at the London School of Hygiene & Tropical Medicine where she coordinates a large EU-funded (FP6 framework) project on the prevention of obesity in Europe.

Mieke Rijken is Head of the research programme 'Health Care Demands of the Chronically Ill and Disabled' at NIVEL (Netherlands Institute of Health Services Research), Utrecht, The Netherlands.

Dhigna Rubiano is a Research Assistant at the Australian Primary Health Care Research Institute at the Australian National University.

Debbie Singh is Senior Associate at the University of Birmingham Health Services Management Centre and an independent research consultant and evidence reviewer working with health and social service organisations throughout the UK.

Marc Suhrcke is an economist with the WHO Regional Office for Europe in Venice, Italy, where he is in charge of the Health and Economic workstream.

Foreword I:
A health system perspective

Marked success in reducing deaths from acute illnesses in the past half century has resulted in a new emphasis on chronic diseases. As premature death from acute illness is reduced, the prevalence of conditions that accumulate over time rises, particularly in a world in which greater exposure to unnatural environments increases long term vulnerability to ill health. Chronic illness, whether resulting from infections (increasingly viral or fungal), external injuries, developmental abnormalities, autoimmune defects, genetic susceptibilities, or cellular degeneration, are a product of multiple influences on health. No longer is there a culpable 'agent' of disease causation, and 'disease' itself is no longer a straightforward concept.

Diseases, after all, are professionally defined entities without clear biological representations. They can be and are artificially created to suit special interests, and the sum of deaths due to specific diseases in the world exceeds the actual number of deaths. As the case-fatality rate of specific disease decreases, multi-morbidity is the result; diseases now rarely exist in isolation in individuals. Moreover, diseases are but one manifestation of illness; impaired comfort from symptoms, impaired activity from anatomical and physiological derangements, and impaired cognitive and emotional function from biological and psycho-social dysfuntions are legitimate concerns for individuals, subpopulations, and populations.

From the viewpoint of health systems organization, it is well to remember that William Farr, in his contributions to thinking underlying the International Classification of Diseases, set in motion the reigning paradigm that equates ill health with disease, separates person-focused manifestations of health problems with disease-focused ones, and separates primary care from secondary ('specialist') care. The organization of this Classification determined how physicians would be trained and what they would practise – a useful orientation when health services were faced with specific diseases in specific contexts. New recognition of the multiplicity of influences on health, the variability in vulnerability and resilience of different individuals and population groups to threats to illness, and the emerging crisis of harm from iatrogenic causes is calling into question the adequacy of health systems to deal in conventional ways with illness burdens of people and populations. It may even call into question the adequacy of conventional ways of classifying illness.

The current focus on chronic care management is one approach to dealing with this rapidly changing challenge of describing and understanding 'disease' in the 21st century. Whether it is the appropriate one remains to be seen. A disease oriented approach to global health will almost certainly worsen global inequities, because socially disadvantaged people have greater burdens of diseases of all types. Eliminating or controlling diseases one by one is not likely to materially reduce the chances of another in vulnerable populations. It may also be unconscionable when the most serious shortfalls in achieving the Millennium Development Goals are in maternal and child health. Good primary care, which focuses on ALL health conditions with a comprehensive array of services, may be a much better approach to achieve equity in health as well as overall improvement in health.

In this excellent summary of challenges and approaches to dealing with chronic disease in Europe, the editors have done yeoman's work in setting the stage for widespread deliberation of the issues in diseased-focused care. Some chapters frankly advocate (without evidence) for a focus on 'chronic disease' rather than on person-focused care with responsiveness to person-defined needs and priorities. But the introductory chapter and summary, as well as many of the other chapters provide a balanced view; the review indicates a lack of evidence of benefit of a focus on specific chronic diseases. We are still a long way away from knowledge, wisdom and political will to achieve effective, equitable, and efficient health services systems that improve the health of populations and subpopulations.

Professor Barbara Starfield MD, MPH
John Hopkins Bloomberg School of Public Health
April 2008

Foreword II

In the history of mankind few, if any, pandemics will have led to as much suffering and premature deaths as is emerging from the global epidemic of chronic disease. A combination of prevailing life-style factors including diet, lack of physical activity and smoking have contributed to the rising incidence of chronic disease in all parts of the globe, accounting for the majority of premature deaths in all but the lowest income countries. The speed at which obesity, diabetes and vascular disease have become common causes of death in societies which, only a generation ago, were struggling with significant levels of under-nutrition, illustrates the speed at which social and cultural change has impacted health. Even at current levels, the impact of chronic disease is profound, but more worrisome is that all predictions indicate that the prevalence of these diseases is likely to grow, particularly in middle income countries, substantially increasing the overall burden of these diseases.

All countries will need to manage this very substantial healthcare burden better as the potential impact of these diseases on economic growth in these countries is very significant. At the level of individual families, the loss of a parent from chronic disease can have profound consequences on the family unit. In the workplace, employers will need to carry the increasing financial burden of chronic disease, and society as a whole, particularly through healthcare systems, will need to understand better how to deal with this emerging problem. Healthcare providers have not yet found mechanisms to adapt to the chronic disease burden either by developing disease prevention programmes or disease management pathways suitable for chronic rather than acute disease. More novel and creative approaches to public health will be needed if we are to amend the societal and cultural factors that underlie most if not all these diseases.

This book represents a very timely contribution to our understanding of the scale and impact of chronic disease and, in particular, provides important insights into approaches to care pathways for such patients. For clear reasons of focus, it has concentrated on the healthcare management structures in Europe for chronic disease, but many of these lessons will apply widely around the world. It considers not simply the burden of disease in human terms, but also the clear economic impact on families, business and governments and makes a compelling case for a change in the approach of healthcare systems to help deal with this serious emerging problem. These diseases require an important mix of both appropriate healthcare provision and disease prevention strategy and this balance is carefully considered in this volume.

This book represents an important call to action "for all those involved in healthcare systems and public health". Many of the existing structures within our healthcare systems are highly inappropriate for most chronic diseases and few serious attempts have been made to manage many of the lifestyle factors that have created this epidemic in the first instance. Governments, employers, healthcare providers and individuals need to be attentive to the main messages in this important volume. The pace at which this epidemic is gathering momentum suggests we have little time to waste.

Professor Sir John Bell
Regius Professor of Medicine, University of Oxford
and President Academy of Medical Sciences

Acknowledgements

This volume is one of a series of books produced by the European Observatory on Health Systems and Policies. We are grateful to all the authors for their hard work and enthusiasm in this project and to Barbara Starfield and Sir John Bell for contributing the Forewords.

In addition to the contributions of the authors (see List of contributors), this work draws on a series of eight case studies provided by: Nicholas J Glasgow, Nicholas Zwar, Mark Harris, Iqbal Hasan and Tanisha Jowsey (Australia); Izzat Jiwani and Carl-Ardy Dubois (Canada); Michaela L. Schiøtz, Anne Frølich and Allan Krasnik (Denmark); Debbie Singh and Daragh Fahey (England); Isabelle Durand-Zaleski and Olivier Obrecht (France); Ulrich Siering (Germany); Eveline Klein-Lankhorst and Cor Spreeuwenberg (The Netherlands); and Ingvar Karlberg (Sweden). These case studies will be appearing in a companion volume, for which we are grateful to Cecile Knai for co-editing.

We gratefully acknowledge the contributions of those who participated in a workshop held in London to discuss contents, direction and individual draft chapters of the volume. These were, in addition to the case study writers and the chapter authors: Allessandra Badellin, Armin Fidler, Bernard Merkel, Carmel Martin, Chris Ham, Christian Lüthje, Christine Hancock, Clare Siddall, Jill Farrington, Kenneth Thorpe, Kevin McCarthy, Margot Felix, Richard Saltman, Tit Albreht, Johan Calltorp and Ian Basnett. The workshop discussions provided an invaluable source for guiding this work further.

We are especially grateful to the National Institute for Health Research (NIHR), UK for their award of a Career Scientist Award to Ellen Nolte without which this work would not have been possible.

We also gratefully acknowledge the time taken by the final reviewers of this volume, Philip Berman and Antonio Duran. We greatly benefited from their very helpful comments and suggestions.

Finally, this book would not have appeared without the able and patient support throughout the project of our colleagues in the Observatory. In particular, we would like to thank Caroline White and Sue Gammerman, who, with the invaluable assistance of Maria Teresa Marchetti, Pieter Herroelen and Alain Cochez organised and managed all administrative matters related to this work, and in particular for organising the workshop in London. We are also very grateful to Jonathan North for managing the production process and to Jane Ward for copy-editing the manuscript.

chapter one

Caring for people with chronic conditions: an introduction

Ellen Nolte and Martin McKee

Introduction

One of the greatest challenges that will face health systems globally in the twenty-first century will be the increasing burden of chronic diseases (WHO 2002). Greater longevity, "modernization" of lifestyles, with increasing exposure to many chronic disease risk factors, and the growing ability to intervene to keep people alive who previously would have died have combined to change the burden of diseases confronting health systems.

Chronic conditions are defined by the World Health Organization (WHO) as requiring "ongoing management over a period of years or decades" and cover a wide range of health problems that go beyond the conventional definition of chronic illness, such as heart disease, diabetes and asthma. They include some communicable diseases, such as the human immunodeficiency virus and the acquired immunodeficiency syndrome (HIV/AIDS), that have been transformed by advances in medical science from rapidly progressive fatal conditions into controllable health problems, allowing those affected to live with them for many years. They also extend to certain mental disorders such as depression and schizophrenia, to defined disabilities and impairments not defined as diseases, such as blindness and musculoskeletal disorders (WHO 2002), and to cancer, the subject of a separate volume published by the European Observatory (Coleman et al. 2008). While others have offered different definitions for chronic illness (Conrad and Shortell 1996; Unwin et al. 2004), the common theme is that these conditions require a complex response over an extended time period that involves coordinated inputs from a wide range of health professionals and access to essential medicines and monitoring systems, all of which need to be optimally embedded within a system that promotes patient empowerment.

Yet healthcare is still largely built around an acute, episodic model of care that is ill-equipped to meet the requirements of those with chronic health problems. Chronic conditions frequently go untreated or are poorly controlled until more serious and acute complications arise. Even when chronic conditions are recognized, there is often a large gap between evidence-based treatment guidelines and current practice. For example, McGlynn et al. (2003) demonstrated that only approximately 45% of service users with diabetes who had accessed healthcare in the United States by the end of the 1990s had received the recommended care; this proportion was somewhat higher for patients with congestive heart failure, but, at 64%, still suboptimal. Similarly, a systematic review of quality of clinical care in general practice in Australia, New Zealand and the United Kingdom found that, even in the best-performing practices only 49% of patients with diabetes had had undergone routine foot examinations and only 47% of eligible patients had been prescribed beta blockers after heart attack (Seddon et al. 2001).

In response to the emerging challenge posed by chronic diseases, several countries have experimented with new models of healthcare delivery that can achieve better coordination of services across the continuum of care. Yet although better coordination of care delivery has a logical appeal, the available evidence on the value of different approaches remains uncertain (Conrad and Shortell 1996; Ouwens et al. 2005). Furthermore, the diversity of European healthcare systems means that there is unlikely to be a universal solution to the challenges posed by chronic disease. What may be possible in one healthcare system may be impossible, at least in the short term, in another ostensibly similar system if the two differ in critical aspects. Each system must find its own solution, although it can also draw on the lessons learned by others.

This book aims to support this process by systematically examining some of the key issues involved in the care of those with chronic conditions. It explores potential implications for different stakeholders in chronic care so as to identify contextual, organizational, professional, funding and patient-related factors that enable or hinder implementation of strategies to address chronic conditions. It aims to provide a platform for identifying best practices and the prerequisites for implementing them.

The challenges

Advances in healthcare that keep people alive while controlling, although not curing, their conditions have led to growing numbers of people surviving with chronic illness. At the same time, the proportion of older people in the population is also growing, further increasing the number of those with chronic health problems because of accumulated exposure to chronic disease risk factors over their lifetime. The consequences are not trivial. In 2006, 20% to over 40% of the population in the European Union aged 15 years and over reported a long-standing health problem and one in four currently receives medical long-term treatment (TNS Opinion & Social 2007). There are also a growing number of people with multiple health problems. These are most common among older people, with an estimated two-thirds of those who have reached pensionable age having at least two chronic conditions (van den Akker et al. 1998; Wolff et al. 2002; Deutsches Zentrum für Altersfragen 2005).

The implications for health systems and society as a whole are considerable. People with chronic health problems are more likely to utilize healthcare, particularly when they have multiple problems. For example, in England, people with chronic illness account for 80% of general practice consultations and approximately 15% of people who have three or more problems account for nearly 30% of inpatient days (Wilson et al. 2005). Chronic diseases place a substantial economic burden on society. Estimates for the United States place the costs of chronic illness at around three-quarters of the total national health expenditure (Hoffman et al. 1996). Some individual chronic diseases, such as diabetes, account for between 2 and 15% of national health expenditure in some European countries (Suhrcke et al. 2005).

Chronic conditions have become vastly more complex to manage as new, more potent, but also often potentially more hazardous, drugs become available. However, these drugs are often being given to people whose characteristics, in particular their age, would have excluded them from the trials that demonstrated their effectiveness (Britton et al. 1999). It is not known whether evidence about many medications can be generalized to the types of patient that have been excluded from trials because of their age or health problems (Tinetti et al. 2004). Thus, the disparities between results reported in trials and those obtained in routine clinical practice mean that much of the reputed evidence base for clinical decisions is of limited value (Hampton 2003). A further complication is that many people with chronic illness will be receiving treatment for several conditions and will thus be consuming a complex combination of pharmaceutical preparations whose combined efficacy and scope for interaction have never been adequately tested. In Europe, between 4 and 34% of people aged 65 years and older use five or more prescription medications (Junius-Walker et al. 2007). Boyd et al. (2005) showed how, by following existing clinical practice guidelines, a hypothetical 79-year-old woman with chronic obstructive pulmonary disease, type 2 diabetes, osteoporosis, hypertension and osteoarthritis would be prescribed 12 separate medications, a mixture that risks multiple adverse reactions among drugs and diseases. The consequences of a complex medication regimen can be illustrated by the case of a 76-year-old woman with heart failure (Jelley 2006):

> "[L]ater she developed diabetes . . . we controlled her blood pressure with tablets which worsened her renal function. A statin lowered her cholesterol, but her liver function went haywire . . . Beta blockers made her breathing worse and her warfarin had to be stopped after a gastric bleed . . . there always seemed to be a new symptom or drug side effect to deal with. . . ."

The risk of adverse drug reactions increases with multiple (co-)morbidities, the use of some types of drug (e.g. warfarin) and the number of drugs taken (Hajjar et al. 2007). The use of multiple medications also increases the risk of inappropriate prescribing: among adults with two or more chronic conditions, between one-fifth and a quarter (from 16% in Germany to 32% in the United States) reported a medical or medication error such as wrong dosage, wrong medication or erroneous laboratory tests (Schoen et al. 2007). Multiple medications may increase the risk of problems associated with ageing, such as cognitive impairment and falls (Hajjar et al. 2007), and increases in complexity of treatment regimens has been associated with substantially lower adherence, further impairing effective treatment (WHO 2003).

While these factors highlight the challenges facing patients, carers and health professionals alike in managing chronic health problems, multimorbidity per se is only one facet of patient complexity, which also reflects determinants beyond biological factors that impact on health status and influence the effectiveness of specific treatments, such as socioeconomic, cultural and environmental factors and patient behaviour (Safford et al. 2007). Consequently, while patient complexity can be challenging when addressing treatment goals for one condition, it will become ever more complex when attempting to prioritize treatment targets for multiple conditions (Ritchie 2007).

The goals of chronic care are not to cure but to enhance functional status, minimize distressing symptoms, prolong life through secondary prevention and enhance quality of life (Grumbach 2003). It is clear that these goals are unlikely to be accomplished by means of the traditional approach to healthcare that focuses on individual diseases and is based on a relationship between an individual patient and a doctor. While it is equally clear that what is needed is a model of care that takes a patient-centred approach by working in partnership with the patient and other healthcare personnel to optimize health outcomes, it is much more difficult to define the best model. Each approach is highly dependent on context, with terminology used in one setting having a quite different meaning in another one. Therefore, many organizational interventions, such as stroke units, are evaluated as "black boxes", in which the intervention is defined by the name given to it, often with little understanding about the critical factors for success or failure.

Chronic illness confronts patients with a spectrum of needs that requires them to alter their behaviour and engage in activities that promote physical and psychological well-being, to interact with healthcare providers and adhere to treatment regimens, to monitor their health status and make associated care decisions, and to manage the impact of the illness on physical, psychological and social functioning (Clark 2003). Yet, increasing responsibility taken by patients for self-management can create particular challenges for those with multiple conditions, as they may experience aggravation of one condition by treatment of another. For example, a patient with chronic respiratory disease may struggle to adhere to exercise programmes designed for their diabetes (Bayliss et al. 2003).

Patients vary in their preferences for care and the importance they place on health outcomes. Thus, some will prioritize maintenance of functional independence over intense medical management while others will be willing to tolerate the inconvenience and risk of adverse effects associated with complex multiple medication regimens if this is linked to longer survival, even if at the expense of quality of life (Tinetti et al. 2004). The ability of patients to develop individualized treatment plans is, therefore, of critical importance for effective care. The growth of the consumer society, coupled with the explosion in information available on the Internet, is creating more empowered patients, a phenomenon acting to increase the responsiveness with which health services are delivered. However, this may also compromise equitable access to care, as the digital divide enables those who are most privileged to take greatest advantage of the new opportunities provided while those in most need are left behind (Stroetmann et al. 2002). The situation is exacerbated as populations change, with increased global migration creating groups who, despite the goal of universal coverage, may fall between the cracks, especially if their migration has been illegal (Healy and McKee 2004). Unfortunately, our understanding of the scale and nature of any impact of these changes on access to care remains limited.

The shifting balance of care

Taken together, these developments can be seen as evidence of a growing complexity of healthcare. They are influencing profoundly the way that healthcare is being delivered. These influences can be considered under several headings (Royston 1998).

First, the growing opportunities for early intervention, coupled with a greater recognition in some countries of the benefits of reducing the burden of disease as a means of relieving pressure on health systems, is shifting the balance between treatment and prevention. In the United Kingdom, for example, a 2002 Treasury study on future needs for healthcare constructed a variety of scenarios differing largely in the extent to which the health of the population improves. The difference in costs in 2022 between the most optimistic and pessimistic scenarios was approximately £30 billion (€50 billion), approximately half of the 2002 National Health Service (NHS) expenditure (Wanless 2002). Yet the issue is not one of simply shifting resources from treatment to prevention; rather it is one of finding ways to integrate the two, with prevention strategies that take full advantage of developments in healthcare while reorienting healthcare to embed prevention at all stages.

Second, there is a changing balance between hospitals and alternative care settings (Hensher and Edwards 2002). Hospitals have the advantage of confining the patient in one place, waiting for a series of investigations or a sequence of treatments to be undertaken. The patient is seen when it is convenient for the healthcare providers. Organizationally, this makes it easy to deliver complex packages of care, but it also brings major disadvantages for the patient, whose liberty is restricted. Even for those people requiring continuing care, hospitals may not be the most appropriate setting to receive it. Patients with advanced cancer may be better placed in a hospice; those with moderate disabilities may be able to manage better in their own homes but with enhanced nursing or other support. Again, this introduces a degree of complexity, as the needs of the patient are assessed and alternative modes of care provided.

Third, there is a changing balance in the degree of professional and patient involvement in care. In a less-deferential society, patients are less willing to accept instructions without explanations. At the same time, it is recognized that many chronic conditions where the course of the disease may be labile, such as asthma or diabetes, require significant participation by informed patients (Wagner et al. 1996). This, in turn, calls for support from healthcare providers to inform and enable patients to self-manage their illness and may also necessitate an ongoing collaborative process between patients and professionals to optimize long-term outcome.

Fourth, as already noted, there is a changing balance between evidence and intuition in the clinical encounter, with a growing quest for evidence to under-pin clinical practice, and for mechanisms to ensure that the evidence is acted upon, that performance is assessed and action taken to improve it. This balance is, however, dynamic as initial enthusiasms for protocol-driven care confront the reality of individual patient characteristics, thus exposing the limits of determinism (McKee and Clarke 1995).

Fifth, in the face of evidence of growing inequities in societies, there is the shifting balance between services that simply respond to demand and those that proactively seek need, even when it is not voiced as demand, in the knowledge that those whose needs are greatest may be least able to access the care that they need.

Sixth, there is the growing potential of information technology. Patients accustomed to booking holidays or shopping on the Internet are increasingly puzzled by the continuing reliance on postal communication by health services. In theory, booking an appointment should be easy. Yet there is a crucial differ-ence. The Internet model of holiday booking, involving the booking of a set of return tickets and a hotel, is analogous to a single episode of care, for example an attendance for a routine medical examination. However, the traveller in search of a tailor-made holiday, visiting a sequence of destinations suited to his or her individual needs, and using a variety of travel modes (a model more analogous to a patient with a multiple chronic diseases), will require the services of travel agent. Given that most patient journeys more closely resemble the bespoke holiday market, it is unsurprising that healthcare information systems often struggle to deliver what they promise.

Finally, there is the challenge of developing a workforce to respond to the changing healthcare environment. This is a vast area, drawing together many of the previous six issues but added to by the problem of how to provide training in the increasingly diverse settings for healthcare.

Conceptual framework

To explore the challenges outlined above, the study will use a conceptual frame-work that draws, broadly, on the Chronic Care Model (CCM) developed by Wagner and colleagues (1999). This model presents a structure for organizing healthcare to improve outcomes among patients with chronic illness and will be described in detail in Chapter 4. In brief, the model comprises four interacting system components considered key to providing good care for chronic illness: self-management support, delivery system design, decision support and clini-cal information systems. These are set in a health system context that links an appropriately organized delivery system with complementary community resources and policies.

Clearly, issues related to chronic illness that can be addressed under each of these headings are potentially boundless and our aim is not to duplicate work that has already been undertaken, such as the increasing volume of reviews of the effectiveness of the different components of the CCM that form part of many disease management and related care programmes (see for example (Renders et al. 2001; Bodenheimer et al. 2002; Weingarten et al. 2002; Ofman et al. 2004; Ouwens et al. 2005; Tsai et al. 2005; Zwar et al. 2006). Instead, we use the headings to examine in depth some of the key features related to the growing complexity of healthcare that have so far received less attention.

The focus of the study is on the health system/services arrangements for people with established chronic health problems/diseases. Consequently, contributions to this book are based on chronic conditions/diseases, defined (using the WHO definition) as requiring ongoing management over a period of years or decades, and where there may be intercurrent acute episodes associated with a chronic condition or other acute illnesses. We consider all activities that stretch from minimizing the probability that those with risk factors will develop established chronic disease all the way through to the management of highly complex cases, as illustrated in Figure 1.1. The focus is on the healthcare sector, and social and/or community service models are only discussed where there is an integrative link with healthcare and/or they provide useful lessons learnt.

The ensuing work has evolved from a process of analysis at two levels, similar to previous Observatory studies, such as our recent work on *Human Resources for Health* (Dubois et al. 2006; Rechel et al. 2006). On one level, a series of key themes are examined, based on a synthesis of the theoretical and empirical evidence from a wide range of mostly high-income countries. On a second level, detailed analyses have been undertaken in individual countries that examine approaches to chronic illness care in different healthcare settings; these are published in a companion volume (Nolte et al. 2008).

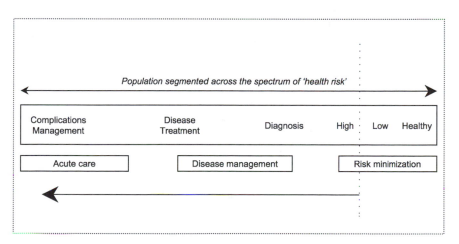

Figure 1.1   Health system activities covered in this book.

Source: Adapted from Petersen and Kane 1997.

Outline of the book

Given the breadth and complexity of the topic, it is important to say what this book is not. It is not a practical manual on how to implement a disease management programme, first because there are many such guides elsewhere but, second, and more importantly, a key lesson from the analyses presented in this book is that the differing contexts in which people work require that solutions be tailored to national circumstances. Instead, we set out the evidence about what has been found to work, or not work, in different circumstances in the hope that this will be of use to those engaged in tackling the challenge of complex chronic disease. In contrast to some other volumes on often quite specific aspects of chronic disease, therefore, we have taken a broad perspective, setting the context within which policies are being made, addressing the prerequisites for effective policies and examining how decisions made for other purposes, such as how to pay for healthcare, may impact on managing chronic disease.

The book is divided into three broad sections. The first sets out the epidemiological evidence on the changing burden of chronic disease in the European region and explores the economic case for investing in chronic disease management. The second section examines some of the key challenges posed by the rising complexity of healthcare, including prevention, using headings adapted from the CCM. The third section looks at the role of the broader health system, examining systems for financing chronic care and how the overall policy environment enables or hinders the introduction and implementation of effective approaches to chronic care.

Looking in more detail, Chapter 2 examines the burden of chronic disease facing the European region. It pays particular attention to morbidity patterns, drawing together epidemiological data on leading chronic conditions, such as stroke, diabetes, chronic obstructive pulmonary disease and asthma, and selected mental disorders, such as depression. One key challenge the chapter highlights is that of identifying reliable, appropriate and comparable data that allow for a comprehensive assessment of the burden of disease across the European region and that can inform local and national policies. It argues that changing demographic patterns and increasing evidence on the health and societal costs of chronic diseases make it crucial to overcome the methodological challenges in assessing and monitoring the chronic disease burden.

Chronic diseases pose a sizeable burden for national economies, with some studies estimating the associated costs at up to 7% of a country's gross domestic product (Oxford Health Alliance Working Group 2005). This is partly a result of direct medical costs, from increased utilization of health services, medication and potentially costly interventions (e.g. Jonsson 2002; Reynolds et al. 2004) but also reflects indirect costs, for example through decreased work productivity (Oxford Health Alliance Working Group 2005). Chapter 3 explores the economic and business case for tackling chronic disease, in order to provide the evidence base required for an informed debate weighing the costs associated with coordinated care programmes (Congressional Budget Office 2004) against the expected societal benefit. A key concern is an observed disconnect between the economic and the business case, which is likely to result in the provision of what is, from a societal perspective, a suboptimal level of active chronic disease management if not addressed by appropriate financing and delivery mechanisms.

Chapter 4 explores approaches to addressing the healthcare needs of those with chronic health problems. It reviews different approaches to chronic care, which have variously been described as "integrated care", coordinated care', "managed care", "disease management", "case management", "patient-centred care", "chronic (illness) care", "continuity of care" and others. It then describes selected theoretical frameworks and existing delivery models designed to provide care to those with varied levels of need. It goes on to examine the evidence base, taking advantage of the accumulating evidence on the relative effectiveness of different models and component features of chronic care (Bodenheimer et al. 2002; Weingarten et al. 2002; Ouwens et al. 2005; Singh 2005a; Singh and Ham 2006).

Although this book is mainly concerned with the management of chronic disease, it is clear that an effective response includes preventing chronic diseases from occurring in the first place. The leading risk factors are mostly known, and so are effective interventions to reduce exposure; yet the response to the challenge remains inadequate in many countries (Yach et al. 2004). Chapter 5 provides an overview of trends in the leading determinants of chronic diseases and provides examples of effective prevention efforts in both the clinical and the population-based context. It illustrates how prevention is truly "everyone's business", with government, the private sector, the healthcare system and the individual patient all having substantial responsibilities for applying evidence-based prevention to the growing burden of chronic diseases.

Chronic illness confronts patients with a spectrum of needs that requires them to alter their behaviour and engage in activities that promote physical and psychological well-being, to interact with healthcare providers and adhere to treatment regimens, to monitor their health status and make associated care decisions, and to manage the impact of the illness on physical, psychological and social functioning (Clark 2003). Chapter 6 explores approaches to engage and/or empower patients towards self-management. It describes theoretical approaches that underpin many self-management support interventions and analyses the nature and effectiveness of self-management support in chronic disease, highlighting the challenges of providing such support to people with multiple conditions or those disadvantaged because of their ethnic or socio-economic background. It identifies a clear need for more research to understand better the impact of support programmes on health outcomes and on the sustainability of improvements over the long term. It also shows that, while self-management support is recognized as an important element of chronic care, few countries seem to be developing or implementing systematic strategies to promote this process. This underlines how important it will be for health policy makers, insurers and providers to create systems that enable all patients to manage their conditions effectively as part of a coordinated strategy.

It has been suggested that the key to effectively controlling chronic disease is the creation of systems that involve many different professionals and specialists working as teams to ensure that the right patients get the right type of care at the right time (Norris et al. 2003; Singh 2005b). Yet while the benefits for patients may be obvious, it is less clear how restructuring of the delivery system impacts on those who have to implement it, namely the healthcare workers. Chapter 7 explores the crucial role of human resources in the provision of essential services to people with long-term conditions. It examines consequences of organizational restructuring for the composition and deployment of the healthcare workforce as well as the impact on job design and work practices (e.g. role substitution, job expansion, job diversification, team work, skill mix). It illustrates key levers that can motivate change and enable the successful and sustainable implementation of approaches to chronic care from a workforce perspective. These include conceptualizing a human resources continuum, where service users take a key role, redefining professional roles, developing generic competencies and reconfiguring the practice environment.

An important component of chronic disease management is decision support that will help healthcare providers to ensure effective treatment (Wagner et al. 1996). Chapter 8 shows how decision support embraces a broad array of interventions, increasingly reliant on electronic systems for their delivery, with the common purpose of increasing the quality of chronic disease care through the standardization of the delivery of care in accordance with best evidence-based practice while containing costs. It focuses in particular on computerized clinical decision support systems, identifying evidence of gains in both quality and safety of care associated with such systems. It notes the many challenges systems are facing in implementing these systems, highlighting the implications for, for example, funders of health services, who will have to balance the costs related to the use of new technologies and new activities against the rather uncertain knowledge about whether these new expenditures will be offset by savings elsewhere in the system.

The CCM recognizes that "improvement in the care of patients with chronic illness will only occur if the system leaders . . . make it a priority and provide the leadership, incentives and resources necessary to make improvements happen" (Epping-Jordan et al. 2004). Chapter 9 sets out the different means by which funders can pay for healthcare, exploring the theoretical advantages and disadvantages of each approach while recognizing the rather more limited evidence base. It then considers the organizational facilitators and barriers to setting up those payment systems that will be expected to achieve optimal results before moving on to look in detail at the lessons emerging from the few evaluations that have been conducted, primarily in the United Kingdom and the United States.

Chapter 10 concludes by exploring existing challenges to better coordination and integration, seeking to identify ways of overcoming them. Examining the various approaches taken by different countries, it identifies three key elements that ought to be in place for an effective response to chronic disease: sustained financing, skilled and motivated health professionals, and supportive information systems. However, it also finds that putting these elements in place will not be sufficient in itself. The complexity of chronic diseases and the potential responses to them mean that solutions will not emerge spontaneously but instead require a comprehensive, consistent and contextually appropriate framework that ensures that the necessary actions are taken to reconfigure organizational structures, remove barriers to change, and invest in training and information technology. Success is not impossible, but the difficulties should not be underestimated.

The audience for this book

Few people will go through life unaffected by chronic disorders, whether as sufferers, informal carers, health professionals and managers, or developing policies in the health and other sectors. This book will, inevitably, be of most interest to the last two groups, but we hope that there will also be something useful in it for the others. The nature of healthcare is changing, in many cases quite rapidly. Yet many health systems are still configured in ways that are more appropriate for the demands of the mid twentieth century rather than the mid twenty-first. Effective responses will require initiatives at all levels to ensure that the right resources (skilled staff, technology, pharmaceuticals and knowledge) can be assembled in the right place at the right time, while establishing support and incentives for everyone to work together to achieve this shared aim. There are no easy answers, and those working in different health systems must find models that are appropriate to their own circumstances. Yet there is also considerable scope for shared learning from each other's successes (and failures). This book, and the companion volume of case studies, seek to contribute to this process.

References

Bayliss, E.A., Steiner, J.F., Fernald, D.H., Crane, L.A. and Main, D.S. (2003) Descriptions of barriers to self-care by persons with comorbid chronic diseases, *Ann Fam Med*, 1: 15–21.

Bodenheimer, T., Wagner, E.H. and Grumbach, K. (2002) Improving primary care for patients with chronic illness: the chronic care model, Part 2, *JAMA*, 288: 1909–14.

Boyd, C., Darer, J., Boult, C. et al. (2005) Clinical practice guidelines and quality of care for older patients with multiple comorbid diseases, *JAMA*, 294: 716–24.

Britton, A., McKee, M., Black, N. et al. (1999) Threats to applicability of randomised trials: exclusions and selective participation, *J Health Serv Res Policy*, 4: 112–21.

Clark, N.M. (2003) Management of chronic disease by patients, *Ann Rev Public Health*, 24: 289–313.

Coleman, M.P., Alexe, D., Albreht, T. and McKee, M. (2008) *Responding to the Challenge of Cancer in EUROPE*. Ljubljiana: Government of Slovenia and European Observatory on Health Systems and Policies.

Congressional Budget Office (2004) *An Analysis of the Literature on Disease Management Programs*. Washington, DC: US Congressional Budget Office.

Conrad, D.A. and Shortell, S.M. (1996) Integrated health systems: promise and performance, *Front Health Serv Manage*, 13: 3–40.

Deutsches Zentrum für Altersfragen (2005) *Gesundheit und Gesundheitsversorgung. Der Alterssurvey: Aktuelles auf einen Blick, ausgewählte Ergebnisse*. Bonn: Bundesministeriums für Familie, Senioren, Frauen und Jugend. http://www.dza.de/download/Gesundheit.pdf (accessed 12 December 2006).

Dubois, C.-A., McKee, M. and Nolte, E. (2006) Human resources for health in Europe: future trends, opportunities, and challenges, in C.-A. Dubois, M. McKee and E. Nolte (eds) *Human Resources for Health in Europe*. Buckingham/New York: Open University Press/McGraw-Hill Education.

Epping-Jordan, J.E., Pruitt, S.D., Bengoa, R. and Wagner, E.H. (2004) Improving the quality of health care for chronic conditions, *Qual Saf Health Care*, 13: 299–305.

Grumbach, K. (2003) Chronic illness, comorbidities, and the need for medical generalism, *Ann Fam Med*, 1: 4–7.

Hajjar, E., Cafiero, A. and Hanlon, J. (2007) Polypharmacy in elderly patients, *Am J Geriatr Pharmacother*, 5: 345–51.

Hampton, J.R. (2003) Guidelines: for the obedience of fools and the guidance of wise men? *Clin Med*, 3: 279–84.

Healy, J. and McKee, M. (2004) *Accessing Health Care: Responding to Diversity*. Oxford: Oxford University Press.

Hensher, M. and Edwards, N. (2002) The hospital and the external environment: experience in the United Kingdom, in M. McKee and J. Healy (eds) *Hospitals in a Changing Europe*. Buckingham, UK: Open University Press.

Hoffman, C., Rice, D. and Sung, H. (1996) Persons with chronic conditions. Their prevalence and costs, *JAMA*, 276: 1473–9.

Jelley, D. (2006) Which patients with which needs are leading the patient-led NHS? *BMJ*, 332: 1221.

Jonsson, B. (2002) Revealing the cost of type II diabetes in Europe, *Diabetologia*, 45: S5–12.

Junius-Walker, U., Theile, G. and Hummers-Pradier, E. (2007) Prevalence and predictors of polypharmacy among older primary care patients in Germany, *Fam Pract*, 24: 14–19.

McGlynn, E.A., Asch, S.M., Adams, J. et al. (2003) The quality of health care delivered to adults in the United States, *N Engl J Med*, 348: 2635–45.

McKee, M. and Clarke, A. (1995) Guidelines, enthusiasms, uncertainty, and the limits to purchasing, *BMJ*, 310: 101–4.

Nolte, E., Knai, C. and McKee, M. (eds) (2008) *Managing Chronic Conditions: Experience in Eight Countries*. Copenhagen: European Observatory on Health Systems and Policies.

Norris, S.L., Glasgow, R.E. and Engelgau, M.M. (2003) Chronic disease management. A definition and systematic approach to component interventions, *Dis Manage Health Outcomes* 11: 477–88.

Ofman, J.J., Badamgarav, E., Henning, J.M. et al. (2004) Does disease management improve clinical and economic outcomes in patients with chronic diseases? A systematic review, *Am J Med*, 117: 182–92.

Ouwens, M., Wollersheim, H., Hermens, R., Hulscher, M. and Grol, R. (2005) Integrated care programmes for chronically ill patients: a review of systematic reviews, *Int J Qual Health Care*, 17: 141–6.

Oxford Health Alliance Working Group (2005) *Economic Consequences of Chronic Diseases and the Economic Rationale for Public and Private Intervention*. Oxford: Oxford Health Alliance [draft report].

Petersen, K. and Kane, D. (1997) Beyond disease management: population-based health management, in W. Todd and D. Nash (eds) *Disease Management. A Systems Approach to Improving Patient Outcomes*. Chicago, IL: American Hospital Publishing.

Rechel, B., Dubois, C.-A. and McKee, M. (2006) *The Health Care Workforce in Europe: Learning From Experience*. Copenhagen: World Health Organization 2006, on behalf of the European Observatory on Health Systems and Policies.

Renders, C.M., Valk, G.D., Griffin, S. et al. (2001) Interventions to improve the management of diabetes mellitus in primary care, outpatient and community settings, *Cochrane Database Syst Rev*, 1: CD001481.

Reynolds, M.W., Frame, D., Scheye, R. et al. (2004) A systematic review of the economic burden of chronic angina, *Am J Manag Care*, 10(Suppl): S347–57.

Ritchie, C. (2007) Health care quality and multimorbidity, *Med Care*, 45: 477–9.

Royston, G. (1998) Shifting the balance of healthcare into the 21st century, *Eur J Oper Res*, 105: 267–76.

Safford, M., Allison, J. and Kiefe, C. (2007) Patient complexity: more than comorbidity. The vector model of complexity, *J Gen Intern Med*, 22(Suppl 3): 380–90.

Schoen, C., Osborn, R., Doty, M. et al. (2007) Toward higher-performance health systems: adult's health care experiences in seven countries, 2007, *Health Aff*, 26: w717–34.

Seddon, M.E., Marshall, M.N., Campbell, S.M. and Roland, M.O. (2001) Systematic review of studies of quality of clinical care in general practice in the UK, Australia and New Zealand, *Qual Health Care*, 10: 152–8.

Singh, D. (2005a) *Transforming Chronic Care. Evidence about Improving Care for People with Long-term Conditions*. Birmingham: University of Birmingham, Surrey and Sussex PCT Alliance.

Singh, D. (2005b) *Which Staff Improve Care for People with Long-term Conditions? A Rapid Review of the Literature*. Birmingham: University of Birmingham and NHS Modernisation Agency.

Singh, D. and Ham, C. (2006) *Improving Care for People with Long-term Conditions. A review of UK and International Frameworks*. Birmingham: University of Birmingham, NHS Institute for Innovation and Improvement.

Stroetmann, V.N., Husing, T., Kubitschke, L. and Stroetmann, K.A. (2002) The attitudes, expectations and needs of elderly people in relation to e-health applications: results from a European survey, *J Telemed Telecare*, 8(Suppl 2): 82–4.

Suhrcke, M., McKee, M., Sauto Arce, R., Tsolova, S. and Mortensen, J. (2005) *The Contribution of Health to the Economy in the European Union*. Brussels: European Commission.

Tinetti, M., Bogardus, S. and Agostini, J. (2004) Potential pitfalls of disease-specific guidelines for patients with multiple conditions, *N Engl J Med*, 351: 2870–4.

TNS Opinion & Social (2007) *Health in the European Union. Special Eurobarometer 272e.* Brussels: European Commission.

Tsai, A.C., Morton, S.C., Mangione, C.M. and Keeler, E.B. (2005) A meta-analysis of interventions to improve care for chronic illnesses, *Am J Manag Care*, 11: 478–88.

Unwin, N., Epping Jordan, J. and Bonita, R. (2004) Rethinking the terms non-communicable disease and chronic disease, *J Epidemiol Community Health*, 58: 801.

van den Akker, M., Buntinx, F., Metsemakers, J., Roos, S. and Knottnerus, J. (1998) Multimorbidity in general practice: prevalence, incidence, and determinants of co-occurring chronic and recurrent diseases, *J Clin Epidemiol*, 51: 367–75.

Wagner, E.H., Austin, B.T. and Von Korff, M. (1996) Organizing care for patients with chronic illness, *Milbank Q*, 74: 511–44.

Wagner, E.H., Davis, C., Schaefer, J., Von Korff, M. and Austin, B. (1999) A survey of leading chronic disease management programs: Are they consistent with the literature? *Manage Care Q*, 7: 56–66.

Wanless, D. (2002) *Securing our Future Health: Taking a Long-term View*. London: HM Treasury.

Weingarten, S.R., Henning, J.M., Badamgarav, E. et al. (2002) Interventions used in disease management programmes for patients with chronic illness: which ones work? Meta-analysis of published reports, *BMJ*, 325: 925.

WHO (2003) *Adherence to Long-Term Therapies. Evidence for Action*. Geneva: World Health Organization.

WHO (2002) *Innovative Care for Chronic Conditions: Building Blocks for Action*. Geneva: World Health Organization.

Wilson, T., Buck, D. and Ham, C. (2005) Rising to the challenge: will the NHS support people with long-term conditions? *BMJ*, 330: 657–61.

Wolff, J., Starfield, B. and Anderson, G.F. (2002) Prevalence, expenditures, and complications of multiple chronic conditions in the elderly, *Arch Intern Med*, 162: 2269–76.

Yach, D., Hawkes, C., Gould, C.L. and Hofman, K.J. (2004) The global burden of chronic diseases: overcoming impediments to prevention and control, *JAMA*, 291: 2616–22.

Zwar, N., Harris, M., Griffiths, R. et al. (2006) *A Systematic Review of Chronic Disease Management*. Sydney: Australian Primary Health Care Institute.

two

The burden of chronic disease in Europe

Joceline Pomerleau, Cécile Knai and Ellen Nolte

Introduction

Chronic diseases pose a major challenge to population health in Europe and worldwide. They are an important cause of premature mortality and, because they also cause disability, they have a major impact on the expectancy of life lived in good health. As populations age and new treatments allow those with once fatal diseases to survive, the prevalence of chronic diseases is rising in many countries (Yach et al. 2004). This is particularly the case in Europe, where fertility rates are declining; as a consequence there is now a much higher proportion of the population living with chronic diseases and, in many cases, multiple diseases.

Several reports have assessed the burden of disease in Europe and elsewhere (WHO 2005a; WHO Regional Office for Europe 2005b; Mathers and Loncar 2006). This chapter seeks to advance existing work, focusing on selected chronic conditions, to provide a broad picture while highlighting the key challenges involved in quantifying the burden of chronic disease. It will draw on a wide range of data sources, thereby promoting a better understanding of the available evidence. Although the focus of this chapter will be on the European region, we will refer to other high-income countries where appropriate. We conclude by discussing strategies to overcome some of the current methodological challenges in assessing the disease burden.

Assessing the disease burden: the challenge

One of the main challenges in assessing the disease burden is the relative lack of comparable and representative data. Assessments often have to draw, to a considerable extent, on mortality data as these are routinely available in most countries. However, mortality data only capture those causes of disease that have a fatal outcome and inevitably underestimate the burden of disease attributable to conditions that rarely cause death, such as mental illness, or that may not be listed as the immediate cause of death but which contribute to mortality, such as diabetes (Jougla et al. 1992).

Attempts to overcome these limitations have involved the development of summary indicators such as disability-adjusted life years (DALYs) which combine information on mortality and non-fatal health outcomes, advanced mainly by the Global Burden of Disease study (Murray et al. 2002). DALYs essentially represent the sum of years of life lost and years of life lived with disability; the burden of disease measures the gap between the current health status of a given population and an ideal situation where everyone in the population lives to old age in full health.[1] It makes it possible to estimate the contribution of different health problems, including chronic diseases, to the overall disease burden in a given population.

In practice, burden of disease assessments tend to focus on major disease categories only, often using broad classifications such as non-communicable diseases (NCD), communicable diseases and injuries, and/or selected disease categories within these, such as cardiovascular disease, cancer, diabetes or HIV/AIDS (Mathers and Loncar 2006). Yet, although the term "chronic disease" might be interpreted as a component of NCDs, these two categories are by no means identical.[2] Thus, NCDs also include a range of conditions that are not considered "chronic" (i.e. acute conditions) while chronic diseases may also include selected communicable diseases such as HIV/AIDS. It, therefore, remains a challenge to assess the burden of chronic disease in the European region based on existing data sets.

Against this background, we do not attempt in this chapter to portray the total burden of chronic disease in Europe. Instead, we focus on a few selected conditions, chosen because of the multiple challenges they pose to health systems. On this basis we have included **cerebrovascular disease**, an important contributor to the burden of death and disease and a major cause of long-term disability; **diabetes mellitus**, the prevalence of which is predicted to increase dramatically in the next few decades; **chronic obstructive pulmonary disease** (COPD) and **asthma**, the former being the fourth leading cause of death in the world yet still underrecognized and asthma constituting the most common chronic disease in children (Pauwels and Rabe 2004); and **unipolar depressive disorders**, which are projected to become the second major contributor to the disease burden worldwide by 2020. We acknowledge that this selection excludes other important chronic conditions, such as congestive heart failure, dementia, arthritis or renal failure; this is mainly a result of the difficulty in obtaining reliable and comparative data, a problem we illustrate for congestive heart failure (Box 2.1) and dementia (Box 2.2, below). We also recognize the importance of socioeconomic factors in relation to the disease burden; it is often greater among those at the lower end of the social scale (Marmot et al. 1991, 2001; Kaplan and Keil 1993). However, constraints on space and, most importantly, limitations on data availability in many European countries precluded us from examining this aspect in detail.

Box 2.1 Congestive heart failure

Congestive or chronic heart failure (CHF) is a complex syndrome that impairs the ability of the heart to function as a pump to support physiological circulation (Mosterd and Hoes 2007). Several pathologies frequently coexist with CHF, including hypertension and diabetes mellitus. CHF is a major and growing public health issue that affects all Western countries (Cowie et al. 1997; Mosterd and Hoes 2007). However, public awareness of the condition remains low (Remme et al. 2005), and there are few comparative and nationally representative data from across Europe (Mehta and Cowie 2006). A recent review of the epidemiological evidence suggests little indication of a decline in the incidence of heart failure since the 1980s (Mosterd and Hoes 2007) although mortality from CHF appears to have been declining over recent years (Murdoch et al. 1998; Najafi et al. 2006). The true extent is difficult to assess as death from heart failure is substantially underestimated by official statistics. It has been estimated that possibly at least one-third of deaths attributed to coronary heart disease may also be related to CHF (Murdoch et al. 1998). Because of the ageing of the population, coupled with improved survival because of improved treatment, the projected burden of CHF is set to increase (Stewart et al. 2003). This poses a considerable challenge to healthcare systems, with one study estimating the costs attributable to caring for people with CHF at 1–2% of healthcare resources in industrialized countries, which is likely to increase given the projected rise in the CHF burden (Bundkirchen and Schwinger 2004).

Population ageing and chronic disease

Before examining in detail the burden of selected chronic conditions, it is important to emphasize that the burden of disease worldwide is dynamic (Mathers and Loncar 2006). One factor is the changing age structure of the population. In many populations, the number of old people, and especially the very old, is increasing. For Europe, the proportion of older people (aged 65 years and older) is projected to grow from just under 15% (in 2000) to 23.5% by 2030, while the proportion of those aged 80 years and over is expected to more than double (from 3% in 2000 to 6.4% in 2030) (Kinsella and Phillips 2005). The likelihood of developing a potentially disabling chronic condition rises with increasing age because of the progressive accumulation of exposure to risk factors over a lifetime (Ben-Shlomo and Kuh 2002; Janssen and Kunst 2005). However, there is increasing evidence supporting the "compression of morbidity" thesis put forward by Fries (1983), which suggests that as populations adopt healthier lifestyles and therapeutic advances continue, the period of illness (morbidity) that individuals experience prior to death is compressed.
Studies in several countries demonstrate that people are indeed both living longer and spending less time in poor health (Parker and Thorslund 2007). For

example, a recent systematic review demonstrated how disability and functional limitations among older adults in the United States have declined consistently during the 1990s (Freedman et al. 2002). Part of this improvement results from therapeutic advances, as older people are increasingly enabled to function with multiple disorders by complex combinations of treatment. Freedman et al. (2007) reported that between 1997 and 2004 a rising prevalence of chronic conditions among older Americans (aged 65 and over) was accompanied by declines in the proportion reporting disability as a result of those conditions, a phenomenon also reported for the Swedish population (Parker and Thorslund 2007). Therefore, while disability might be declining, other health problems might be increasing.

This is further supported by a recent report by the OECD that reviewed trends in the prevalence of (severe) disability, defined as one or more limitations in basic activities of daily living, among those aged 65 and over (Lafortune et al. 2007). It identified evidence for declining disability prevalence in some countries, such as Denmark, Finland, Italy, the Netherlands and the United States and stable rates in Australia and Canada, while for others the evidence was more mixed (France, United Kingdom) or indicated an increase (Belgium, Sweden). Based on the expected demographic changes, including population ageing and greater longevity, the analysis projected an increase in the number of older people with severe disability by 2030 even for those countries which recorded a sustained decline over recent years, although the relative increase in projected numbers remained lower than what would be expected if there was no change in current age-specific prevalence rates.

Yet while ageing of populations is an important driver of increases in chronic disease, it is important to emphasize that the perception that chronic illness is an "old people's" fate no longer applies, with increasing numbers of young and middle-aged people developing some form of chronic health problem. It is estimated that in 2002 60% of all DALYs attributable to NCDs were lost before the age of 60 (WHO 2004a). Recent evidence from the United States points to a rapid increase in the number of children and teengagers with chronic health conditions since the 1960s (Perrin et al. 2007), in particular as a response to growing levels of obesity. Rising rates of childhood chronic conditions imply subsequent higher rates of related conditions among adults (van der Lee et al. 2007).

This brief overview, illustrating how population ageing is an important although not the sole driver of the burden of chronic disease, already points to the varied challenges facing contemporary society. The next section will examine, in detail, specific chronic health problems to highlight further the complexity to which health systems will have to respond in order to address the rising burden of chronic disease effectively in Europe and beyond.

The burden of selected chronic diseases

Cerebrovascular disease

Cerebrovascular disease, or stroke, ranks among the leading causes of death worldwide; in 2002, stroke accounted for approximately 15% (men, 11%;

women, 19%) of all deaths and approximately 7% (6% and 8%, respectively) of the total disease burden in Europe (WHO 2004a). Stroke is a leading neuro-logical cause of long-term disability, with over half of those still alive after six months being left to depend on others for everyday activities (Wolfe 2000) and at least one-quarter remaining moderately or severely disabled three years after stroke (Patel et al. 2006). Stroke has also been associated with depression (Hackett et al. 2005) and been shown to increase the risk of dementia (Liebetrau et al. 2003) and of falls and fractures (Poole et al. 2002), further adding to the overall disease and disability burden.

Mortality from stroke has been falling throughout most of the twentieth cen-tury and particularly so since the 1960s (Bonita 1992; Ebrahim and Harwood 1999). The reasons for this decline are not yet fully understood. Declining inci-dence has been identified as one contributor, as has improved survival after stroke, attributed to reductions in case-fatality, although the evidence is not consistent (Thorvaldsen et al. 1997; Feigin et al. 2003). Data from the US-based Framingham study indicate a decline in the incidence of stroke over the past 50 years, but there was no decline in severity of stroke and an observed fall in case-fatality was only significant for men (Carandang et al. 2006). Changes in stroke incidence have been attributed to changing patterns of exposure to, or control of, risk factors for stroke, changing completeness of case ascertainment because of improved awareness and diagnostic practice, and period and cohort effects (Feigin et al. 2003). Elevated blood pressure is a major modifiable risk factor for stroke and an observed fall in blood pressure levels among young people since the beginning of the twentieth century has been associated with falling stroke incidence (McCarron et al. 2002), as has increased treatment of high blood pressure (Rothwell et al. 2004).

Current projections by the WHO (2006a) suggest that the mortality and dis-ease burden attributable to stroke in their European Region will decrease in both sexes and all ages by 2030. However, others have argued that stroke prevalence and the overall population burden of stroke is likely to increase further since older people are the most stroke-prone age group and constitute the fastest growing segment of the population (Feigin et al. 2003; Terent 2003; Carandang et al. 2006). Moreover, emerging evidence of a recent increase in mean blood pressure in young people in countries such as the United States (Din-Dzietham et al. 2007), along with the rise in childhood obesity in several countries, indi-cate that recent favourable trends in stroke incidence may not be maintained. A recent analysis showed that one in eight deaths from stroke may be attributed to high blood glucose levels (Danai et al. 2006), highlighting how the diabetes "epidemic", which will be described below, may impact on the future burden of stroke.

Figure 2.1 illustrates wide variation in the mortality and disease burden attributed to stroke in selected European countries in 2002. The highest burden is concentrated in the countries that have emerged from the Soviet Union, with death and DALY rates in the Russian Federation and the central Asian Republics of Kyrgyzstan and Kazakhstan up to ten times the levels seen in Switzerland, Israel and France. The regional variation in the burden of cerebrovascular dis-ease is further illustrated by utilization data, such as hospital discharge rates, which tend to be higher in north-eastern and central Europe, with, in 2005, very

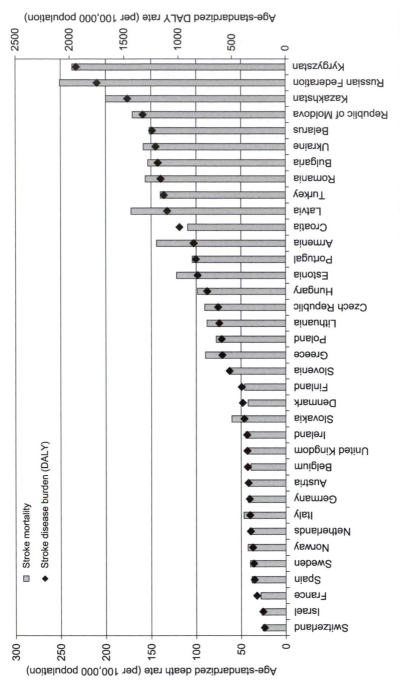

Figure 2.1 Burden of death and disease attributable to stroke in selected countries in the World Health Organization European Region, 2002.

Source: From WHO 2004b.

high rates of over 1000 discharges per 100,000 population observed for Hungary, Belarus and Lithuania compared to only between 200 to 230 per 100,000 in Switzerland, France, the Netherlands and the United Kingdom (WHO 2007). This large variation in utilization is likely to reflect higher incidence of stroke in some of the countries, as for example reported for Ukraine and the Russian Federation (Feigin et al. 2003). Utilization data such as hospital discharge rates are however difficult to interpret in part because of differences in definitions, for example whether or not long-term beds are included, which for a potentially disabling condition such as stroke is likely to reflect on reported utilization.

The implications for health systems are not insignificant: A recent review of data on stroke prevalence found the age-standardized prevalence for people aged 65 years or more ranging from 4.6% in selected regions of the United States to just over 7% in Italy (L'Aquila) and Newcastle, United Kingdom (Feigin et al. 2003). The proportion of strokes associated with disability or impairment varied between 55% of all strokes in New Zealand and 77% in Yorkshire, United Kingdom.

Diabetes mellitus

Diabetes mellitus is a major problem worldwide, affecting approximately 180 million people (WHO 2006b). Although not among the leading causes of death recorded in Europe, diabetes has a major impact on the global burden of disease through its detrimental impact, if not controlled, on the heart, blood vessels, eyes, kidneys and nerves, so accelerating death and disability from other conditions. In 2002, approximately 1.5% of the total disease burden was attributed to diabetes in Europe (men, 1.2%; women, 1.8%) (WHO 2004a). The number of DALYs lost through diabetes tends to increase with age up to 80 years. Rates tend to be higher among men under the age of 60 but higher for women at older ages.

The prevalence of diabetes worldwide in 2000 was estimated to be 2.8% and is expected to increase to 4.4% by 2030 (Wild et al. 2004). In the United States, the age-adjusted prevalence is already 6.3% (Engelgau et al. 2004), with one in three persons born in 2000 anticipated to develop diabetes at some point in their life (Narayan et al. 2003). This increase is mainly in type 2 diabetes although type 1 diabetes is also increasing swiftly, at approximately 3% per year, especially in central and eastern Europe and among young children (Green and Patterson 2001).

Diabetes prevalence is projected to increase in Europe within the next two decades (International Diabetes Federation 2003), partly a result of rising obesity levels. There is a strong association between obesity, increasingly affecting children, and incidence of type 2 diabetes (Haines et al. 2007). Large relative increases in diabetes prevalence are expected to be seen in countries undergoing economic and nutrition transition such as Belarus, Slovenia, Slovakia, the Czech Republic, Poland and Turkey, but also in others, for example Switzerland (International Diabetes Federation 2003).

In 2003, estimates for the prevalence of all forms of diabetes mellitus among those aged 20–79 years ranged from approximately 3.4% (Ireland) to 10.2%

(Germany) (Figure 2.2) (International Diabetes Federation 2003). There appears to be no clear regional pattern, except perhaps for a clustering of relatively high prevalence rates in central and north-eastern Europe. Data such as those shown in Figure 2.2 have to be interpreted with caution, however, as they are based on surveys that vary in terms of diagnostic criteria (self-report, physician diagnosed, laboratory diagnosed) and estimates are not standardized for differences in age structure between populations (International Diabetes Federation 2003).

The DECODE study of cohorts, established in nine European countries in the 1990s estimated a prevalence of under 10% among those under 60 years of age and 10–20% in those aged 60–79 years (DECODE Study Group 2003). Importantly, it confirmed that much diabetes is undiagnosed among those under 50 years of age, suggesting that the "true" burden of diabetes as measured by disease prevalence in Europe is likely to be higher than estimates shown here.

There are important variations in mortality and disease burden attributable to diabetes mellitus within Europe. Age-standardized death rates per 100,000 population ranged from 4.0 (Greece) to 17.9 (Portugal) in 2002, with higher levels reported for Israel (36.1) and Armenia (46.8) (Figure 2.3; WHO 2004b). It has to be emphasized, though, that officially reported deaths from diabetes are likely to underestimate the "true" burden in a given population because of underrecording of diabetes as an underlying cause of death, particularly among older people (Jougla et al. 1992). The most common cause of death among people with diabetes is cardiovascular disease, accounting for up to two-thirds of all deaths (Danai et al. 2006).

Diseases of the respiratory system

Respiratory diseases, and particularly COPD and asthma, place a considerable burden on many populations and are among the leading causes of premature death in the European region. Respiratory diseases are responsible for over 4% of total deaths and disease burden in the WHO European region (WHO 2004a).

Chronic obstructive pulmonary disease

COPD refers to a condition previously described as chronic bronchitis (inflammation and narrowing of the airways) and emphysema (weakening of the structure of the lung) (Loddenkemper et al. 2003). It is increasingly common with age. It is currently the fourth leading cause of death in the world (WHO 2006c). Mortality increases sharply with age in both sexes; rates are higher in men than women.

COPD is a common health problem across Europe, but is often underdiagnosed (Pauwels 2000; Pauwels and Rabe 2004) as many sufferers accept breathlessness and limited exercise tolerance as features of ageing and regard smoker's cough as normal. A study conducted in Manchester (United Kingdom) that reported non-reversible airflow obstruction in 11% of adults aged over 45 years suggested that of these 65% had not had COPD diagnosed (Devereux 2006). In western Europe, the overall prevalence of COPD (based on spirometry, a measure of lung function, to confirm diagnosis) is 4–11%, based on data from

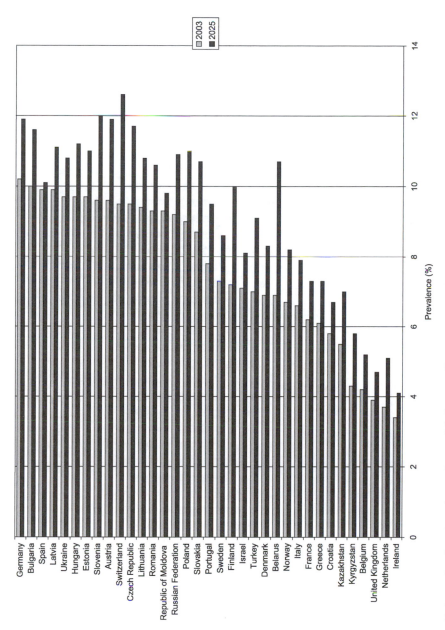
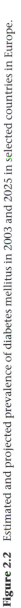

Figure 2.2 Estimated and projected prevalence of diabetes mellitus in 2003 and 2025 in selected countries in Europe.

Source: From International Diabetes Federation 2003.

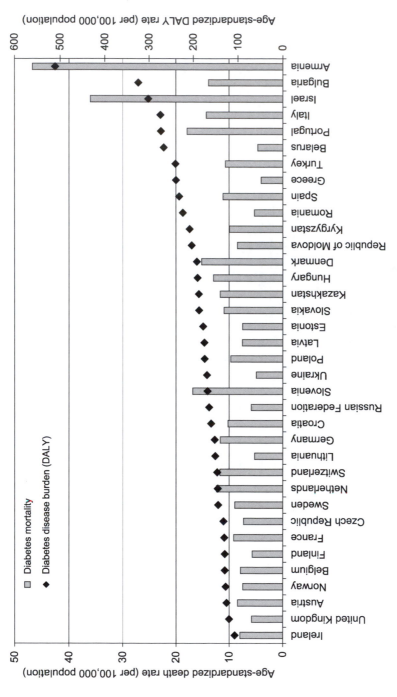

Figure 2.3 Burden of death and disease attributable to diabetes in selected countries in the World Health Organization European Region, 2002.

Source: From WHO 2004b.

Denmark (individuals aged 20–90 years), England (60–75 years), Finland (30 years and older), Italy (25 years and older), Norway (16–70 years), Spain (40–69 years) and the United Kingdom (16–65 years) (Devereux 2006; Halpin and Miravitlles 2006). Data from other regions of Europe are very limited.

COPD places a considerable burden on affected individuals, including poor physical functioning and distressing symptoms that require frequent hospital admission. The burden of COPD is estimated to be 393 DALYs per 100,000 population, with particularly high rates in individuals aged 70 years and over (WHO 2004a). At the age of 60–79 years, rates are almost twice as high in men as in women, reflecting the leading role of smoking as a causative factor.

COPD mortality is increasing worldwide despite advances in its management in recent decades; most patients are not diagnosed until their mid-fifties (Halpin and Miravitlles 2006). At the European level, the predicted number of deaths attributable to COPD is expected to increase from almost 270,000 in 2005 to over 338,000 deaths by 2030, while the absolute burden of COPD is projected to fall from approximately 3,440,000 to 2,950,000 DALYs (WHO 2006a). However, both death and DALYs are expected to decrease in all age groups and both sexes, with the exception of women aged 70 years and over who will see increases in COPD mortality and DALYs.

The contribution of COPD to the overall mortality and burden of disease in European countries varies considerably (Figure 2.4). For example, while it is estimated that in Latvia COPD causes approximately 5.1 deaths and 70 DALYs per 100,000 population, in Kyrgyzstan it associated with 80.9 deaths and 1088 DALYs per 100,000 population.

Asthma

Although asthma has a relatively low fatality rate compared with other chronic diseases, it is estimated that, worldwide, deaths from asthma will increase by almost 20% in the next 10 years if action is not taken to address it (WHO 2006d).

At the European level, asthma is responsible for approximately 0.4% of all deaths and 1% of the global burden of disease, equivalent to approximately 43,000 deaths and 1,358,000 DALYs (WHO 2006a). The relative importance of asthma increases with age and is particularly apparent in elderly men and middle-aged women.

Available data suggest that approximately 30 million people in the European region are affected by asthma (Masoli et al. 2004). Prevalence of clinical asthma, (here defined as 50% of the prevalence of wheezing (self-reported) in the previous 12 months in children aged 13–14 years), ranges from approximately 1.3 to 18.4% (Figure 2.5). In the United States, asthma prevalence among children and adolescents has been estimated at around 9%, double the figure reported in the 1980s (Moorman et al. 2007). These trends are relevant for projecting the future burden attributable to this condition since asthma persists to adulthood in at least 25% of children (Sears et al. 2003).

In adults, asthma prevalence ranges from less than 5% to more than 10% (Loddenkemper et al. 2003). A survey of asthma prevalence in France, Germany,

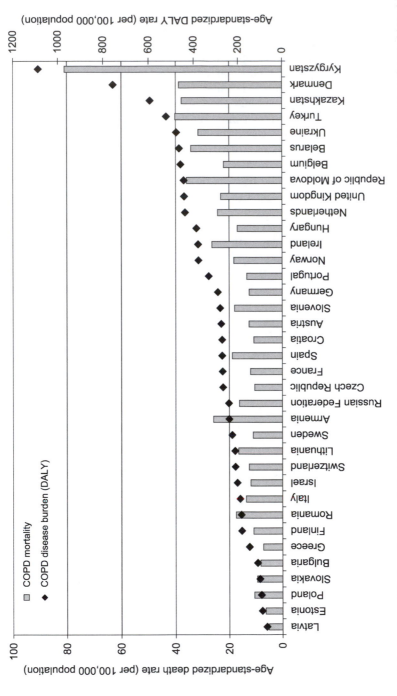

Figure 2.4 Burden of death and disease attributable to chronic obstructive pulmonary disease (COPD) in selected countries in the World Health Organization European Region, 2002.

Source: From WHO 2004b.

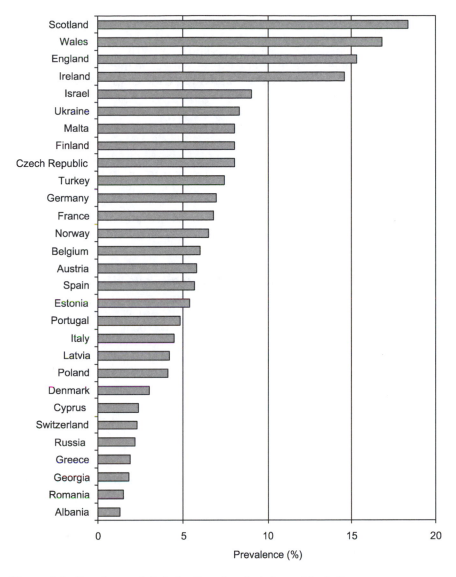

Figure 2.5 Prevalence of clinical asthma in selected countries in Europe.

Source: From Masoli et al. 2004.

Italy, the Netherlands, Spain, Sweden, and the United Kingdom suggests that, on average, 15.1% of children and 20.5% of adults with the condition experience severe persistent asthma (Rabe et al. 2000). These individuals are less responsive to standard asthma therapy and have been shown to experience greater morbidity and a lower quality of life than those whose disease can be controlled adequately by therapy (ENFUMOSA-Study-Group 2003).

Projected trends in the burden of death and disability from asthma differ slightly from those described above for COPD. In terms of mortality, falls in age-standardized death rates are projected in the period 2005–2030 in both sexes and at all ages except in men aged 80 years and over (WHO 2006a). The burden of disease attributable to asthma is also expected to fall in men and women aged 30 years and over, but not in younger individuals; increases in DALYs are projected of approximately 1–2% in boys and girls aged 0–4 years, of 3% in those aged 5–14 years and 6–7% in those aged 15–29 years.

Age-standardized deaths and DALYs attributable to asthma in European countries appear to vary considerably: age-standardized death rates per 100,000 population range from 0.2 in Greece to 9.1 in the Russian Federation and standardized DALY rates per 100,000 population vary from 66 in Romania to over 330 in the United Kingdom and Ireland (Figure 2.6; WHO 2004b). The Global Burden of Asthma Report 2004 (Masoli et al. 2004) suggested that central Asian republics have some of the highest case-fatality rates (asthma deaths per 100,000 asthmatics) in the European region.

Neuropsychiatric diseases: unipolar depressive disorders

The prevalence of mental disorders is high in the European region (Anderson et al. 2001; Demyttenaere et al. 2004; Kessler et al. 2005; Kessler 2007), with unipolar depressive disorders being the most common (see also Box 2.2). It is estimated that 33.4 million Europeans are affected by major depression each year and that one in five individuals will develop depression during their lifetime (WHO 2003).

The Global Burden of Disease study estimated the overall incidence and prevalence of unipolar depressive disorders in Europe for the year 2000 (Ustun et al. 2004). Although subject to a considerable degree of uncertainty, the estimated figures provide useful information for the region. The age-standardized incidence of major depressive episodes was estimated to be highest in southeast Europe, the Caucasus and central Asia for both men and women, at 3286 and 5353 per 100,000, respectively. For men, the estimated incidence tended to be somewhat lower in the Baltic countries and northeast Europe, at 2923 per 100,000, and lowest in southern and western Europe, the Nordic countries and parts of central Europe, at 2610 per 100,000. For women, the estimated incidence was fairly similar in these regions, though, at 4470 and 4482 per 100,000, respectively, and considerably higher than among men (Ustun et al. 2004).

Mental disorders are increasingly affecting children and adolescents in Europe (WHO 2003). This is particularly alarming as it is now recognized that many mental disorders seen in adulthood have their origins in childhood. It has been estimated that approximately 2 million young people in the European Region are affected by mental disorders, ranging from depression to schizophrenia. Approximately 4% of those aged 12–17 years and 9% of those aged 18 years are affected by depressive disorders (WHO 2005c). Depression is associated with suicide in the young, a major problem in many countries and the third leading cause of death among young people. Certain populations, including eastern European men, are at a particular risk of suicide; in western Europe the risk of suicide in adolescents also appears to be increasing (WHO 2005c).

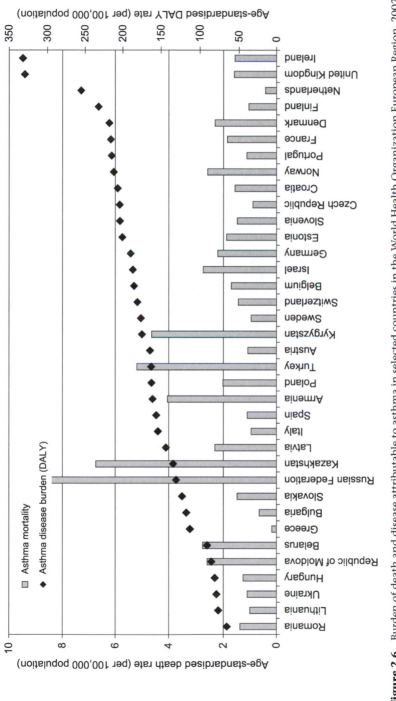

Figure 2.6 Burden of death and disease attributable to asthma in selected countries in the World Health Organization European Region, 2002.

Source: From WHO 2004b.

Box 2.2 Dementia

Dementia is an increasingly prevalent mental disorder in Europe. A generic term, dementia refers to chronic or progressive dysfunction of cortical and subcortical function that results in complex cognitive decline. Alzheimer's diseases is the most common form of dementia in Europe and North America (Ritchie and Lovestone 2002). Dementia is one of the most important causes of disability in older people and is set to rise with the increasing proportion of older people. Current estimates suggest that there are 7.4 million people living with dementia in Europe, accounting for approximately 30% of the total worldwide (Wimo et al. 2003). In developed countries, dementia prevalence is estimated at 1.5% at 65 years, doubling every four years to approximately 30% among those aged 80 years (Ritchie and Lovestone 2002). Within Europe in 2000, prevalence among those 65 years or older is estimated to vary between 6% in eastern Europe and 8% in northern Europe (Wimo et al. 2003). More recent estimates derived from a Delphi exercise involving international experts have placed the prevalence of dementia in Europe among those 60 years or older at 3.8% in eastern Europe and 5.4% in western Europe, somewhat higher than that estimated for the developed western Pacific, at 4.2%, but lower than in North America, at 6.4% (Ferri et al. 2005). Consistent with other analyses, Ferri et al. (2005) projected an increase in the number of people (age 60+ years) with dementia in Europe from 7.7 million in 2001 to 10.8 million in 2020 (31–51% increase in different regions in Europe). The aetiology of dementia is not yet well understood. Confirmed risk factors include increasing age, the occurrence of dementia in a family member and genetic predisposition (Ritchie and Lovestone 2002). More recently, increased body mass index has been associated with an increased risk of dementia (Gorospe and Dave 2006), which, if confirmed, may have considerable implications for the future given rising obesity levels.

In 2002, unipolar depressive disorders accounted for 6.2% of the regional global burden of disease (1064 DALY per 100,000 population) but only for 0.02% of all deaths (0.21 deaths per 100,000 population) (WHO 2004a).

Current projections suggest that age-standardized death rates for unipolar depressive disorders may decrease slightly in both men and women (from 0.15 to 0.13 per 100,000 population) between 2005 and 2030, yet given the high level of morbidity involved, the burden of disease attributed to this health problem is projected to increase in both sexes (age-standardized rate per 100,000 increasing in men from 777 to 785 and in women from 1312 to 1337) (WHO 2006a).

Figure 2.7 shows between-country variations in the burden of unipolar depressive disorders in Europe. Age-adjusted DALY rates per 100,000 range from 660 to 1430 DALYs. Rates are lowest in Spain and Greece (less than 700) and highest in Finland, Israel, Slovenia, Belgium and France (greater than 1250) (WHO 2004b).

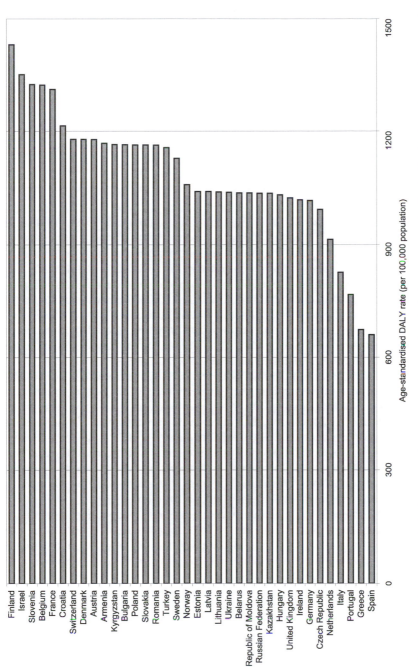

Figure 2.7 Burden of disease attributable to unipolar depressive disorder in selected countries in the World Health Organization European Region, 2002.

Source: From WHO 2004b.

Prevalence estimates vary because of variations in case definition, assessment tools and the populations covered. A pooled analysis of community studies in five European countries gave an overall estimate of the prevalence of depressive disorders among adults aged 18–65 years at 8.6%, ranging from 6.6% in men and 10.1% in women (Ayuso-Mateos et al. 2001). Estimates of 12-month prevalence of depression among the working population in 13 European countries ranged from 3.2% in Italy to 10.1% in Norway, with a "European" median of 6.9% (Sobocki et al. 2006). Prevalence rates were reported to be consistently higher among women and to slightly vary with age, with the estimated European medians being 5.8% for men and 8.3% for women in those aged 18–34 years and 5.2% for men and 8.5% for women in those aged 35–49 years. Prevalence tended to fall for those aged 50–64, to 3.4% in men and 6.6% in women.

Comorbidity and multimorbidity

Previous sections have set out the present and projected future burden of disease attributable to a range of leading chronic conditions. However, as noted above, it is important to recognize that these conditions often do not occur in isolation. Indeed, increased longevity, coupled with advances in healthcare, has meant that there are growing numbers of people with multiple disease processes, creating a range of diverse and sometimes contradictory needs that pose considerable challenges to those affected and to the delivery of health services (Piette et al. 2004). For example, depression and arthritis in people with diabetes impair functioning and cause substantial barriers to implementing lifestyle changes and adhering to therapeutic regimens (Piette and Kerr 2006).

Multimorbidity has been defined as the simultaneous occurrence of several medical conditions in the same person (Fortin et al. 2005). The term multimorbidity is often used interchangeably with comorbidity, although the latter refers more specifically to conditions that occur as a consequence of one leading ("index") condition such as diabetes (Feinstein 1970) (although others have offered different taxonomies, see for example Piette and Kerr (2006) and van Weel and Schellevis (2006)). However, in either case, the available epidemiological evidence is fairly restricted, posing challenges to those seeking a comprehensive assessment of the extent of this problem.

A recent overview of the available evidence reports a wide range of estimates of the prevalence of multimorbidity in four industrialized countries in the 1990s, although these are difficult to compare because of differences in data sources, for example population surveys or administrative databases, and age ranges covered (Fortin et al. 2005). Keeping these limitations in mind, among those aged 65 years and over the reported prevalence of the presence of two or more chronic health problems was at least 50%, increasing markedly with age. That study also undertook a separate analysis of data obtained from family practices in Quebec, Canada, estimating that two or more chronic health problems were present in 69% of those aged 18–44 years, 93% of those aged 45–64 years and 99% of those aged 65 and over. It found that almost 50% of patients between the ages of 45 and 64 years had five or more chronic conditions (Fortin et al. 2005). These seemingly high figures are likely to be explained,

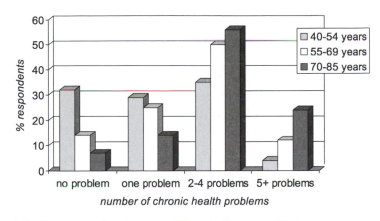

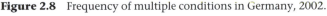

Figure 2.8 Frequency of multiple conditions in Germany, 2002.

Source: From Deutsche Zentrum für Altersfragen 2005.

at least in part, by the design of the study, with data collected in a primary care setting.

In contrast, data from a population-based study of eight countries undertaken during the 1990s found prevalence rates of those with one chronic condition, based on self-reported data of the adult population aged 18 years and over, to range from 14% in the Netherlands to 28–29% in France and Norway (pooled estimate of eight countries, 25%; Alonso et al. 2004). Those reporting two chronic conditions ranged from 7% in the Netherlands to 18% in Italy and the United States (pooled estimate, 13%). These figures are much lower than those reported by Fortin et al. (2005). The former study relied on self-reported data, and also considered a limited range of health problems as "chronic condition" only (Alonso et al. 2004). However, the Canadian study considered a much broader range of conditions; furthermore, data were collected from patients seeking care, thus possibly overestimating the prevalence of multimorbidity in the general population.

Additional evidence on the extent of multimorbidity comes from the individual country case studies in the volume that accompanies this book, although methodological constraints (as noted above) make it difficult to compare these data. Those reported are not dissimilar to those reported by Alonso et al. (2004) and Fortin et al. (2005). For example, in the Netherlands, 61% of men aged 60–79 years reported at least two chronic conditions (average 2.4); this increased to 74% among men who were 80 years or older (average 3.2) (van den Jeths et al. 2004). In Germany, some 62% people aged 55–69 years reported at least two chronic conditions, and this proportion increased to approximately 80% among those aged 70–85 years (Figure 2.8).

Interpreting the evidence

This chapter has relied to a great extent on mortality statistics to evaluate patterns of health in European populations. The advantage is that mortality data are routinely available in most countries and that death is a unique event that is clearly defined (Ruzicka and Lopez 1990). There are, however, important caveats regarding statistics of causes of death, concerning validity and completeness of both death and population denominator data. While mortality data in the European region are generally considered as of good quality, there are some countries in transition that have been experiencing problems in ensuring complete registration of all deaths, mainly those of the least-developed parts of central Asia (McKee and Chenet 2002) and regions that have been afflicted by war, as in the Caucasus (Badurashvili et al. 2001) and southeast Europe (Bozicevic et al. 2001). Despite some improvements since the 1990s, problems remain, with recent figures estimating completeness of mortality data from vital registration systems to range between 60% in Albania and 66–75% in the Caucasus to 84–89% in Kazakhstan and Kyrgyzstan (Mathers et al. 2005). These estimates relate to adult deaths only, and completeness of child death registration is likely to be lower in many parts of the region. In addition, in several countries, the vital registration system does not cover the total resident population but excludes certain geographical areas, such as Chechnya in the Russian Federation or the Transdnistria region in Moldova (WHO 2007).

Importantly, however, as indicated above, mortality data capture only those causes of morbidity that have a fatal outcome and they are, therefore, only an approximate measure of the burden of disease in a given population. This is because mortality data available for statistical analysis routinely report a single underlying cause of death only (Kelson and Farebrother 1987; Mackenbach et al. 1987). This creates problems when certifying deaths at old age, as multiple conditions coexist and attribution of death to just one of them may be almost impossible. Although methodologically more complex, applying multiple cause of death codings, which considers all (contributing) causes of death, could help to provide more comprehensive insights and facilitate studies of the relationships among conditions (Jougla et al. 2001). Consequently, estimating the "true" burden of mortality from chronic illness in the European region will remain a challenge if it is based on existing routine statistics in their current format.

In contrast to mortality, routine collection of markers of morbidity such as incidence and prevalence rates remains relatively scarce, with the possible exception of infectious diseases, which are generally captured in national monitoring and control systems, albeit to varying degrees (MacLehose et al. 2002). Available information on morbidity attributable to chronic diseases is often limited to local studies, such as the WHO MONICA Project, or registries for specific diseases, such as cancer registries. These can provide useful additional information but can sometimes be misleading, for example where registration is not population based. Population surveys, by comparison, are often not comparable across regions, and even when they are, will usually reflect only the "general" population while excluding specific subpopulations such as the institutionalized or those who are difficult to reach.

Estimates of prevalence or incidence are also influenced by the criteria used to identify health problems. For example, the DECODE Study examined the effect of different diagnostic practices on prevalence estimates for diabetes and impaired glucose regulation in 13 populations from nine European countries (DECODE Study Group 2003). It found that using fasting glucose as the sole diagnostic criterion potentially underestimated the prevalence of both problems in several populations, particularly in women and in older men. Similarly, there is as yet no consensus on the precise definition of COPD, as is also the case for multimorbidity. Consequently, while it is generally agreed that COPD should be diagnosed using spirometry, the criteria used to define airflow obstruction vary and may produce prevalence estimates that differ by 200% (Celli et al. 2003). Also, similarities in the presentation of asthma and COPD, and the fact that these conditions coexist in many patients, create diagnostic uncertainty.

Assessing the "true" disease burden is particularly problematic for conditions that are not easily identified, as in the case of dementia. Many people in the early stages of dementia are undiagnosed; for example in the United Kingdom, it is estimated that only about a third to a half of sufferers ever receive a formal diagnosis (National Audit Office 2007). Fear and ignorance of the disease among people affected as well as attitudes of health professionals, namely a perception that little can be done, along with a lack of urgency in investigation and intervention, have been identified as key barriers to early diagnosis.

As for multimorbidity, there is lack of agreement on how to measure it and, more importantly perhaps, most assessments are based on a simple count of the number of conditions without taking account of their severity (Fortin et al. 2005). This type of information is, however, crucial for assessing the "true" burden of illness if it is to inform healthcare planning.

The way forward

This chapter has illustrated the many challenges associated with assessing, comparing and contrasting the level, distribution, and nature of the chronic disease burden in Europe. Clearly it will be essential to continue efforts to tackle the technical and methodological problems and to ensure the development and collection of robust, consistent indicators required to inform policies to respond to burden of chronic diseases in Europe and elsewhere. Initiatives such as the European Health Survey System, currently being developed by Eurostat and the European Commission's Health and Protection Directorate-General, is a potential way forward, with the recent Special Eurobarometer report *Health in the European Union* as one important step in this direction (European Commission 2004, 2007), albeit with small samples of uncertain representative power in each country. Governments and international agencies are calling for greater accountability and transparency, as are civil society, the donor community, scientists and the public, in order to measure progress and performance of health systems. This calls for information that goes beyond simple descriptive statistics to including aspects of health system performance such as quality, efficiency, equity and quantification of uncertainty.

Primary collection of data on chronic diseases is of critical importance to elucidate the disease burden in a given population and thus devise appropriate strategies for prevention and management. Inadequate quality and poor availability of health statistics may result from poor measurement instruments, insufficient or suboptimal data collection methods and lack of analysis and methods to produce comparable estimates (Boerma and Stansfield 2007). Several chronic conditions and their risk factors lack an appropriate "test" that can be used in surveys to estimate population prevalence (Boerma and Stansfield 2007). In discussing the development of the ISARE project to generate a database of various health, demographic and socioeconomic indicators at subnational level in Europe, Wilkinson et al. (2008) have highlighted the difficulties encountered in supplying data even when there is willingness to do so.

Murray (2007) identified several issues to be addressed to achieve good practice in the use of health statistics. There is a need to channel efforts to improving the measurement of a small set of priority indicators in order to enhance political visibility while using limited resources most effectively. The definition of priority indicators should meet certain criteria so as to enhance their usefulness to inform policy. These include being clear on what the proposed indicator is intended to measure, the public health significance of the indicator, how well the indicator measures the quantity of interest, how readily interpretable the indicator value is, whether there is a practical measurement strategy and how well the indicator captures equity (Murray 2007).

Murray (2007) has also argued for explicit data audit trails to address existing controversies about health statistics, to increase transparency and to encourage better primary data collection and analytical methods. Audit trials should be available to the public and make explicit the process for primary data collection, post-data collection adjustments, choice of models, including covariates used for predictions, and all other documentation necessary to understand data presented to the public.

However, while enhancing data collection systems and methodological approaches to overcome inevitable data limitations is certainly an important step forward in assessing the "true" burden of disease in a given population, it is important to emphasize the need to go beyond simply creating health information systems. What is needed is a willingness among policy makers to invest in "intelligence", a system in which knowledge generation, synthesis and implementation are crucially integrated in the healthcare system in order to enable systematic and comprehensive assessment of population health needs and to inform strategic responses to the rising burden of chronic illness in Europe and elsewhere.

Conclusions

This chapter has described the major contribution that chronic diseases make to the overall burden of disease and death in the WHO European Region. With cardiovascular diseases and cancers continuing to be the leading causes of mortality in the region, and complex conditions such as diabetes and depression projected to impose a growing and costly burden, the need for reliable, appropriate and comparable data to inform local and national policies and initiatives is all the more pressing. With changing demographic patterns and increasing evidence of the health and societal costs of chronic diseases, it will be all the more crucial to address the methodological challenges in assessing and monitoring the chronic disease burden.

Notes

1. Estimates of the disease burden are based on a range of assumptions and their limitations have been discussed in detail elsewhere (Lopez et al. 2006; Mathers and Loncar 2006). A key issue is how to define and measure disability and then to select the weights to apply to particular health states. The effect of disability weighting is that conditions which, while disabling, rarely cause death (in particular mental illness) are ranked as more important than they would be using mortality alone. A related issue is the value placed on a year of life at different stages in life, with the Global Burden of Disease study placing more weight on a year of life of a young adult than on that of a child or older person. This has the effect of reducing the burden of disease arising from deaths in childhood.
2. We here use the definition put forward by the United States National Library of Medicine's controlled vocabulary used for indexing articles, which defines chronic diseases as those "which have one or more of the following characteristics: they are permanent, leave residual disability, are caused by non-reversible pathological alteration, require special training of the patient for rehabilitation, or may be expected to require a long period of supervision, observation, or care" (Timmreck 1986). This definition includes a range of health problems such as diabetes, cerebrovascular and heart disease, depression, chronic obstructive pulmonary disease, progressive multiple sclerosis, chronic heart and renal failure as well as HIV/AIDS. Cancer has traditionally been excluded from this definition because of the generally non-chronic nature of the disease; however, this is changing with the expansion of effective treatment, and the WHO (2005a) now explicitly considers cancer as a chronic disease.

References

Alonso, J., Ferrer, M., Gandeck, B. et al. (2004) Health-related quality of life associated with chronic conditions in eight countries: results from the International Quality of Life Assessment (IQOLA) project, *Qual Life Res*, 13: 282–98.

Anderson, R., Minimo, A., Hoyert, D. and Rosenberg, H. (2001) *Comparability of Cause of Death Between ICD-9 and ICD-10: Preliminary Estimates. National Vital Statistics Report*, Vol. 49/2. Maryland, MD: National Center for Health Statistics.

Ayuso-Mateos, J.L., Vasquez-Barquero, J.L., Dowrick, C. et al. (2001) Depressive disorders in Europe: prevalence figures from the ODIN study, *Br J Psychiatry*, 179: 308–16.

Badurashvili, I., McKee, M., Tsuladze, G. et al. (2001) Where there are no data: what has happened to life expectancy in Georgia since 1990? *Public Health*, 115: 394–400.

Ben-Shlomo, Y. and Kuh, D. (2002) A life course approach to chronic disease epidemiology: conceptual models, empirical challenges, and interdisciplinary perspectives, *Int J Epidemiol*, 31: 285–93.

Boerma, J. and Stansfield, S. (2007) Health statistics now: are we making the right investments? *Lancet*, 369: 779–86.

Bonita, R. (1992) Epidemiology of stroke, *Lancet*, 339: 342–4.

Bozicevic, I., Oreskovic, S., Stevanovic, R. et al. (2001) What is happening to the health of the Croatian population? *Croat Med J* 42: 601–5.

Bundkirchen, A. and Schwinger, R. (2004) Epidemiology and economic burden of chronic heart failure, *Eur Heart J Suppl*, 6(D): 57–60.

Carandang, R., Seshadri, S., Beiser, A. et al. (2006) Trends in incidence, lifetime risk, severity, and 30-day mortality of stroke over the past 50 years, *JAMA*, 296: 2939–46.

Celli, B., Halbert, R., Isonaka, S. and Schau, B. (2003) Population impact of different definitions of airway obstruction, *Eur Respir J*, 22: 268–73.

Cowie, M., Mosterd, A. and Wood, D. (1997) The epidemiology of heart failure, *Eur Heart J*, 18: 208–25.

Danai, G., Lawes, C., van der Hoorn, S., Murray, C.J. and Ezzati, M. (2006) Global and regional mortality from ischaemic heart disease and stroke attributable to higher-than-optimum blood glucose concentration: comparative risk assessment, *Lancet*, 368: 1651–9.

DECODE Study Group (2003) Age- and sex-specific prevalences of diabetes and impaired glucose regulation in 13 European countries, *Diabetes Care*, 26: 61–9.

Demyttenaere, K., Bruffaerts, R., Posada-Villa, J., et al. (2004) Prevalence, severity, and unmet need for treatment of mental disorders in the World Health Organization World Mental Health Surveys, *JAMA*, 291: 2581–90.

Deutsche Zentrum für Altersfragen (2005) *Gesundheit und Gesundheitsversorgung. Der Alterssurvey: Aktuelles auf einen Blick, ausgewählte Ergebnisse*. Bonn: Bundesministeriums für Familie, Senioren, Frauen und Jugend. Gesundheit und Gesundheitsversorgung, http://www.statistik.at/web_de/services/publikationen/4/index.html (accessed 12 December 2006).

Devereux, G. (2006) ABC of chronic obstructive pulmonary disease. Definition, epidemiology and risk factors, *BMJ*, 332: 1142–4.

Din-Dzietham, R., Liu, Y., Bielo, M. and Shamsa, F. (2007) High blood pressure trends in children and adolescents in national surveys, 1963 to 2002, *Circulation*, 116: 1488–96.

Ebrahim, S. and Harwood, R. (1999) *Stroke. Epidemiology, Evidence, and Clinical Practice*. Oxford: Oxford University Press.

ENFUMOSA-Study-Group (2003) The ENFUMOSA cross-sectional European multicentre study of the clinical phenotype of chronic severe asthma, *Eur Respir J*, 22: 470–7.

Engelgau, M.M., Geiss, L.S., Saaddine, J.B. et al. (2004) The evolving diabetes burden in the United States, *Ann Intern Med*, 140: 945–950.

European Commission (2004) *Building a European Health Survey System: Improving Information on Self-perceived Morbidity and Chronic Conditions. Report of the Working Party on Morbidity and Mortality*. Luxembourg: European Commission Health and Consumer Protection Directorate-General. http://ec.europa.eu/health/ph_information/implement/wp/morbidity/docs/ev_20040120_rd04_en.pdf (accessed 24 October 2007).

European Commission (2007) *The European Health Survey System*. Luxembourg: European Commission Health and Consumer Protection Directorate-General. http://ec.europa.eu/health/ph_information/dissemination/reporting/ehss_en.htm (accessed 13 June 2008).

Feigin, V., Lawes, C., Bennett, D. and CS, A. (2003) Stroke epidemiology: a review of population-based studies of incidence, prevalence, and case-fatality in the late 20th century, *Lancet Neurol*, 2: 43–53.

Feinstein, A. (1970) The pre-therapeutic classification of co-morbidity in chronic disease, *J Chronic Dis*, 23: 455–69.

Ferri, C., Prince, M., Brayne, C. et al. (2005) Global prevalence of dementia: a Delphi consensus study, *Lancet*, 366: 2112–17.

Fortin, M., Bravo, G., Hudon, C., Vanasse, A. and Lapointe, L. (2005) Prevalence of multimorbidity among adults seen in family practice, *Ann Fam Med*, 3: 223–8.

Freedman, V., Martin, L. and Schoeni, R. (2002) Recent trends in disability and functioning among older adults in the United States, *JAMA*, 288: 3137–46.

Freedman, V., Schoeni, R., Martin, L. and Cornman, J. (2007) Chronic conditions and the decline in late-life disability, *Demography*, 44: 459–77.

Fries, J.F. (1983) The compression of morbidity, *Milbank Mem Fund Q Health Soc*, 61: 397–419.

Gorospe, E. and Dave, J. (2006) The risk of dementia with increased body mass index, *Age Ageing*, 36: 23–9.

Green, A. and Patterson, C.C. (2001) Trends in the incidence of childhood-onset diabetes in Europe 1989–1998, *Diabetologia*, 44(Suppl 3): B3–8.

Hackett, M., Yapa, C., Parag, V. and Anderson, C. (2005) Frequency of depression after stroke, *Stroke*, 36: 1330–40.

Haines, L., Wan, K., Lynn, R., Barrett, T. and Shield, J. (2007) Rising incidence of type 2 diabetes in children in the UK, *Diabetes Care*, 30: 1097–101.

Halpin, D.M.G. and Miravitlles, M. (2006) Chronic obstructive pulmonary disease. The disease and its burden to society, *Proc Am Thoracic Soc*, 3: 619–23.

International Diabetes Federation (2003) *Diabetes Atlas: eatlas*. Brussels: International Diabetes Federation. http://www.idf.org/e-atlas (accessed 24 October 2007).

Janssen, F. and Kunst, A. (2005) Cohort patterns in mortality trends among the elderly in seven European countries, 1950–99, *Int J Epidemiol*, 34: 1149–59.

Jougla, E., Papoz, L., Balkau, B., Maguin, P. and Hatton, F. (1992) Death certificate coding practices related to diabetes in European countries: the "EURODIAB Subarea C" study, *Int J Epidemiol*, 21: 343–51.

Jougla, E., Rossolin, F., Niyonsenga, A. and Chappert, J. (2001) *Comparability and Quality Improvement of the European Causes of Death Statistics*. Nantes: INSERM.

Kaplan, G. and Keil, J. (1993) Socioeconomic factors and cardiovascular disease: a review of the literature, *Circulation*, 88: 1973–98.

Kelson, M. and Farebrother, M. (1987) The effect of inaccuracies in death certification and coding practices in the European Economic Community (EEC) on international cancer mortality statistics, *Int J Epidemiol*, 16: 411–14.

Kessler, R. (2007) The global burden of anxiety and mood disorders: putting the European Study of the Epidemiology of Mental Disorders (ESEMeD) findings into perspective, *J Clin Psychiatry*, 68(Suppl 2): 10–19.

Kessler, R., Demler, O., Frank, R. et al. (2005) Prevalence and treatment of mental disorders, 1990 to 2003, *N Engl J Med*, 352: 2515–23.

Kinsella, K. and Phillips, D. (2005) Global aging: the challenge of success, *Population Bull*, 60: 5–42.

Lafortune, G., Balestat, G. and Disability Study Expert Group Members (2007) *Trends in Severe Disability among Elderly People: Assessing the Evidence in 12 OECD Countries and the Future Implications*. Paris: OECD.

Liebetrau, M., Steen, B. and Skoog, I. (2003) Stroke in 85-year-olds: prevalence, incidence, risk factors, and relation to mortality and dementia, *Stroke*, 34: 2617–22.

Loddenkemper, R., Gibson, G.J. and Sibille, Y. (2003) *European Lung White Book*. Sheffield, UK: European Respiratory Society.

Lopez, A.D., Mathers, C.D., Ezzati, M., Jamison, D.T. and Murray, C., J L (2006) *Global Burden of Disease and Risk Factors*. New York: Oxford University Press and World Bank.

Mackenbach, J., Van Duyne, W. and Kelson, M. (1987) Certification and coding of two underlying causes of death in the Netherlands and other countries of the European Community, *J Epidemiol Comm Health*, 41: 156–60.

MacLehose, L., McKee, M. and Weinberg, J. (2002) Responding to the challenge of communicable disease in Europe, *Science*, 295: 2047–50.

Marmot, M., Smith, G., Stansfeld, S. et al. (1991) Health inequalities among British civil servants: the Whitehall II study, *Lancet*, 337: 1387–93.

Marmot, M., Shipley, M., Brunner, E. and Hemingway, H. (2001) Relative contribution of early life and adult socioeconomic factors to adult morbidity in the Whitehall II study, *J Epidemiol Community Health*, 55: 301–7.

Masoli, M., Fabian, D., Holt, S. and Beasley, R. (2004) *Global Initiative for Asthma. The global Burden of Asthma Report.* Southampton, UK: University of Southampton.

Mathers, C. and Loncar, D. (2006) Projections of global mortality and burden of disease from 2002 to 2030, *PLoS Med*, 3: e442.

Mathers, C., Ma Fat, D., Inoue, M., Rao, C. and Lopez, A. (2005) Counting the dead and what they died from: an assessment of the global status of cause of death data, *Bull World Health Organ*, 83: 171–7.

McCarron, P., Davey Smith, D. and Okasha, M. (2002) Secular changes in blood pressure in childhood, adolescence and young adulthood: systematic review of trends from 1948 to 1998, *J Hum Hypertens*, 16: 677–89.

McKee, M. and Chenet, L. (2002) Patterns of health, in M. McKee, J. Healy and J. Falkingham (eds) *Health Care in Central Asia*, pp.57–66. Buckingham: Open University Press.

Mehta, P. and Cowie, M. (2006) Gender and heart failure: a population perspective, *Heart*, 92(Suppl III): 14–18.

Moorman, J., Rudd, R., Johnson, C. et al. (2007) National surveillance for asthma. United States, 1980–2004, *MMWR*, 56: 1–14, 18–54.

Mosterd, A. and Hoes, A. (2007) Clinical epidemiolgy of heart failure, *Heart*, 93: 1137–46.

Murdoch, D., Love, M., Robb, S. et al. (1998) Importance of heart failure as a cause of death, *Eur Heart J*, 19: 1829–35.

Murray, C. (2007) Towards good practice for health statistics: lessons from the Millennium Development Goal health indicators, *Lancet*, 369: 862–73.

Murray, C.J.L., Salomon, J.A., Mathers, C.D. and Lopez, A.D. (eds) (2002) *Summary Measures of Population Health. Concepts, Ethics, Measurement and Applications.* Geneva, World Health Organization.

Najafi, F., Dobson, A. and Jamrozik, K. (2006) Is mortality from heart failure increasing in Australia? An analysis of official data on mortality for 1997–2003, *Bull World Health Organ*, 84: 722–8.

Narayan, K.M., Boyle, J.P., Thompson, T.J., Sorensen, S.W. and Williamson, D.F. (2003) Lifetime risk for diabetes mellitus in the United States, *JAMA*, 290: 1884–90.

National Audit Office (2007) *Improving Services and Support for People with Dementia.* London: The Stationery Office.

Parker, M. and Thorslund, M. (2007) Health trends in the elderly population: getting better and getting worse, *Gerontologist*, 47: 150–8.

Patel, M., Tilling, K., Lawrence, E. et al. (2006) Relationships between long-term stroke disability, handicap and health-related quality of life, *Age Ageing*, 35: 273–9.

Pauwels, R.A. (2000) COPD. The scope of the problem in Europe, *Chest*, 117: 332–5.

Pauwels, R.A. and Rabe, K.F. (2004) Burden and clinical features of chronic obstructive pulmonary disease (COPD), *Lancet*, 364: 613–20.

Perrin, J., Bloom, S. and Gortmaker, S. (2007) The increase of childhood chronic conditions in the United States, *JAMA*, 297: 2755–9.

Piette, J. and Kerr, E. (2006) The impact of comorbid chronic conditions on diabetes care, *Diabetes Care*, 29: 725–31.

Piette, J., Richardson, C. and Valenstein, M. (2004) Addressing the needs of patients with multiple chronic illnesses: the case of diabetes and depression, *Am J Manage Care*, 10: 152–62.

Poole, K., Reeve, J. and Warburton, E. (2002) Falls, fractures, and osteoporosis after stroke. Time to think about protection? *Stroke*, 33: 1342–6.

Rabe, K.F., Vermeire, P.A., Soriano, J.B. and Maier, W.C. (2000) Clinical management of asthma in 1999: the Asthma Insights and Reality in Europe (AIRE) study, *Eur Respir J*, 16: 802–7.

Remme, W., McMurray, J., Rauch, B. et al. (2005) Public awareness of heart failure in Europe: first results from SHAPE, *Eur Heart J*, 26: 2413–21.

Ritchie, K. and Lovestone, S. (2002) The dementias, *Lancet*, 360: 1759–66.

Rothwell, P., Coull, A., Giles, M. et al. (2004) Change in stroke incidence, mortality, case-fatality, severity, and risk factors in Oxfordshire, UK from 1981 to 2004 (Oxford Vascular Study), *Lancet*, 363: 1925–33.

Ruzicka, L. and Lopez, A. (1990) The use of cause-of-death statistics for health situation assessment: National and international experiences. *World Health Stat Q*, 43: 249–58.

Sears, M., Greene, J., Willan, A. et al. (2003) A longitudinal, population-based, cohort study of childhood asthma followed to adulthood, *N Engl J Med*, 349: 1414–22.

Sobocki, P., Joensson, B., Angst, J. and Rehnberg, C. (2006) Cost of depression in Europe, *J Ment Health Policy Econ*, 9: 87–98.

Stewart, S., MacIntyre, K., Capewell, S. and McMurray, J. (2003) Heart failure and the aging population: an increasing burden in the 21st century? *Heart*, 89: 49–53.

Terent, A. (2003) Trends in stroke incidence and 10-year survival in Soederhamn, Sweden, 1975–2001, *Stroke*, 34: 1353–8.

Thorvaldsen, P., Kuulasmaa, K., Rajakangas, A. et al. (1997) Stroke trends in the WHO MONICA project, *Stroke*, 28: 500–6.

Timmreck, T. (1986) *Dictionary of Health Services Management*. Owings Mills, MD: National Health Pub.

Ustun, T.B., Ayuso-Mateos, J.L., Chatterji, S., Mathers, C. and Murray, C.J. (2004) Global burden of depressive disorders in the year 2000, *Br J Psychiatry*, 184: 386–92.

van den Jeths, A.B., Timmermans, J.N., Hoeymans, N., Woittiez, I.B. (2004) Ouderen nu en in de toekomst. Gezondheid, verpleging en verzorging 2000–2020. [The Elderly Now and in the Future. Health, Care and Caring for 2000–2020.] Bilthoven: RIVM. www.rivm.nl/bibliotheek/rapporten/270502001.pdf (accessed 24 October 2007).

van der Lee, J., Mokkink, L., Grootenhuis, M., Heymans, H. and Offringa, M. (2007) Definitions and measurement of chronic health conditions in childhood, *JAMA*, 297: 2741–51.

van Weel, C. and Schellevis, F. (2006) Comorbidity and guidelines: conflicting interests, *Lancet*, 367: 550–51.

WHO (2003) *Mental Health in the WHO European Region. Factsheet EURO/03/03*. Copenhagen: World Health Organization Regional Office for Europe.

WHO (2004a) *Health Statistics and Health Information Systems. Revised Global Burden of Disease (GBD) 2002 Estimates*. Geneva: World Health Organization. http://www.who.int/healthinfo/bodgbd2002revised/en/index.html (accessed 9 January 2007).

WHO (2004b) *WHO Statistical Information System. Causes of Death and Burden of Disease Estimates by Country (2002)* Geneva: World Health Organization. http://www.who.int/healthinfo/statistics/bodgbddeathdalyestimates.xls (accessed 10 January 2007).

WHO (2005a) *Preventing Chronic Diseases. A Vital Investment: WHO Global Report*. Geneva: World Health Organization.

WHO (2005b) *The European Health Report 2005. Public Health Actions for Healthier Children and Populations*. Copenhagen: World Health Organization.

WHO (2005c) *The Health of Children and Adolescents in Europe. Factsheet EURO/06/05*. Copenhagen: World Health Organization, Regional Office for Europe. http://www.euro.who.int/document/mediacentre/fs0605e.pdf (accessed 11 January 2007).

WHO (2006a) *Health Statistics and Health Information Systems. Projections of Mortality and Burden of Disease to 2030*. Geneva: World Health Organization. http://www.who.int/healthinfo/statistics/bodprojections2030/en/index.html (accessed 10 January 2007).

WHO (2006b) *Diabetes: Factsheet 312*. Geneva: World Health Organization. http://www.who.int/mediacentre/factsheets/fs312/en/ (accessed 11 January 2007).

WHO (2006c) *Chronic Obstructive Pulmonary Disease*. Geneva: World Health Organization.

http://www.who.int/respiratory/copd/burden/en/index.html (accessed 11 January 2007).

WHO (2006d) *Asthma: Factsheet 307*. Geneva: World Health Organization. http://www.who.int/mediacentre/factsheets/fs307/en/index.html (accessed 11 January 2007).

WHO (2007) *Health for all Database*. Copenhagen, World Health Organization Regional Office for Europe.

Wild, S., Roglic, G., Green, A., Sicree, R. and King, H. (2004) Global prevalence of diabetes, *Diabetes Care*, 27: 1047–53.

Wilkinson, J., Berghmans, L., Imbert, F. et al. (2008) Health indicators in the European regions ISARE II., *Eur J Public Health*, 18: 178–83.

Wimo, A., Winblad, B., Aguero-Torres, H. and von Strauss, E. (2003) The magnitude of dementia occurence in the world, *Alzheimer Dis Assoc Disord*, 17: 63–7.

Wolfe, C. (2000) The impact of stroke, *Br Med Bull*, 56: 275–86.

Yach, D., Hawkes, C., Gould, C. and Hofman, K. (2004) The global burden of chronic diseases, *JAMA*, 291: 2616–22.

three

Economic aspects of chronic disease and chronic disease management

Marc Suhrcke, Daragh K. Fahey and Martin McKee

Introduction

Health policy makers face many competing calls on their attention. Inevitably, their focus is often dominated by the urgent and the measurable, hence the priorities given to, for example, outbreaks of communicable disease or the reduction in waiting lists. In contrast, despite the enormous contribution that it makes to the overall burden of disease, the phenomenon of chronic diseases tends to be seen as being neither urgent nor easily measurable. Indeed, until the seminal work of the Global Burden of Disease study, which added morbidity to the traditional measurement of mortality, the scale of the problem posed by chronic diseases was, to many policy makers, largely invisible. The problem was compounded by the absence of easy solutions. During the twentieth century, huge health gains were achieved with technically relatively simple solutions, such as mass vaccination or the integrated management of childhood illness. In contrast, as illustrated in Chapters 4 and 10, effective management of chronic diseases demands the creation of complex systems that bridge the different disciplinary perspectives and confront entrenched cognitive and financial barriers to cooperation, plus the support of appropriate information technology. Worse, from the perspective of the politician whose time horizon is dominated by the electoral cycle, the results of innovation are likely to be seen long in the future, when someone else will be able to take the credit.

This chapter recognizes the strong disincentives to initiate effective action but seeks to counterbalance them by highlighting the economic arguments for doing so. It presents evidence showing that the economic cost of chronic disease in Europe is high and that there may well be a strong economic argument for a society to invest in chronic disease management.

The starting point for the first part of the chapter, on the assessment of the cost of chronic disease, is a recent publication by the European Commission (Suhrcke et al. 2005) that has assembled much of the existing body of research on this topic. Before looking at this evidence, however, it is necessary to consider what is meant by "economic costs" and, in particular, how they are relevant to the discussion of chronic disease.

The second part examines the economics of chronic disease management. We begin by discussing briefly the reasons for undertaking such economic evaluations, providing a framework that describes the different categories of costs and benefits that are relevant and complementing the conceptual discussion with selected empirical examples. Inevitably, the examples chosen draw heavily on the much greater volume of research on this topic from the United States, compared with Europe. Nevertheless, where possible, we review what has been done or is planned to be done in terms of evaluations – economic and non-economic – in Europe, given the quite different health systems contexts.

The economic burden of chronic diseases in Europe

This section reviews different concepts of economic costs, highlighting their variety and the potential confusion between them and illustrating them with selected empirical examples. A more complete account of the empirical evidence on the costs of chronic disease can be found in Adeyi et al. (2007) and Suhrcke et al. (2006); Suhrcke et al. (2007) have focused on evidence from eastern Europe and central Asia. We distinguish five cost concepts, each with distinctive implications for measurement: costs of illness, microeconomic costs/consequences, macroeconomic costs/consequences, "welfare" or "true" economic costs and public policy-relevant versus policy-irrelevant costs.

Cost of illness

Cost-of-illness studies estimate both the quantity of resources (in monetary terms) used to treat a disease and the negative economic consequences of illness, measured as lost productivity to society or to a specific sector. They represent a useful first step in assessing the economic burden of ill health in general and of chronic disease in particular, with most studies suggesting that the burden is substantial. Cost-of-illness studies can also provide the foundation for subsequent economic evaluations of specific interventions or policy measures to reduce the burden of disease. Cost-of-illness studies separate costs into three components.

Direct costs. These are the costs of medical care in relation to prevention, diagnosis and treatment of disease. They include costs such as ambulances, inpatient or outpatient care, rehabilitation, community health services and medication. Of the cost components, this is the least controversial measurement, although it is also not without problems.

Indirect costs. The loss of human resources caused by morbidity or premature death reflect indirect costs. The measurement of indirect costs is a matter of much debate. Some cost-of-illness studies consider the loss of future earnings (the human-capital approach) and thereby restrict the estimate to the working population. Others use the willingness-to-pay method, which assesses what people are willing to pay for relatively small changes in the risk of death. These figures, which are not restricted to the working population, make it possible to derive the value that people assign to life.

Intangible costs. These capture the psychological dimensions of illness including pain, bereavement, anxiety and suffering. This cost category is typically hardest to measure.

Table 3.1 provides examples of these components.

Table 3.1 Examples of direct, indirect and intangible costs

Type of cost	Example
Direct costs	
Healthcare	Ambulance
	Clinician assessment and management (e.g. physicians, nurses)
	Ongoing care (e.g. nurse assistants, carers)
	Procedures (e.g. surgery)
	Investigations (e.g. blood tests)
	Medicines
	Equipment (e.g. dialysis, wheelchairs)
	Educational (e.g. leaflets, websites)
	Lifestyle (e.g. exercise on prescription, dietetics)
Rehabilitation	Physical (e.g. physiotherapy, occupational therapy)
	Mental (e.g. counselling)
	Social (e.g. employment training, support for independence and activities of daily living)
Social care	Home assessments and upgrades
	Meals on wheels
	Housing (e.g. sheltered housing)
Indirect costs	
Wider economy	Reduced productivity of patient and carer
	Unemployment benefits
Individual	Reduced income
	Loss of future earnings from selling assets
	Carers leaving education early to care for sick relative
Intangible costs	Pain
	Bereavement
	Anxiety
	Stigma
	Frustration
	Depression

In practice, most studies assess direct and indirect costs only.[1] A selective literature review undertaken for an earlier study showed that the cost of chronic diseases and their risk factors, as measured by cost-of-illness studies, is sizeable, ranging from 0.02% to 6.77% of a country's gross domestic product (GDP) (Suhrcke et al. 2006). For cardiovascular disease, the total cost varies between 1 and 3% in most developed countries for which results are available, although when interpreting the figures it is important to note that the numerical results from cost-of-illness studies are typically not directly comparable across countries, disease categories and time. Table 3.2 presents estimates of direct costs of cardiovascular disease for 25 countries of the European Union. Table 3.3 shows cost-of-illness estimates for a limited set of other conditions and risk factors.

Cost-of-illness studies are limited by certain conceptual and methodological constraints. Some have argued that the cost-of-illness approach represents a public health view of "costs", rather than an economic view (Sindelar 1998). From a public health perspective, society should be as healthy as possible, which would reduce expensive medical treatments. From this perspective,

Table 3.2 Healthcare costs for cardiovascular disease by EU country, 2003

Country	Cost per capita (€)	Percentage of total healthcare expenditure
Germany	423	15
United Kingdom	368	18
Sweden	318	12
Netherlands	273	11
Luxembourg	255	8
Austria	247	11
Finland	235	12
Denmark	215	7
Italy	204	11
Belgium	201	8
France	194	8
Greece	140	11
Ireland	108	4
Spain	97	7
Portugal	93	8
Czech Republic	83	14
Slovenia	80	8
Cyprus	67	7
Estonia	55	17
Hungary	52	9
Slovakia	52	18
Poland	46	16
Lithuania	43	16
Latvia	24	11
Malta	22	2
TOTAL EU	230	12

Source: Petersen et al. (2005).

Table 3.3 Selected cost-of-illness studies in which cost is expressed as percentage of national health expenditure

Condition/risk factor	Country	Percentage of national health expenditure	Year
Coronary heart disease	United Kingdom	11	1999
Schizoprenia	France	2	1992
	United Kingdom	1.7	1992–03
	Netherlands	1.6	1989
Depression	United Kingdom	0.9	1990–01
Mental illness	United States	7	1990
Obesity	France	2	1992
	Portugal	3.5	1996
Diabetes	Various	2.5–15	Various
Tobacco	Germany	5.6	1993

Source: Suhrcke et al. (2005), where full details of studies are given.

cost-of-illness studies should assign a monetary value to all the morbidity and mortality that is associated with a disease or a risk factor and measure the medical expenditures that would be saved if there had been no illness. In contrast, an economic perspective does not start from the assumption that society should be as healthy as possible. Economists assess the cost of a given situation by comparing it with its next best (and feasible) alternative situation (the "counterfactual"). Implicitly, cost-of-illness studies assume that the counterfactual is the absence of chronic disease, mortality or the risk factor that gives rise to disease. This is often too ambitious a counterfactual, either because it cannot be achieved even with the most intensive possible interventions or it may be undesirable from a welfare perspective because the resources required could be used more effectively in other ways.

A significant further limitation of cost-of-illness studies, irrespective of whether they take a public health or economic perspective, is that the methodologies commonly applied do not address causality. While they include costs that are seemingly associated with chronic disease and risk factors they do not establish that chronic disease or risk factors actually *cause* the costs to occur.[2] This is of particular relevance in relation to unhealthy behaviours, where the assignment of costs to a specific disease is problematic. From a policy perspective it is, however, critical to understand the "true" causes in order to be able to target interventions most effectively.[3]

Microeconomic costs/consequences

Microeconomic studies assess the effect of health on economic outcomes while taking into account other relevant factors. Microeconomic analysis can evaluate the mechanisms by which health influences economic outcomes and can assess the relative contributions of these mechanisms. Ideally, such studies also attempt to address the two most salient econometric challenges involved:

measurement error in the (often self-reported) health proxy that is used and the potential reverse causality (with a better economic situation contributing to better health).

The importance of at least trying to assess the direction of causality should not be underestimated. This is of immediate relevance to policy makers as it helps to specify entry points for policy interventions. For individuals, micro-economic evidence of this kind may illustrate the price they are paying in addition to the disease burden they are suffering.

The key routes through which ill health may impact on final economic output are through its effects on education, saving and investment, labour productivity and labour supply (Suhrcke et al. 2005). Much of the empirical evidence is on labour productivity and supply, not necessarily because they are more important but because these two factors are generally easier to measure. Why, and how far, does ill health in general and chronic disease in particular affect these two key economic factors?

Labour productivity. Healthier individuals could reasonably be expected to produce more per hour worked. Thus, productivity could increase directly as a result of enhanced physical and mental activity. At the same time, individuals who are more physically and mentally active could make better and more efficient use of technology, machinery or equipment. A healthier labour force could also be expected to be more flexible and adaptable to changes (e.g. changes in task profiles or the organization of labour).

Labour supply. The impact of health on labour supply is theoretically ambiguous. Good health reduces the number of days an individual spends sick, which consequently results in an increase in the number of healthy days available for either work or leisure. But health also influences the decision to supply labour through its impact on wages, preferences and expected life horizon. The effect of health on labour supply through each of these intermediate mechanisms is not always obvious. On the one hand, if wages are linked to productivity, and healthier workers are more productive, health improvements will be expected to increase wages and thus the incentives to increase labour supply (substitution effect). On the other hand, being healthy might allow higher lifetime earnings and, therefore, allow people to retire early (income effect).

There is considerable evidence to suggest that both mechanisms operate, especially with chronic diseases (and their related risk factors).

Labour productivity

In the absence of measures of physical output, economists use wages and (partly) earnings as indicators of labour productivity. Several studies demonstrate that poor health is associated with decreases in wages and earnings (Chirikos and Nestel 1985; Currie and Madrian 1999; Hansen 2000; Contoyannis and Rise 2001; Pelkowski and Berger 2004). Although the magnitude of the effect differs among studies using different proxy measures for health, the results do not differ qualitatively. Other studies use measures such as height and body mass index as proxies for health and find that, in general, greater height, which tends to reflect health in childhood, has a positive impact on wages and earnings while a higher body mass index depresses them, although more so for women than for men (Averett and Korenman 1996; Cawley 2000; Mitra 2001; Finkelstein et al. 2005; Brunello and d'Hombres 2007). It is, however, plausible that these associations could, in part, be accounted for by the social meaning attributed to height, and by social stigma in the case of obesity, rather than by a direct effect of health on productivity (Averett and Korenman 1996).

Labour supply

There is also considerable research showing that better health increases labour supply in developed countries, as measured by employment, hours worked, and the probability of retiring from the labour force. It is, however, important to recognize that findings will be sensitive to institutional frameworks, such as pension regulations, availability of disability benefits and occupational insurance arrangements, which can protect against or exacerbate the economic impact of poor health. Ill health matters, not only for those in employment but also for their household members, who adapt their employment in response to illness among their household members (Ettner 1996; Spiess and Schneider 2004). For the European Union and the United States, it was found that men reduce their work levels and are more likely to exit the labour force when their wives become ill, while women are more likely to work when their husbands fall ill, presumably to compensate for lost household income (Berger 1983; Charles 1999; Jiménez-Martín et al. 1999). However there is a need for caution when applying research in the United States to Europe, as labour participation decisions are sensitive to the availability of health insurance and disability benefits (Coile 2003).

Macroeconomic costs/consequences

A further cost dimension, of particular interest to policy makers, relates to the aggregate economy and seeks to capture the extent to which ill health (or here specifically chronic diseases) can make a difference (if any) to the level or the growth rate of national per capita income. Health in general – measured as life expectancy or adult mortality – has generally been found to be a robust and strong predictor of economic growth (Barro 1991, 1996; Levine and Renelt 1992; Barro and Lee 1994; Barro and Martin 1995; Sachs and Warner 1995, 1997; Easterly and Levine 1997; Bhargava et al. 2001; Sala-i-Martin et al. 2004; Acemoglu and Johnson 2006). Since chronic disease constitutes a major part of the overall health burden and accounts for a major part of adult mortality, it might be expected to have a negative impact on economic growth. Quantifying this impact is, however, fraught with methodological challenges.[4] The relationship between health and the economy also differs between rich and poor countries: once a certain level of economic development is reached, there is no longer a clear association between per capita incomes and life expectancy.

Barro (1996), using a worldwide sample of rich and poor countries, estimated that a five-year increase in life expectancy was associated with a 0.3–0.5% higher annual GDP growth rate in subsequent years. This finding could, in principle, be used indirectly to infer a relationship between chronic disease mortality and growth. Other studies, again using a worldwide sample of countries, have assessed the impact of specific diseases, including malaria (Gallup and Sachs 2001), HIV/AIDS (Dixon et al. 2001), malnutrition (Weil 2005) and tuberculosis (Delfino and Simmons 1999), on growth, controlling for a set of other standard determinants of growth.

These studies do not, of course, look at chronic diseases. Suhrcke and Urban (2006) looked at the impact of cardiovascular deaths among the working-age population on economic growth. Using a worldwide sample of countries for which data were available, they found that the result was dependent on the initial economic situation of the country. Dividing the sample into (broadly) low/middle-income countries and high-income countries they found a 1% increase in the mortality rate decreased the growth rate of per capita income in the subsequent five years by approximately 0.1% in high-income settings. The finding was based on panel data at five-year-intervals between 1960 and 2000 and took account of other factors including initial income, openness and secondary schooling. The authors used a dynamic panel growth regression framework, taking into account potential problems from reverse causality or omitted variables that might influence both cardiovascular mortality and growth simultaneously. While 0.1% may appear small in terms of growth, the absolute level is quite substantial when summed over the long term. In contrast, there was no significant influence of cardiovascular mortality on growth in the sample from low/middle-income countries.

The findings of that analysis must, however, be interpreted with great caution, in particular as they relate to countries of low and middle incomes, where most cause-specific adult mortality data are very limited in terms of quality and completeness. At the same time, the findings for this group of countries appear plausible because cardiovascular disease only began to emerge as a substantial contributor to mortality towards the later part of the period observed (1960–2000). The increase is arguably in response to economic progress, rather than it being a determinant thereof. If the results for high-income countries can be taken as a guide, cardiovascular disease is likely to assume a greater role as a determinant of economic growth as the chronic disease burden in developing countries progresses further.

"Welfare" or "true" economic costs

Valuing the macroeconomic losses incurred as a result of chronic disease by means of a broader measure than per-person GDP would explicitly recognize that the "true" purpose of economic activity is to maximize social welfare and not just GDP. This concept begins with the uncontroversial premise that GDP is an imperfect measure of social welfare: specifically it fails to incorporate the value of health. One different approach is the willingness-to-pay method, which makes it possible to attribute an approximate monetary value to changes in mortality. Extending this approach to chronic diseases is a fairly straightforward and instructive exercise, the results of which are likely to demonstrate more clearly the importance of chronic disease.

A great deal, if not all, of the reservations about putting a monetary value on life and health stems from a misunderstanding of what such a value actually means, and some of that misperception may reflect unfortunate use of terminology. In fact, we cannot – and do not seek to – place a monetary value on our own or on other individuals' *lives*. Instead, we are valuing what are often comparatively small changes in the *risk* of mortality, which is a very different matter. While, under normal circumstances, no one would trade his or her life for a sum of money, most people will be prepared to choose between equipment at different prices that offer different levels of safety, between different ways of crossing a street but taking different lengths of time, or between jobs that involve different mortality risks but different wages. The fact that these choices are made indicates that people do implicitly put a price on their risk of mortality.

While the value of an increase or decrease in the risk of mortality is not directly observable, it can be inferred from the actual choices people make when facing trade-offs between mortality risk and financial compensation. The most common procedure is to use labour market data about the wage premium that workers demand if they are to do a more dangerous job. Once the risk premium is estimated, the implied value of a statistical life can readily be calculated and then used to value the "costs" of mortality (and, with modifications, of ill health).

By way of caution, it is important to bear in mind that, while the underlying concept is theoretically sound and generally accepted among economists, serious problems need to be overcome when applying it empirically. Estimates of the value of a statistical life vary by a large factor, even within a given country. This is attributable, for example, to the use of different methodologies to calculate the risk premium or to using data on different populations. A simplified application of the welfare cost approach to the valuation of the costs of chronic disease is provided elsewhere (WHO 2005).

Public policy: relevant versus irrelevant costs

From an economic perspective, not all of the costs described above are relevant for public policy. Costs are considered relevant if they justify public policy intervention on the grounds of efficiency. In the idealized world that fits the following assumptions, there are no costs that justify public policy interventions:

- all costs and benefits are "internal" (or "private"): all the costs and benefits associated with a given choice are taken into account and borne by the person making that choice
- rationality: individuals maximize some objective function (e.g. their utility function) under the constraints they face, weighing the cost they would expect to incur with the expected benefits of the choice in question, the ultimate decision maximizing net benefits (or utility)
- perfect information: individuals have complete information about the expected consequences of their actions
- preferences are "time-consistent": put simply, individuals face no serious problems of self-control.

In reality, however, one or more of these assumptions almost always does not hold true, with the result that the market, left alone, does not achieve the outcome most desirable for society. In this case, at least some of the costs of chronic disease do justify public policy intervention. This is because the costs are either not borne by the individual directly concerned ("external costs") or they are incurred by an individual person making a particular choice (i.e. private) as a consequence of non-rational behaviour, imperfect information or because of intra-personal conflicts. The higher the share of the internal or external costs relevant to public policy, the greater is the justification for government to intervene to improve net social welfare (if it can).

Suhrcke et al. (2006) discuss extensively the potential market failures that arise in relation to chronic disease risk factors. In brief, their main conclusions are as follows.

- The presence of health or social costs of an individual's unhealthy behaviours that are borne by society at large ("externalities") or by family members ("quasi-externalities") may justify intervention, although the former, in particular, are typically not considered to be large in comparison with internal costs.
- There is widespread recognition that some members of the population, in particular children, are not (yet) the rational actors that economic theory assumes. Therefore, interventions that protect children are more likely to be supported.
- Information is a public good and as such it will generally be undersupplied compared with what is socially optimal. Hence, there is, in principle, a case for governments to intervene to provide information, especially in developing countries.
- A recently defined justification for intervention, grounded in behavioural economics, is the idea of time-inconsistent preferences (giving rise to "intra-personal" externalities or "internalities"): individuals seek instant gratification (for example, the calming effect of nicotine) at the expense of their long-term best interests (for example, the resulting risk of lung cancer).

Although more research is needed, these arguments can justify accepting some of the large internal costs of chronic diseases as relevant to public policy, in addition to any external costs that may exist.

Cost concepts: summary

It is important to note that this section has discussed only whether there are market failures that would – in principle – justify a public policy intervention. This by itself says nothing about whether, in reality, governments would have the means to correct the market failure at a cost that is outweighed by the return. Many interventions might not fulfil this criterion, in which case the optimal choice is to live with the status quo. Evidence of "value for money" (such as cost-effectiveness evidence) is needed. The link between the debate on market failure and evidence of cost-effectiveness also runs the other way: evidence of cost-effectiveness on its own is not a sufficient argument to justify a role for public policy. This is because, in the absence of a market failure, a highly cost-effective intervention may be undertaken privately.

The costs and benefits of chronic disease management

The fact that chronic diseases impose a significant economic burden, measured in the different ways set out in the preceding section, does not by itself necessarily imply that investment in chronic disease management is an economically sensible way forward. Such an assessment depends less on the costs of the existing disease burden but rather on that part of the disease costs that can be averted through the intervention (hence, the benefits of the intervention) set against the costs of carrying out the intervention. This is what a proper "economic evaluation" should assess, and it cannot be assumed that the net benefits will be positive. Unfortunately, economic evaluations of chronic disease management in Europe are scarce. Therefore, this section will focus on a conceptual discussion, illustrated with empirical examples where available, often drawing on work from the United States, bearing in mind the limits to the transferability of such evidence.

Costs and benefits of a given chronic disease management intervention differ according to the perspective taken. Table 3.4 provides a typology of the different costs and benefits from the four main perspectives commonly adopted: the patient, the health plan/provider, the employer and society.

If the maximization of societal welfare is the overarching policy objective, as in theory it should be, then the societal perspective is the "right" perspective to assume. However, to explain actual decision making it is often useful to understand the perspective of the different players, to see how they oppose and/or substitute each other, recognizing that this may ultimately produce a less than optimal societal output. This should also provide public policy makers with indications of how to alter incentives for private actors in a way that stimulates them to approximate better to the optimal societal outcome.

Costs of chronic disease management

As we assume that the patient will be enrolled in a health insurance scheme, the only direct costs carried by the patient will be those that the health insurance organization (i.e. the plan/provider) passes on to him or her, through increased premiums or out-of-pocket payments, as a result of reduced wages in response to greater employer payments for health insurance.

The provider of the chronic disease management programme faces three types of cost: (fixed) set-up costs (e.g. for information technology systems, staffing costs for the management of the programme), operating costs (primarily for human resources to deliver services in a coordinated manner) and adverse selection costs (arising from increased enrolment of high-cost patients in response to the improved reputation of a given programme).

The costs to the employer depend on the institutional arrangements. In the context of the United States, the health plan may be in a position to require

Table 3.4 Costs and benefits of chronic disease management

	Benefits	Costs
Patient	Improved length/quality of life (net of non-monitoring costs of changing behaviours)	Higher premium for health insurance (if the employer responds in this way) Out-of-pocket expenses (e.g. copayments) Possible reduced wages due to greater employer payments for health insurance
Plan provider	Lower use of acute services over time (if the patient remains with the plan) Higher premium for disease management programme (if the health plan can charge for it)	Set-up costs (e.g. computer technology) Operating costs (e.g. nurses, drugs, primary care physicians) Adverse selection costs (to a given plan)
Employer	Possible productivity gains (if the patient remains with the company) Possible reduced wages in exchange for better health benefits	Higher premium paid for disease management programme (if the health plan can charge for it)
Net to society	Improved length/quality of life (net of non-monetary costs of changing behaviours and indirect patient costs) Potential long-term cost savings owing to lower use of acute services over time Potential productivity gains	Setup costs Operating costs Adverse selection costs

Source: Beaulieu et al. (2003).

higher premiums in return for access to the chronic disease management programme. The situation is different in Europe, where all countries provide virtually universal coverage through statutory funding systems. Where a combination of competing insurance funds coexist with specific chronic disease management programmes, as in Germany, risk-equalization mechanisms have been put in place (Busse 2004). Issues could, however, arise in relation to private insurance (Mossialos and Thomson 2002). This may be:

- *substitutive*, where it is purchased by those outside the statutory system, typically because they have high incomes
- *complementary*, offering cover for care already within the statutory system but with greater choice of provider
- *supplementary*, covering areas excluded from the statutory system, such as some types of dentistry.

However, any consequences will be minimal, either because of the mix of subscribers (typically much healthier than average) or the nature of the package (complementary and supplementary schemes often exclude chronic disorders).

Benefits of chronic disease management

There are three primary benefits that may be derived from improved chronic disease management:

- improved health (i.e. quantity and quality of life years gained), experienced by the patient
- long-term cost savings from complications avoided and healthcare utilization reduced, experienced by the plan, the providers and potentially employers)
- workplace productivity gains, experienced by patients and their employers.

As there is often misunderstanding, it is important to emphasize that the outcome "improved health" does represent an *economic* benefit as much as a *health* benefit. Improved health increases the lifetime consumption possibilities of individuals, thereby directly augmenting utility – the maximization of which is seen by economists to be the ultimate objective of human endeavour. The economic benefit is thus clearly not limited to the more narrow perspective of cost savings or labour productivity gains. Therefore, a first essential input into the economic evaluation of any health programme is evidence of its effectiveness in terms of health improvement, measured, for instance, by the quantity and/or quality of life of the patient(s). After all, health improvement should be the primary purpose of any health intervention, and hence also the primary criterion for judging its value. If, in addition, the programme leads to cost saving and/or labour productivity gains, these are welcome side effects, but they should not be the main criterion for judging the economic desirability of a health programme. If the intervention succeeds in achieving a certain health improvement at a cost that is lower than the resulting benefit,[5] then the investment is economically worthwhile irrespective of whether there are additional cost savings and/or labour productivity effects.

As discussed at length in the other chapters in this book, advocates of active chronic disease management seek better health outcomes than are achieved with the current more-fragmented approach. While the idea has a great deal of intuitive appeal, can it be shown whether chronic disease management in real life is actually making a positive difference to health, irrespective of any monetary considerations?

As the country case studies in the companion volume to this book demonstrate, relatively few evaluations have been undertaken in European countries. For reasons discussed elsewhere in this book, research from the United States may be of limited relevance to the situation in Europe, not least because of the very much worse baseline that American disease management programmes are starting from. However, even in the United States, much of the evidence is inconclusive. Overall, it is reasonable to conclude that there is a real scarcity of scientifically solid and systematic evaluations of chronic disease management programmes. This may partly be explained by the relatively short time period that has elapsed since chronic disease management programmes have been established in many of the countries considered here. Other factors include the serious methodological challenges involved in isolating the effects of the often complex, multicomponent chronic disease management programmes, as well as the limited investment in health services research in many European countries. Finally, policy makers may be reluctant to commission comprehensive and unbiased evaluations of programmes that they "believe" are effective, or where they have been persuaded of this by those seeking to sell proprietary, almost exclusively American, models.

In the absence of randomized controlled trials, which have so far been applied only rarely to interventions designed to manage chronic diseases, it is difficult to ascertain whether the change in health status that might have been observed during the observation period can unambiguously be attributed to the specific chronic disease management examined. There is, however, considerable unrealized scope from research using observational data (Linden and Adams 2006; Linden et al. 2006a, 2006b).

The evaluation of chronic disease management programmes does require careful preparation and ideally has to be built into the development of the programme from the outset. Few countries have so far actively adopted the idea that evaluation (not to mention a full economic evaluation) should be an integral component of public health programmes. Rare exceptions include the Netherlands, Canada, Australia and the United Kingdom. Furthermore, the fact that evaluations have been carried out does not, by itself, say anything about their quality and hence their informative value. Very few have collected actual health outcomes, concentrating instead on the admittedly easier to obtain process indicators (such as resource use or admission rates).

On the basis of the evaluations reported in the companion volume, there is considerable evidence that some chronic disease management programmes do indeed improve health outcomes. Outcomes of diabetes mellitus in the Group Health Centre in Ontario, Canada, an ambulatory care centre with a group practice and multidisciplinary teams using electronic medical records, have been evaluated. The clinical outcomes measured, alongside the nine process outcomes, comprised blood pressure, serum glycosylated haemoglobin (HbA1c) and serum lipids. Improvements have been particularly noticeable with respect to blood pressure targets and HbA1c outcomes. The study in France also reported that where "formal evaluations were available, the results were very positive with fewer drug prescriptions, fewer hospitalisations and lower mortality rate compared to a control group."

The more comprehensive trials of improved care coordination for people with chronic and complex illness in Australia produced more mixed results. While in the first round of trials, outcomes in intervention groups were not better in terms of quality of life or hospitalization rates, readmission or length of stay (Esterman and Ben-Tovim 2002), the evaluation of the subsequent extended primary care package provides some evidence that care plans are associated with better provision and outcomes of care for diabetes (Zwar et al. 2007). Moreover, following the introduction of the National Integrated Diabetes Program, improvements in intermediate outcomes were seen in a cohort of patients on diabetes registers (Georgiou et al. 2006). Further encouraging results came from the evaluation of demonstration projects on self-management as part of the Sharing Healthcare Initiative. Observational studies reported positive effects on health outcomes and quality of life and reduced use of health services (Australian Department of Health and Ageing 2005).

If it is accepted that, on the whole, chronic disease management programmes produce health benefits for the patients involved, a view supported by the more comprehensive evidence from the United States, what about the other two types of expected benefit: cost saving and labour productivity effect?

While it is plausible that the health benefits of chronic disease management programmes result in labour productivity gains in respect of patients who are in the labour force, we are not aware of any definite evidence of such a causal (or even associative) link, and nor is such evidence reported in the case studies, although there is some evidence from the United States (Testa and Simonson 1998; Ng et al. 2001; Ramsey et al. 2002). There is, however, some very limited information on the impact on healthcare costs, but what exists does not encourage optimism that substantial cost savings will be realized. For instance, most evaluations in England, "have found little reduction in hospital admissions". Likewise, in the evaluation of a regional transmural diabetes management programme in the Netherlands (Matador), there was no impact on total costs (despite a marked reduction in hospitalization rates).

Although these findings cannot be generalized, it does suggest that, although there is some evidence from the United States to the contrary (Fendrick et al. 1992; Persson 1995; Bodenheimer et al. 2002; Sidorov et al. 2002; Short et al. 2003), the hope that chronic disease management programmes will be cost-cutting instruments is overoptimistic.

Fireman et al. (2004) have, however, identified three ways in which chronic disease management programmes might at least in principle yield savings to the health system: quality improvement, utilization management and productivity improvement.

Quality improvement. Chronic disease management can improve health by increasing use of effective medications and improving self-care, thereby preventing enough exacerbations and complications to save money.

Utilization management. Disease management can reduce overuse through a supportive approach that is acceptable to patients. Predictably high-cost patients are given a case manager who coaches self-care and discourages inappropriate use of the emergency room, facilitates timely discharge from the hospital, prevents duplicative tests and steers patients to less-costly services.

Productivity improvement. Disease management can offload work from doctors to less-costly practitioners, delivering care by telephone and via the Internet instead of traditional office visits. Although disease management typically supplements usual care, it could boost productivity if delivered in ways that substitute for – or reengineer – usual care.

However, in their empirical evaluation of four conditions included in disease management programmes delivered by Kaiser Permanente in Northern California, they do not find cost savings even though there are improvements in quality and health outcomes.

Nevertheless, even if chronic disease management (or other interventions) do not save money, they can still represent excellent value for money from a societal perspective if they buy better health at a cost that is "worth it". Typically, however, the improvement in health will require additional resources, not less. At least during the initial years when a chronic disease management programme is being established, it will require very significant additional start-up costs (e.g. costs for the production and dissemination of guidelines, salaries, information technology).

As the above discussion illustrates, there is a potential conflict between the objective of the health plan/provider to realize a financial profit (i.e. to save money) – the "business case" – on the one hand and the societal objective of achieving a health improvement at a reasonable (but typically positive) cost on the other hand – the broader "economic case".[6] This is a problem because what seems to be a relatively poor business case for chronic disease management reduces or even eliminates the incentives for the health plan/provider to establish programmes that may bring a net benefit to society as a whole. The reasons for such a disconnect are rooted in the current financing structure and delivery systems of health systems, and it is beyond the scope of this chapter to analyse these in greater detail (see Chapter 9). The greatest disconnect between the business case and the broader economic case is the fact that the private benefits derived by patients enrolled in a chronic disease management are not transferred to the health plans and providers. Given the benefits patients expect from chronic disease management, it can be anticipated that the employers or purchasers acting on their behalf would be willing to pay a premium for participation in a good-quality chronic disease management programme, but that does not appear to happen. Employers also have an incentive to pay premiums that will allow sick workers to be enrolled in chronic disease management programmes, in the expectation of direct benefits in the form of reduced work absences and/or higher productivity, although this of course raises many complex issues including the possibility of covert discrimination in employment procedures against those with such disorders.

One of several problems that prevent such transfers from occurring is that the relationship with the patient would have to continue for perhaps ten years or more, until positive results emerge, in order for the plan/provider or the employer to be able to reap the benefits from any investment in chronic disease management. As such a long-term commitment is rather the exception than the rule, and as it may not be able to be enforced in the present institutional environment (a situation that is exacerbated by the tendency, in several countries, to introduce the right to shift between health insurance funds, which is only partly overcome by risk-equalization mechanisms), the difference between societal and business returns remains. The only way to justify chronic disease management is then on the basis of cost saving, and, as we argued above, such savings are only likely to be realized after a prolonged period of time, if at all.

Overall, there are a number of "Catch-22" situations in the current arrangements. The health insurer needs to find a way to charge the patient, employer and government for the benefits. This is important not only for the insurance company but also for society as a whole, because of the burden of chronic diseases and the societal cost savings from certain chronic disease management programmes. Clearly this is not such a problem in many countries in Europe, where funding comes from compulsory social insurance or national taxes.

However even in these situations, there can be considerable power and auto-nomy devolved to providers, making it incumbent on them to achieve financial balance. For example, in England, health services are commissioned and pro-vided by primary care trusts and practice-based commissioners. They are given a weighted budget annually to cover populations of approximately 200,000. They face severe penalties if they fail to achieve financial balance annually. Given that their average chief executive remains in post for three years, it is not sur-prising that they are more interested in investing in solutions where the benefits can be seen quite quickly, such as improved acute services, than in facing the high initial costs for a long-term gain in chronic disease management pro-grammes. Although the government tries to compensate by setting up systems of inspection to ensure that enough is being done to tackle chronic diseases, none of this is considered important if the organization is not achieving financial balance.

These findings have a number of policy implications that require more exten-sive country-specific elaborations in future research. Most obviously, and as has been noted over the years by many commentators, there is a strong argument for ensuring that reimbursement systems pay providers on the basis of the qual-ity of the services they offer, rather than the number of services provided. The challenges are substantial and, in reality, many are insurmountable, as illus-trated by the so-called "payment-by-results" system in the English National Health Service, which is, in reality, "payment by activity". Nevertheless, there is considerable scope to move to a situation where payments begin to reward health outcomes, or at least the use of processes that can, on the basis of sound evidence, be expected to achieve better outcomes. There is also an economic argument for explicit direct subsidies by government as a means of better aligning business and societal interests.

Conclusions

This chapter has discussed the economic costs of chronic disease and the eco-nomic aspects of chronic disease management from a conceptual perspective, providing some empirical evidence from Europe. As for the former, we emphasized the need to make clear what type of costs we are talking about when we talk about "costs", and from which perspective. Whatever the particular cost concept applied, there is much evidence to suggest that chronic diseases are imposing a substantial cost burden on society. There is also evidence that at least part of these costs justify government intervention to prevent and control chronic disease.

While there is increasing recognition that improving health can provide direct economic *benefits* at both the individual and perhaps even at the macro-economic level, there is far less information on the *costs* of the different ways of achieving better health, and, hence, on the "return on investment". This applies to both preventive and curative approaches, and, as we have argued in this chapter, this seems to apply with a vengeance to chronic disease management: the economic evaluation of chronic disease management is a significantly underresearched issue. In great part, this is because the essential building block of such evaluations, that is the proof of effectiveness of such programmes, is not very advanced in the countries considered, with a few exceptions. Looking ahead, therefore, our key recommendation is to undertake much more research on whether and how far chronic disease management programmes are making a difference to health outcomes. Should this be supported by the resulting evidence on a larger scale, that in itself would also be a major step forward for any future economic assessment. Unless this evidence gap is filled, we see very little hope that what is seen as a promising way to tackle the growing challenge of chronic diseases will gain widespread political and financial support in European countries.

We distinguished the business case from the (societal) economic case and found a worrying disconnect between the two, which unless it is overcome through appropriate financing and delivery mechanisms will result in the provision of a socially suboptimal level of active chronic disease management, a consequence that will be hard to tolerate in light of the ever more pressing need to tackle the high and growing burden of chronic disease our societies will inevitably face. The question of how better to align the financial and economic incentives involved in chronic disease management should be high on the research agenda, and this is an issue that will be addressed in some detail in Chapter 9.

Notes

1. The costs associated with a disease or a risk factor can be measured either by the "prevalence approach" (assessing costs at a single point in time) or the "incidence approach" (assessing the costs over a lifetime). The former is by far the most common one. The more data-extensive incidence or "life cycle" approach estimates the present value of the cost of adding to society a person who contracts the specific disease or takes up a certain unhealthy behaviour (Rice 1994). Another important parameter is whether the study uses an "epidemiological" or an "econometric" approach. The logic of the former is that it apportions a fraction of the overall medical costs to either a disease or a risk factor (using methods very similar to those that quantify mortality attributable to a specific disease or risk factor). The less widely practised econometric approach uses regression analysis to quantify (direct and indirect) costs while controlling, to the extent possible, for other observable characteristics that are likely to affect cost and be correlated with the disease or the risk factor. Doing so, in fact, brings the cost-of-illness approach rather close to the microeconomic one discussed below.
2. This criticism applies specifically to the epidemiological approach of cost-of-illness measurement, which becomes clear from the way the costs are derived. An estimate of the costs of hospitalization directly related to, say, physical inactivity is calculated by multiplying the following three components: the percentage out of each disorder that can be attributed to physical inactivity, the number of hospitalizations by disorder and the average cost per hospital stay. Attribution of the percentages is not always straightforward, particularly so for the attribution of a given disorder to a specific risk factor (Sindelar 1998).
3. A further limitation – already mentioned – is the limited comparability of the results across different studies of the same disease/risk factor or across different diseases/risk factors. Although such comparisons are tempting, given the seemingly similar categories used, the details of each study differ too much in most cases (Godfrey 2004).

4. These include a persistent problem of multicollinearity, the difficulty of disentangling symptoms from causes, a wide divergence from more robust microeconomic analyses and the limited utility of results based on cross-country averages for inferring country-specific lessons. See Pritchett (2006) for a more extensive discussion of the limits of cross-country growth analytics.
6. A particularly useful illustration of this conflict is by Beaulieu et al. (2003) in the context of diabetes care at two major health plans in the United States; unfortunately, no similar information is available for Europe, Australia or Canada. Beaulieu et al. found that improved care for diabetics has large potential net benefits for society as a whole but the net return to health plans and providers was negative in the first few years and minimal (if at all) over a decade interval.

References

Acemoglu, D. and Johnson, S. (2006) *Disease and Development: The Effect of Life Expectancy on Economic Growth*. Chicago, IL: University of Chicago. http://economics.uchicago.edu/Acemoglu_042506.pdf (accessed 17 May 2006).

Adeyi, O., Smith, O. and Robles, S. (2007) *Public Policy and the Challenge of Chronic Noncommunicable Diseases*. Washington DC: World Bank.

Australian Department of Health and Ageing (2005) *Australia. National Evaluation of the Sharing Health Care Demonstration Projects June 2005*. Canberra: Department of Health and Ageing, Australia.

Averett, S. and Korenman, S. (1996) The economic reality of the beauty myth, *J Hum Resour*, 31: 304–30.

Barro, R. (1991) Economic growth in a cross-section of countries, *Q J Econ*, 106: 407–43.

Barro, R. (1996) *Health and Economic Growth*. Washington, DC: Pan American Health Organization. http://www.paho.org/English/HDP/HDD/barro.pdf (accessed 3 October 2006).

Barro, R. and Lee, J.W. (1994) Sources of economic growth, *Carnegie Rochester Conf Series Public Policy*, 40: 1–46.

Barro, R. and Sala-i-Martin, X. (1995) *Economic Growth*. New York: McGraw-Hill.

Beaulieu, N., Cutler, D. and Ho, K. (2003) *The Business Case for Diabetes Disease Management at Two Managed Care Organizations*. Boston, MA: Harvard University Press. http://www.economics.harvard.edu/faculty/dcutler/papers.html (accessed 14 January 2007).

Berger, M.C. (1983) Labour supply and spouse's health: the effects of illness, disability and mortality, *Soc Sci Q*, 64: 494–509.

Bhargava, A., Jamison, D.T., Lau, L. and Murray, C. (2001) Modelling the effects of health on economic growth, *J Health Econ*, 20: 423–440.

Bodenheimer, T., Wagner, E.H. and Grumbach, K. (2002) Improving primary care for patients with chronic illness: the chronic care model, Part 2, *JAMA* 288: 1909–14.

Brunello, G. and d'Hombres, B. (2007) Does body weight affect wages? Evidence from Europe, *Econ Hum Biol*, 5: 1–19.

Busse, R. (2004) Disease management programs in Germany's statutory health insurance system, *Health Aff*, 23: 56–67.

Cawley, J. (2000) *Body Weight and Women's Labor Market Outcomes*. Cambridge, MA: National Bureau of Economic Research.

Charles, K.K. (1999) *Sickness in the Family: Health Shocks and Spousal Labor Supply*. Ann Arbor, MI: Gerald R. Ford School of Public Policy, University of Michigan.

Chirikos, T.N. and Nestel, G. (1985) Further evidence on the economic effects of poor health, *Rev Econ Stat*, 67: 61–9.

Coile, C. (2003) *Health Shocks and Couples' Labor Supply Decisions. CRR Working Paper, 08.* Chestnut Hill, MA: Centre for Retirement Research, Boston College.

Contoyannis, P. and Rise, N. (2001) The impact of health on wages: evidence from British household panel survey, *Empir Econ*, 26: 599–622.

Currie, J. and Madrian, B.C. (1999) Health, health insurance and the labour market, in O. Ashenfelter and D. Card (eds) *Handbook of Labour Economics*, Vol. 3, pp 3309–415. Amsterdam: Elsevier Science.

Delfino, D. and Simmons, P.J. (1999) *Infectious Disease And Economic Growth: The Case of Tuberculosis. Discussion Papers in Economics*, No. 1999/23. York, UK: University of York.

Dixon, S., McDonald, S. and Roberts, J. (2001) AIDS and economic growth in Africa: a panel data analysis, *J Int Dev*, 13: 411–26.

Easterly, W. and Levine, R. (1997) Africa's growth tragedy: policies and ethnic divisions, *Q J Econ*, 112: 1203–1250.

Esterman, A.J. and Ben-Tovim, D.I. (2002) The Australian coordinated care trials: success or failure? The second round of trials may provide more answers, *Med J Aust*, 177: 469–70.

Ettner, S.L. (1996) The opportunity costs of elder care, *J Hum Resour*, 31: 189–205.

Fendrick, A.M., Javitt, J.C. and Chiang, Y.P. (1992) Screening and treatment of diabetic retinopathy in Sweden, *Int J Technol Assess Health Care*, 4: 694–707.

Finkelstein, E.A., Ruhm, C.J. and Kosa, K.M. (2005) Economic causes and consequences of obesity, *Annu Rev Public Health*, 26: 239–57.

Fireman, B., Bartlett, J. and Selby, J. (2004) Can disease management reduce health care costs by improving quality? *Health Aff*, 23: 63–75.

Gallup, J.L. and Sachs, J. (2001) *The Economic Burden of Malaria. Working Paper* No. WG1:10. Cambridge, MA: Commission on Macroeconomics and Health.

Georgiou, A., Burns, J., McKenzie, S. et al. (2006) Monitoring change in diabetes care using diabetes registers: experience from Divisions of General Practice, *Aust Fam Physician*, 35: 77–80.

Godfrey, C. (2004) The financial costs and benefits of alcohol, European Alcohol Policy Conference: Bridging the Gap, *Globe*, 1 & 2: 7–14.

Hansen, J. (2000) The effect of work absence on wages and wage gaps in Sweden, *J Popul Econ*, 13: 45–55.

Jiménez-Martín, S., Labeaga, J.M. and Martínez Granado, M. (1999) *Health Status and Retirement Decisions for Older European Couples, October. IRISS Working Paper Series* No. 1999–01. [Provided by IRISS at CEPS/INSTEAD.] Luxembourg: IRISS.

Levine, R. and Renelt, D. (1992) A sensitivity analysis of cross-country growth regressions, *Am Econ Rev*, 82: 942–63.

Linden, A. and Adams, J.L. (2006) Evaluating disease management programme effectiveness: an introduction to instrumental variables, *J Eval Clin Pract*, 12: 148–54.

Linden, A., Adams, J.L. and Roberts, N. (2006a) Evaluating disease management programme effectiveness: an introduction to the regression discontinuity design, *J Eval Clin Pract*, 12: 124–31.

Linden, A., Adams, J.L. and Roberts, N. (2006b) Strengthening the case for disease management effectiveness: un-hiding the hidden bias, *J Eval Clin Pract*, 12: 140–7.

Mitra, A. (2001) Effects of physical attributes on the wages of males and females, *Appl Econ Lett*, 8: 731–5.

Mossialos, E. and Thomson, S.M. (2002) Voluntary health insurance in the European Union: a critical assessment, *Int J Health Serv*, 32: 19–88.

Ng, Y.C., Jacobs, P. and Johnson, J.A. (2001) Productivity losses associated with diabetes in the US, *Diabetes Care*, 24: 257–61.

Pelkowski, J.M. and Berger, M.C. (2004) The impact of health on employment, wages, and hours worked over the life cycle, *Q Rev Econ Finance* 44: 102–21.

Persson, U. (1995) The indirect costs of morbidity in type 2 diabetes, *Pharmacoeconomics*, 8(Suppl), 1: 28–32.

Petersen, S., Peto, V. and Rayner, M. (2005) *European Cardiovascular Disease Statistics*, 2005 edition. London: British Heart Foundation.

Pritchett, L. (2006) The quest continues, *Finance Dev*, March: 18–22.

Ramsey, S., Summers, K.H., Leong, S.A. et al. (2002) Productivity and medical costs of diabetes in a large employer population, *Diabetes Care*, 25: 23–9.

Rice, D.P. (1994) Cost-of-illness studies: fact or fiction? *Lancet*, 344: 1519–20.

Sachs, J.D. and Warner, A.M. (1995) Economic reform and the process of global integration, *Brookings Papers Econ Activity* 1: 1–95.

Sachs, J.D. and Warner, A.M. (1997) Sources of slow growth in African economies, *J Afr Econ*, 6: 335–76.

Sala-i-Martin, X., Doppelhofer, G. and Miller, R.I. (2004) Determinants of long-term growth: a Bayesian averaging of classical estimates (BACE) approach, *Am Econ Rev*, 94: 813–35.

Short, A.C., Mays, G.P. and Mittler, J. (2003) *Disease Management: A Leap of Faith to Lower-cost, Higher-quality Health Care, Issue Brief* No. 69. Washington DC: Center for Studying Health System Change.

Sidorov, J., Shull, R., Tomcavage, J. et al. (2002) Does diabetes disease management save money and improve outcomes? A report of simultaneous short-term savings and quality improvement associated with a health maintenance organization-sponsored disease management program among patients fulfilling health employer data and information set criteria, *Diabetes Care*, 25: 684–9.

Sindelar, J.L. (1998) Social costs of alcohol, *J Drug Issues*, 28: 763–81.

Spiess, C.K. and Schneider, T. (2004) Midlife care-giving and employment: an analysis of adjustments in work hours and informal care for female employees in Europe, in J. Mortensen, C. Spiess, T. Schneider, J. Costa-Font and C. Patxot (eds) *Health Care and Female Employment: A Potential Conflict? Occasional Paper*, No. 6. Brussels: ENEPRI.

Suhrcke, M. and Urban, D. (2006) *Are Cardiovascular Diseases Bad for Economic Growth? CESIFO Working Paper* No. 1845. Munich: CESIFO.

Suhrcke, M., McKee, M., Sauto Arce, R., Tsolova, S. and Mortensen, J. (2005) *The Contribution of Health to the Economy in the European Union*. Brussels: European Commission.

Suhrcke, M., Nugent, R.A., Stuckler, D. and Rocco, L. (2006) *Chronic Disease: An Economic Perspective*. Oxford: Oxford Health Alliance.

Suhrcke, M., Rocco, L. and McKee, M. (2007) *Health: A Vital Investment for Economic Development in Eastern Europe and Central Asia*, p. 25. Copenhagen: European Observatory on Health Systems and Policies.

Testa, M.A. and Simonson, D.C. (1998) Health economic benefits and quality of life during improved glycemic control in patients with type 2 diabetes mellitus: a randomized, controlled, double-blind trial, *JAMA*, 280: 1490–6.

Weil, D.N. (2005) *Accounting for the Effect of Health on Economic Growth. Working Paper* No. 11455. Washington, DC, National Bureau of Economic Research.

WHO (2005) *Chronic Disease: A Vital Investment*. Geneva: World Health Organization.

Zwar, N.A., Hermiz, O., Comino, E.J. et al. (2007) Do multidisciplinary care plans result in better care for patients with type 2 diabetes? *Aust Fam Physician*, 36: 85–9.

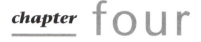
Integration and chronic care: a review

Ellen Nolte and Martin McKee

Introduction

The increasing prevalence of chronic illness is posing considerable challenges to health systems. Chronic illness requires complex models of care, involving collaboration among professions and institutions that have traditionally been separate. Healthcare still builds largely on an acute, episodic model of care that is ill equipped to meet the long-term and fluctuating needs of those with chronic illness. Patients may receive care from many different providers, often in different settings or institutions, even when they have only a single disease, such as diabetes. They are frequently called upon to monitor, coordinate or carry out their own treatment plan, while receiving limited guidance on how to do so. Consequently, in order to provide better support for patients, there is a pressing need to bridge the boundaries between professions, providers and institutions through the development of more integrated or coordinated approaches to service delivery (Plochg and Klazinga 2002). In response, health professionals, policy makers and institutions in many countries are increasingly recognizing the need to respond to those with complex health needs and are initiating new models of service delivery designed to achieve better coordination of services across the continuum of care (Conrad and Shortell 1996; Ouwens et al. 2005).

Yet although this has a logical appeal, the available evidence on the effectiveness of different forms of integration or coordination of care remains uncertain, despite a surge of reviews, systematic and otherwise, of single interventions and complex programmes and models of care (Bodenheimer et al. 2002a; Weingarten et al. 2002; Ofman et al. 2004; Singh 2005a; Tsai et al. 2005; Zwar et al. 2006). One well-known model is the Chronic Care Model (CCM), developed by Wagner et al. (1999), which we will describe in more detail below. There is now sufficient evidence that single or multiple components of the model improve quality of care, clinical outcomes and healthcare resource use; however, it is less clear whether this is a consequence of applying the model as a whole, or whether the same benefits can be achieved using only some of the components (Singh and Ham 2006). Similarly, reviewing the evidence on the effectiveness of collaboration between health and social care, Dowling et al. (2004) showed that while there was some, albeit inconclusive, evidence that collaboration improved service outputs and/or user outcomes, it was not possible to establish a causal link between the various components of the collaboration and its effects.

Alongside the relative paucity of empirical evidence on the consequences of different forms of integration, coordination and care models (Shortell et al. 2000; Singh and Ham 2006), there is the more fundamental challenge arising from the lack of common definitions of underlying concepts and boundaries. Integration and/or coordination have been pursued in many ways in different health systems, and there is a plethora of terminologies that have variously been described as "integrated care", "coordinated care", "collaborative care", "managed care", "disease management", "case management", "patient-centred care", "chronic (illness) care", "continuity of care", "transmural care", "seamless care" and others. Kodner and Spreeuwenberg (2002) even used the biblical story of the Tower of Babel[1] to illustrate this myriad of definitions and concepts, while Howarth and Haigh (2007) describe an "academic quagmire of definitions and concept analyses" surrounding the notion of integration. Systematic understanding of "integrated care" and related notions has been greatly hampered by a lack in specificity and clarity, with commonly used definitions tending to be "vague and confusing" (Kodner and Spreeuwenberg 2002), and by the more general absence of a "sound paradigm through which to examine the process" (Goodwin et al. 2004). This confusion very much reflects the polymorphous nature of a concept that is applied from several disciplinary and professional perspectives and is associated with diverse objectives.

This chapter seeks to contribute to a clearer understanding of the various definitions, concepts, methods and models involved. It does so by tracing the origins of two key concepts, "integrated care" and "disease management", and exploring approaches to what we refer to as "chronic care" in different contexts. We then move on to describe selected typologies, theoretical frameworks and existing delivery models for providing care for those with varying levels of need and we examine the relevant evidence base, taking advantage of the accumulating evidence on the relative effectiveness of different models and components of chronic care. Where appropriate, we illustrate observations with examples from the individual country case studies that have informed this book.

Tracing the origins: the search for the common ground

The lack of common ground underpinning notions of integration is, in part, attributable to the different origins of the various concepts. The terms integrated care and disease management may be taken to reflect two ends of a spectrum of approaches that, ultimately, aim to ensure cost-effective quality care for service users with varied needs.

The notion of integration has its roots in organizational theory and, as it relates to welfare services, is found most prominently in contingency theory, an offshoot of systems theory, as developed by Lawrence and Lorsch (1967; quoted in Axelsson and Axelsson 2006), with its concepts of differentiation and integration, the latter defined as "the quality of the state of collaboration that exists among departments that are required to achieve unity of effort by the demands of the environment". The concept of integrated care has mainly been discussed in the health and social care fields in terms of linking the *cure* and *care* sector (shared care in the United Kingdom, Vernetzung in Germany, and transmurale zorg in the Netherlands). For example, Leutz (1999) defined integration as "the search to connect the healthcare system (acute, primary medical, and skilled) with other human service systems (e.g. long-term care, education, and vocational and housing services) in order to improve outcomes (clinical, satisfaction, and efficiency)". Similarly, Kodner and Spreeuwenberg (2002) defined integration as "a coherent set of methods and models of the funding, administrative, organisational, service delivery and clinical levels designed to create connectivity, alignment and collaboration within and between the cure and care sectors". Hardy et al. (1999) described integrated care as "a coherent set of products and services, delivered by collaborating local and regional health care agencies" and that, through securing "liaison or linkages within and between the health and social care systems", integrated care ensured that service users received comprehensive, multiagency packages of care at the right time and enabled them to move across or through the systems to obtain different types and levels of care.

The application of the concept of integrated care to health and social care is not, however, clear cut. Leichsenring (2004) described several discourses or "sets of academic and political perspectives and approaches" to integrated care that have evolved either from a predominantly healthcare perspective (managed care discourse, public health discourse) or from adopting a broader "whole systems" approach that emphasizes the social services perspective (person-centred discourse); these are complemented by an institutional discourse that focuses on organizational strategies. A strong healthcare perspective is seen in the definition of integrated care coined by the WHO European Regional Office as "a concept bringing together inputs, delivery, management and organization of services related to diagnosis, treatment, care, rehabilitation and health promotion. Integration is a means to improve services in relation to access, quality, user satisfaction and efficiency" (Groene and Garcia-Barbero 2001). Person-centred approaches, in contrast, have evolved from a tradition that emphasizes "demedicalization" by underlining the interdependencies between health and social care in meeting the needs of the individual service user (Leichsenring 2004). The boundaries between these "discourses" remain ambiguous, however. This is, in part, because approaches to integrated care pursued in different systems reflect, to a great extent, the financing and organization of, and responsibilities for, health and social care in a given country. For example, Niskanen (2002), arguing from a healthcare perspective, defined integrated care as including "the methods and strategies for linking and coordinating the various aspects of care delivered by different care levels", that is, by primary and secondary care. However, because he is using Finland as his basis, his definition includes social services since supporting long-term care needs is the duty of the social care sector.

This notion of integrated care in the context of publicly funded systems is somewhat different from that which Shortell et al. (1994), from a United States perspective, referred to as integrated (or organized) delivery systems: "a network of organisations that provides or arranges to provide a coordinated continuum of services to a defined population and is willing to be held clinically and fiscally accountable for the outcomes and the health status of the population served". This definition reflects a strong managed care perspective in that the emphasis is on *defined (but selective) populations* (i.e. enrolled members of a given health plan who pay a predetermined monthly premium) and on *integrating the financing and provision of healthcare*, which in the United States, as in other countries with insurance-based systems, have traditionally been strictly separated (Maynard and Bloor 1998). The concept of integrated delivery in the United States context is not easily comparable with integrated care as interpreted in the European context, where it traditionally refers to the integration of different sectors (i.e. cure and care) rather than different functions (financing and delivery). It should, however, be noted that several elements of what has been described as managed care, such as case management, form integral parts of many integrated care approaches. Consequently, several authors have linked or equated integrated care with managed care (Hunter and Fairfield 1997; Ovretveit 1998; Vondeling 2004).

The unifying "denominator" of integrated care concepts and approaches is their primary aim of improving outcomes for the target population (Ovretveit 1998), traditionally the frail elderly and other population groups with diverse and complex needs. Therefore, according to Leutz (1999), the goal of integration is to benefit populations that have "physical, developmental, or cognitive disabilities – often with related chronic illnesses or conditions." The focus is on service users with multifaceted problems who require assistance with activities of daily living. Social care thus forms an essential component in the spectrum of user need. Kodner and Spreeuwenberg (2002) also defined the overall aim of integrated care as being to "enhance quality of care and quality of life, consumer satisfaction and system efficiency for patients with complex, long-term problems cutting across multiple services, providers and settings".

In contrast, disease management has traditionally targeted persons with a single (chronic) disease or condition. Disease management was first mentioned as a concept in the United States in the 1980s and initially used mainly by pharmaceutical companies offering educational programmes to employers and managed care organizations to promote medication adherence and behaviour change among patients with chronic conditions such as diabetes, asthma and coronary artery disease (Bodenheimer 1999; Boston Consulting Group 2006). A "child of cost controllers" (Bodenheimer 1999), disease management concepts were seen as a means to reduce hospital (re)admissions and hospital days – though the incentive for the pharmaceutical industry to enter the market was driven, in part, by the prospect of increasing sales of their products and also to circumvent a perceived risk of falling profits from prescription drugs purchased by managed care organizations in the early 1990s.

From the mid-1990s, disease management strategies were adopted more widely by the healthcare industry in the United States, in parallel with an emerging body of evidence suggesting the potential for cost savings in the treatment of those with chronic conditions (Krumholz et al. 2006). By 1999, around 200 companies offered disease management programmes for conditions such as diabetes, asthma and congestive heart failure; at the same time, health maintenance organizations, medical groups and hospitals increasingly provided in-house disease management too (Bodenheimer 2000). It has been estimated that between 1997 and 2005 the revenues of disease management organizations in the United States grew by around 40% (from US$78 million to $1.2 billion), with much of the growth occurring in the late 1990s, slowing down somewhat in the early 2000s (Boston Consulting Group 2006).

Payers in the United States, and indeed elsewhere, have now "widely embraced [disease management] initiatives" (Boston Consulting Group 2006). This also includes the United States federal government, which has been developing and piloting a voluntary chronic care improvement programme under the fee-for-service Medicare system for the over 65s (Medicare Health Support, launched in 2005), targeting diverse population groups with heart failure and/or diabetes and delivered by private disease management organizations (McCall et al. 2007). Individual states have also developed and implemented disease management programmes within their Medicaid programmes (Gillespie and Rossiter 2003); over half of the states have some form of disease management in place under Medicaid (Smith et al. 2006). In 2005, two-thirds of employers with 200 or more employees offered disease management through their employment-based health insurance plans, and more than half of employees with such insurance were enrolled in a disease management programme (Geyman 2007). However, the nature and scope of such programmes varies widely, ranging from "small initiatives focused on a narrow subset of members to widespread programs targeting almost all chronically ill members across multiple payer groups" (Boston Consulting Group 2006).

It is important to emphasize that as the disease management "industry" has evolved over time, two key trends have emerged that are relevant to the discussion here. First, amid the variety of programmes operating under the broad label "disease management", there are two basic types of initiative: "on-site" programmes that are directed by the primary provider and delivered within a primary care setting and "off-site" or "carved-out" programmes that focus on specific processes of care or clinical outcomes, mostly patient education and self-management based on information systems (Cavanaugh et al. 2007). Carved-out programmes are normally offered by commercial for-profit vendors, such as specialized disease management organizations, and are marketed to employers and health insurers primarily as a cost-containment strategy (Bodenheimer 2000; Geyman 2007). As carved-out programmes, commercial disease management programmes are not integrated with primary care and normally involve only minimal communication with primary care providers (Geyman 2007). Additionally, they often lack any focus on patient outcomes or they concentrate on short-term outcomes only, one reason why disease management "has a pejorative connotation to some people" (Norris et al. 2003).

At the same time there has been a trend towards developing a broader, population-based approach to disease management (Geyman 2007). Early programmes tended to focus on single conditions or diseases, with commercial programmes targeting patient education and adherence to drug therapies, as mentioned above; more recently, second-generation disease management pro-grammes have evolved that shift the focus to addressing the multiple needs of patients with comorbidities and multiple conditions (Boston Consulting Group 2006; Geyman 2007). Indeed, as Krumholz et al. (2006) have noted "[b]ecause disease management programmes have historically provided narrowly tailored medical solutions focused on one dominant health problem, several . . . alterna-tive models have arisen in an attempt to provide a more integrated approach to care, directing attention to the wide range of patient comorbidities". As with off-site disease management programmes, this has led to the development of administrative databases and disease registration systems designed to identify individuals at risk (Cavanaugh et al. 2007).

As a consequence of these developments, and reflecting the situation with integrated care, there is now a wide range of definitions of disease management that vary in scope, focus, purpose and range of component interventions (Norris et al. 2003). Definitions range from "discrete programs directed at reducing costs and improving outcomes for patients with particular conditions" (Rothman and Wagner 2003) to "a population-based systematic approach that identifies persons at risk, intervenes, measures the outcomes, and provides con-tinuous quality improvement" (Epstein and Sherwood 1996). Ellrodt et al. (1997) defined disease management as "an approach to patient care that coordinates medical resources for patients across the entire delivery system", indicating that the boundaries between "disease management" and "integrated care" have become increasingly blurred.

This confusion is further illustrated by a recent overview of systematic reviews that aimed to assess the effectiveness, definitions and components of integrated care programmes for chronically ill patients (Ouwens et al. 2005). Of the 13 systematic reviews considered, eight were, in fact, reviews of disease manage-ment programmes, each employing a distinct definition of disease manage-ment, with the remainder reviewing some form of care or case management (two), multidisciplinary teams/structures (two), and more generally manage-ment of patients with chronic health problems (one) (Box 4.1). Although very diverse in scope and content, the programmes reviewed shared the common goal of reducing fragmentation and improving continuity and coordination, the very features identified here as characteristic of integrated care approaches.

In conclusion, there is considerable overlap between concepts of "integrated care" and broader perspectives of "disease management". From the review presented here, it may legitimately be argued that the common theme is the ultimate goal of improving outcomes for those with (complex) chronic health problems by overcoming issues of fragmentation through linkage of services of different providers along the continuum of care. However, while concepts of integrated care frequently link with the social care sector, disease management programmes are normally limited to linkages within the healthcare sector.

Box 4.1 "Alternative" care concepts

Care concepts that are frequently, though not always, subsumed under the heading of, or are used interchangeably with, disease management include "case management", "coordinated care" and "multidisciplinary care" (Krumholz et al. 2006). Again, boundaries are not clear cut. Therefore, while disease management frequently targets specific diseases or conditions, case management and multidisciplinary care are generally aimed at those with multiple or complex needs, for example the frail elderly. Although definitions and approaches vary (Roberts 2002; Sargent et al. 2007), one feature of case management is the goal of reducing the use of (unplanned) hospital care (Gravelle et al. 2007) through the development of care or treatment plans that are tailored to the needs of the individual patient who is at high risk socially, financially and medically (Krumholz et al. 2006). Patients are assigned a case manager, often a (specialist) nurse, who oversees and is responsible for coordinating and implementing care (Norris et al. 2002).

Multidisciplinary care has been referred to as an "extension" of case management in that it also normally involves the development of treatment plans tailored to the medical, psychosocial and financial needs of patients, but in contrast to case management utilizes a broader range of medical and social support personnel (including physicians, nurses, pharmacists, dieticians, social workers and others) to facilitate transition from inpatient acute care to long-term outpatient management of chronic illness (Krumholz et al. 2006). Similarly, coordinated care, also used interchangeably with case or care management, involves the development and implementation of a therapeutic plan designed to integrate the efforts of medical and social service providers, often involving designated individuals to manage provider collaboration.

Addressing the needs of people with chronic conditions: an overview of frameworks and models

Building on the experience with and evidence from interventions that aim to address the needs of persons with chronic conditions, numerous frameworks and models have been developed since the 1980s or so designed to optimize care. Given the overlap between concepts of integrated care and disease management, this section begins with an overview of taxonomies of integration before moving on to describe selected frameworks and delivery models that have been most influential in informing approaches to chronic disease management.

Taxonomies of integration

As indicated in the previous section, integrated care is a concept that has been widely but variously used. At the same time, the notion of integration provides a useful way of thinking about a range of approaches that are deployed to increase coordination, cooperation, continuity, collaboration and networking across different components of health service delivery. There have been several attempts to develop a taxonomy of integration in healthcare that would enable systematic assessment of the structures and processes involved, their prerequisites and their effects on healthcare organization and delivery and, ultimately, on user outcomes. A key challenge is that, unlike in many other industries, products and production stages in healthcare, and boundaries between them, are not always easy to define (Simoens and Scott 1999). Importantly, users of health services do not progress linearly through the system towards a common final production stage and, given the probabilistic nature of the treatment process, providers need to be able to cope with uncertain demand at each stage of the process. The integration process in healthcare is, therefore, unlikely to follow a single path and variations are inevitably common. Accordingly, analysts have distinguished different dimensions of integration, with the most common taxonomies differentiating the type, breadth, degree and process of integration.

Type of integration. The literature differentiates functional integration (extent to which key support functions and activities such as financial management, human resources, strategic planning, information management and quality improvement are coordinated across operating units), organizational integration (e.g. creation of networks, mergers, contracting or strategic alliances between healthcare institutions), professional integration (e.g. joint working, group practices, contracting or strategic alliances of healthcare professionals within and between institutions and organizations) and clinical integration (extent to which patient care services are coordinated across the various personnel, functions, activities and operating units of a system) (Shortell et al. 1994; Simoens and Scott 1999; Delnoij et al. 2002).

The breadth of integration. This refers to the range of healthcare services provided. Horizontal integration takes place between organizations or organizational units that are on the same level in the delivery of healthcare or have the same status; vertical integration brings together organizations at different levels of a hierarchical structure (Conrad and Shortell 1996; Simoens and Scott 1999; Axelsson and Axelsson 2006).

The degree of integration. This ranges from full integration, that is the integrated organization is responsible for the full continuum of care (including financing), to collaboration, which refers to separate structures where organizations retain their own service responsibility and funding criteria (Leutz 1999; see also below).

The process of integration. This distinguishes between structural integration (the alignment of tasks, functions and activities of organizations and healthcare professionals), cultural integration (convergence of values, norms, working methods, approaches and symbols adopted by the (various) actors), social integration (the intensification of social relationships between the (various) actors) and integration of objectives, interests, power and resources of the (various) actors (Fabbricotti 2007).

In summary, integration may occur in different and complex structural configurations, reflecting the diverse environments and historical paths taken by health systems and the range of options available to establish and maintain linkages among their various components.

Frameworks and delivery models in chronic care

Drawing on a comparison of initiatives to integrate health and social services in the 1990s in the United States and the United Kingdom, Leutz (1999) noted that strategies tended to focus on a (relatively small) subset of the population with high need while overlooking the needs of the (majority) of chronically ill and disabled people with "less" need (Leutz 2005). Leutz (1999), therefore, proposed an "integration framework" that describes three levels of integration which are set against dimensions of service users' need and operational domains of systems; this would enable a comprehensive approach responding to the varied needs of all persons with chronic and/or disabling conditions.

Dimensions of need were defined in terms of stability and severity of the patient's conditions, duration of illness, urgency of the intervention, scope of services required and the user's (or carer's) capacity for self-direction. The various service domains were structured into (i) systems to identify persons with disabilities (screening), (ii) clinical practices responsive to the needs of these persons, (iii) management of transitions across settings, (iv) information gathering and exchange, (v) case management, (vi) management of funds from multiple payment sources, and (vii) coordination of benefits.

Following this line of reasoning, Leutz (1999) divided service users into three groups: those with mild-to-moderate but stable conditions, a need for a select few routine care services and with high capacity for self-direction or strong informal networks; those with moderate levels of need; and those with long-term, severe, unstable conditions who frequently require urgent intervention from various sectors and who have limited capacity for self-direction. Leutz (1999) argued that the first group would be likely to be served sufficiently by relatively simple, though systematic, "linkage" of different systems. These do, however, require each provider to be aware of and to understand the other providers in terms of health and social care needs, financing responsibilities and eligibility criteria (Figure 4.1). Linkage would operate through the separate structures of existing health and social services systems, with organizations retaining their own service responsibilities, funding and eligibility criteria and operational rules (Goodwin et al. 2004).

The next level, coordination for groups with moderate levels of need, also would operate mainly through systems existing in different sectors but would involve additional explicit structures and processes, such as routinely shared information, discharge planners and case managers, to coordinate care across the various sectors.

At the far end of the spectrum, the last subgroups with long-term, severe, unstable conditions were likely to benefit most from a high level of integration

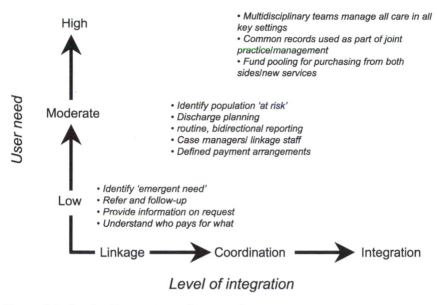

High

• Multidisciplinary teams manage all care in all key settings
• Common records used as part of joint practice/management
• Fund pooling for purchasing from both sides/new services

Moderate

• Identify population 'at risk'
• Discharge planning
• routine, bidirectional reporting
• Case managers/ linkage staff
• Defined payment arrangements

Low

• Identify 'emergent need'
• Refer and follow-up
• Provide information on request
• Understand who pays for what

User need

Linkage ⟶ Coordination ⟶ Integration

Level of integration

Figure 4.1   Levels of integration and user need.

Source: Adapted from Leutz (1999).

of the different service domains (Leutz 1999). Such a "fully" integrated system would assume responsibility for all services, resources and funding, which may be subsumed in one managed structure or through contractual agreements between different organizations (Goodwin et al. 2004).[2]

In the healthcare sector, one example of what has been described as a "fully integrated system" is provided by Kaiser Permanente, a health maintenance organization in the United States.[3] Goodwin et al. (2004) identified a series of key attributes that characterize integrated delivery systems such as that of Kaiser Permanente, including: a population defined by enrolment, contractual responsibility for a defined package of comprehensive healthcare services, financing on the basis of pooling multiple funding streams, a "closed" network (i.e. a selected group of contracted and/or salaried providers), emphasis on primary care and non-institutional services, use of micromanagement techniques to ensure appropriate quality of care and to control costs (e.g. utilization review, disease management) and multidisciplinary teams working across the network with joint clinical responsibility for outcomes.

A key feature of the approach taken by Kaiser Permanente to chronic care is the application of a population management (or care) model that divides the insured population of patients with chronic conditions into three distinct groups based on their degree of need (Bodenheimer et al. 2002a). Patients at level 1 have, in Leutz's terms, a relatively low level of need for healthcare: their chronic condition is reasonably under control, with support for self-management of their condition provided through the primary care team. This population constitutes the majority of the population with chronic conditions.

In contrast, level 2 patients are considered at increased risk because their condition is unstable or because they could deteriorate unless they have structured support through specialist disease management. Finally, level 3 includes individuals with highly complex needs and/or high intensity use of unplanned secondary care (i.e. emergency admissions) who require active management through case managers. This approach has also become known as the Kaiser Permanente "triangle" or "pyramid of care", as illustrated in Figure 4.2.

Kaiser Permanente's approach to management of patients with chronic conditions has evolved over time (Fireman et al. 2004). The focus was, initially, on care and case management of high-risk patients (Bodenheimer et al. 2002a) but it has gradually expanded to include the entire population with chronic disorders at all three levels of healthcare "need".

One other influential service delivery model addressing the needs of high-risk patients in particular, also originating in the United States, is the Evercare model developed in the late 1980s for the Minnesota government by UnitedHealth Group, a for-profit health plan (UnitedHealth Europe 2005). Its overall aim is to combine preventive and responsive care for patients at high risk of deterioration in their health. The Evercare model comprises a form of case management that, initially, targeted vulnerable elderly in Medicare-contracted nursing homes who were at increased risk of unplanned hospital admission (Boaden et al. 2006). The programme uses risk-stratification tools to assess the level of care required and to inform the development of an individual care plan that is coordinated and monitored by a specialist nurse (advanced practice nurse) acting as case manager. More recently, the programme has been extended to older patients living in the community.

The approaches taken by Kaiser Permanente and UnitedHealth Group involve distinct delivery models targeting specific segments of the patient population. Others have developed broader frameworks that, based on the available research

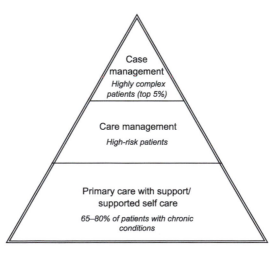

Figure 4.2 Population management levels of care.

Source: Adapted from Department of Health (2005).

evidence, have sought to guide the delivery of effective healthcare to people with chronic conditions by taking an explicit community or systems perspective, frequently involving comprehensive system change (Wagner 1998).

Perhaps the most influential framework has been the Chronic Care Model (CCM) developed by Edward Wagner and colleagues in the United States (Wagner et al. 1999). Recognizing the failures of health systems that remain largely built on an acute, episodic model of care with little emphasis on patient self-management, the CCM aimed to provide a comprehensive framework for the organization of healthcare to improve outcomes for people with chronic conditions (Wagner et al. 2001). It was based on the premise that high-quality chronic care is characterized by productive interactions between the practice team and patients, involving assessment, self-management support, optimization of therapy and follow-up. Drawing on a synthesis of the evidence of effectiveness of various (chronic) disease management interventions, the CCM comprises four interacting system components that are considered key to providing good chronic care: self-management support, delivery system design, decision support and clinical information systems (Wagner et al. 1996, 1999). These are set in a health system context that links an appropriately organized delivery system with complementary community resources and policies (Figure 4.3).

The CCM has been implemented in, or has guided, the (re-)design or reconfiguration of healthcare services in numerous settings across the United States (Pearson et al. 2005; Zwar et al. 2006). Internationally, it has been influential in informing chronic care policies in countries including Australia (Glasgow et al. 2008), Canada (British Columbia; (Jiwani and Dubois 2008)), and England (Department of Health 2005) (Box 4.2), with analysts in Germany

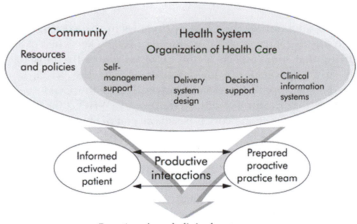

Functional and clinical outcomes

Figure 4.3 The Chronic Care Model.

Source: Reprinted from Effective Clinical Practice, 1: 2–4, Wagner: Chronic disease management: What will it take to improve care for chronic illness, © 1998, with permission from the American College of Physicians.

Box 4.2   International adaptations of the Chronic Care Model

In 2000, the Australian state of New South Wales (NSW) set up a chronic care program that involved a variety of approaches including the appointment of care coordinators for people with chronic conditions and encouraging multidisciplinary team approaches involving physicians, nurses and other allied health professionals (NSW Department of Health 2004). The experience of the first phase of the programme was mixed, however, so a second phase adopted a broader approach, including the development of a NSW chronic care model (NSW Department of Health 2004). Work is underway during this second phase to define the key elements of such a model, which is expected to draw, to a considerable extent, on the Chronic Care Model (Wagner et al. 1999) and the WHO Innovative Care for Chronic Conditions framework to develop a model that is applicable to the local context.

In England, in 2005, the government launched a bespoke NHS and Social Care Model designed to help health and social care organizations to improve care for people with chronic conditions (Singh and Fahey 2008). The model built on approaches such as the Chronic Care Model, the "Kaiser triangle" and the Evercare model, adapted to the values and structures of the NHS in England (Department of Health 2005). It outlines how people with chronic conditions will be identified and will receive care according to their needs. The stated principles driving the NHS and Social Care Model are an improvement in the quality and accessibility of care for people with chronic conditions and containment or reduction of the costs associated with chronic care (Singh and Fahey 2008).

recommending adoption of the CCM's principles in the existing countrywide approach to disease management introduced in 2002 (Gensichen et al. 2006).

Recognizing that some aspects of the CCM are not easily translatable internationally, and in particular to low-resource settings, the WHO, in collaboration with Wagner, applied a global perspective to the CCM to create the Innovative Care for Chronic Conditions framework (WHO 2003; Epping-Jordan et al. 2004). In brief, the framework is based on a set of guiding principles acting at three levels. The *micro level* emphasizes the partnership between patients/families, healthcare teams and community partners. The *meso level* refers to the healthcare organization and community, with a particular emphasis on the need for continuity and coordination as well as for "organized and well-equipped" healthcare teams rather than decision support, in recognition that decision-support tools may not be applicable in low-resource settings. The *macro level*, finally, explicitly considers the policy and financing contexts, which are seen as key factors in any successful system response to chronic conditions (Epping-Jordan et al. 2004).

There are numerous other service delivery models and broader frameworks directly or indirectly targeted at people with chronic conditions (Singh and

Ham 2006). The discussion here has concentrated on some of the more influential models, most prominently the CCM, which have been designed to improve the quality of care and, ultimately, outcomes for those with (complex) chronic conditions. Still, as indicated in the introduction to this chapter, while comprehensive models such as the CCM appear plausible and "the right thing to do", the available evidence on their effectiveness remains uncertain. Indeed, while there is now ample evidence that single or multiple components of the CCM improve selected processes and outcomes of care, it is less clear whether the model as a whole is essential to achieve the same benefits (Singh and Ham 2006). The next section revisits some of the evidence and remaining uncertainties as they relate to the CCM and its components.

What is the evidence?

Bodenheimer et al. (2002b) reviewed studies of diabetes care programmes that featured components of the CCM, building on an earlier Cochrane review by Renders et al. (2000). The most frequent interventions used in the programmes reviewed (and the elements of the CCM they relate to) were patient education and training (CCM component: self-management support); educational materials and meetings for physicians (CCM: decision support); use of case managers, multidisciplinary teams and scheduling of planned visits (CCM: delivery system design); and reminder systems and feedback on physician performance (CCM: clinical information system). Out of 39 studies, 32 found the intervention to improve at least one process or outcome measure. However, the authors noted difficulties in establishing a direct relationship between the number of CCM components and/or specific combinations of CCM components and overall effectiveness. They also noted that the studies included in their review varied in terms of methodological quality and rigour and, importantly, that reported findings were frequently derived from a research setting and were thus not necessarily reproducible in the population at large.

Bodenheimer et al. (2002b) reviewed a further 27 individual studies of interventions related to the CCM and their impact on healthcare utilization and cost in the management of congestive heart failure, asthma and diabetes. Again, self-management support was among the commonest CCM component employed, forming an integral part of all interventions studied. About half of the interventions also used some delivery system redesign, such as the introduction of follow-up by home visits, multispeciality teams, nurse-led clinics and case management (mostly for congestive heart failure and diabetes). The findings were mixed however, with some interventions in each disease category showing positive results (e.g. a reduction in healthcare utilization through reduced hospital admissions or visits to emergency departments) and/or cost reductions, while others did not. The authors acknowledged that it would be difficult to draw any general conclusions since, again, the studies included in their review assessed specific programmes undertaken in research settings rather than a permanent change in the delivery of chronic care; also, where interventions did achieve a cost reduction, this may not be sustainable in the long run.

Weingarten et al. (2002) conducted a meta-analysis of 118 disease management programmes that were evaluated in 102 studies (randomized controlled trials, before–after studies, interrupted time series). The meta-analysis focused on evidence of the effectiveness of different types of intervention used in disease management programmes for patients with chronic conditions. Disease management was defined as "an intervention designed to manage or prevent a chronic disease using a systematic approach to care and potentially employing multiple treatment modalities" (Ellrodt et al. 1997). A systematic approach was further defined as "methodologically developed statements assisting prac- titioner and patient decision making about appropriate healthcare for specific clinical circumstances" such as guidelines, protocols, care plans, standardized education and others (Weingarten et al. 2002): all interventions that may be considered under the CCM headings.

As with findings obtained by Bodenheimer et al. (2002b), patient education formed an integral part in most disease management programmes (92 of 118) studied, whereas provider education (47 of 118) was used widely only for selected conditions (depression, diabetes, hypertension, hyperlipidaemia). The number and combination of interventions varied, with around 40% using only a single intervention while 35% used two interventions, 20% used three and approximately 5% used four (Weingarten et al. 2002). Those using provider education, feedback and/or reminders achieved significant improvements in provider adherence to care guidelines. It was, however, impossible to determine which interventions produced the greatest relative improvement in care, as the studies included in the meta-analysis did not directly compare different interventions. Comparisons were also complicated by the diversity of interven- tions used for each condition. Consequently, the authors argued that there was a paucity of available information to guide programme development and define an optimal strategy.

In a related study, Ofman et al. (2004) revisited the analysis by Weingarten et al. (2002), focusing in particular on the quality of patient care as measured by selected process and outcome measures. While many disease management programmes reviewed were found to be associated with improvements in the quality of care, improvements were greatest for patient satisfaction with treat- ment, patient adherence to treatment recommendations, and measures of dis- ease control. The findings seem to suggest that disease management may be an effective strategy for changing the behaviours of patients and providers. How- ever, the authors warned that improvements in outcomes may be only modest even though evaluation of the effects of disease management programmes in rigorous studies published in the peer-reviewed literature may find statistically significant improvements in processes of care (Ofman et al. 2004). The review further demonstrated that relatively few studies included measures of utiliza- tion, such as emergency department visits or hospitalizations, or costs; of those that did, few found beneficial effects and findings tended to be relatively modest and inconsistent. Also, as the authors note, there is, as yet, relatively little evidence regarding the long-term benefits in terms of economic impact and financial return on investment associated with the development and imple- mentation of disease management programmes (see also Congressional Budget Office (2004) and Chapter 3). This observation is further reinforced by other work, which reported that beneficial effects of disease management on measure of utilization appears to be limited to congestive heart failure and the evidence that disease management may result in a net reduction of direct medical costs is at best inconclusive (Mattke et al. 2007).

There is now a wide range of systematic reviews, reviews of reviews and meta-analyses of the evidence on (chronic disease-) specific interventions and disease management programmes that share selected components of the CCM (e.g. Velasco-Garrido et al. 2003; Gonseth et al. 2004; Neumeyer-Gromen et al. 2004; Knight et al. 2005; Singh 2005a, 2005b; Tsai et al. 2005; Adams et al. 2007). Focusing particularly on the primary care setting, Zwar et al. (2006) recently examined the evidence on the effectiveness of the six CCM elements when tested experimentally. Using a systematic review and a review of reviews, they identified a series of key elements and interventions shown to be effective for selected process and outcome measures, as summarized in Table 4.1.

Table 4.1 Summary of evidence on effectiveness of the components of the Chronic Care Model

Component	Interventions shown to be effective	Outcome measures affected
Patient self-management support	Patient educational sessions Patient motivational counselling Distribution of educational materials	Physiological measures of disease Patient factors: quality of life, health status, functional status, satisfaction with service, risk behaviour, knowledge, service use, adherence to treatment
Delivery system design	Multidisciplinary teams	Physiological measures of disease Professionals adherence to guidelines Patient service use
Decision support	Implementation of evidence-based guidelines Educational meetings with professionals Distribution of educational materials among professionals	Professionals adherence to guidelines Physiological measures of disease
Clinical information systems	Audit and feedback	Professionals adherence to guidelines
Healthcare Organization	Little published experimental evidence	
Community resources	Little published experimental evidence	

Source: adapted from Zwar et al. (2006).

Similar to other reviews, the elements that were identified as impacting most consistently on clinical and patient outcome measures were self-management support and delivery system design, in particular when in combination, with decision support and clinical information systems important factors influencing guideline adherence by health professionals. However, much of the evidence reviewed related to the management of adult patients with type 2 diabetes, potentially limiting the transferability of findings to other chronic conditions. Also, there was little evidence on the impact of the broader CCM system components involving healthcare organization and/or community resources, which the authors attributed, in part, to the challenges faced in designing experimental studies of these elements (Zwar et al. 2006).

Importantly, although the CCM has been widely embraced as key to effective chronic disease management and, as the reviews by Zwar et al. (2006) and others have demonstrated, while its elements have been tested in various combinations and found to lead to some improvement in patient outcomes as outlined above, evidence on the impact of the model as a whole is scarce (Singh and Ham 2006). Indeed, the entire model has only recently been evaluated. For example, using an experimental design, Piatt et al. (2006) assessed the impact on clinical and behaviour outcomes of patients with diabetes of implementing the CCM in a small sample of primary care practices in an under-served area of Pittsburgh, Pennsylvania. The study found marked improvements after 12 months for two of the clinical outcomes and for self-monitoring of blood glucose in the CCM group compared with two other groups (provider intervention; usual care), but all other outcome measures were not significantly improved.

Two linked studies provided an evaluation of the implementation of the CCM by a medical group in Minneapolis, United States. Solberg et al. (2006) asked whether the delivery of care consistent with the six CCM components was correlated with improvements in the quality of care for patients with diabetes, coronary heart disease or depression. Care quality was measured as the proportion of patients who had achieved both of two separate guideline-recommended goals specific to their condition. The analysis showed how both the implementation of most CCM elements and the quality of care for patients with diabetes and coronary heart disease had improved over a period of two years. However, the authors were unable to establish a significant correlation between these changes. They further demonstrated how two of the six CCM elements, self-management support and delivery system design, which elsewhere were suggested to be potentially the most important elements for improving clinical and patient outcomes (e.g. Singh 2005a; Zwar et al. 2006), failed to achieve significant improvements.

The same group also undertook a qualitative evaluation of the implementation process (Hroscikoski et al. 2006). Their analysis identified several barriers to successful implementation, including too many competing priorities, lack of specificity of changes and of agreement about the care process changes desired, and little engagement of physicians. Based on their findings, the authors considered the value of the CCM to lie in its contribution as a practical guide to successful implementation. Specifically, Hroscikoski et al. (2006) noted that "[a]s a conceptual framework, the CCM is useful for thinking about types of care process needing to be addressed". However, as argued by these authors, the

CCM may not provide sufficient practical guidance to assist decision makers with the actual changes to be made to the care process.

In summary, as judged by the published literature, the evidence remains inconclusive on the impact of applying the CCM as a whole on quality of care and patient outcomes, as does the evidence about which components, in what combination, achieve the greatest improvements of what process, output and/ or outcome measures. What seems to be emerging is that the implementation of single interventions in isolation is not sufficient to improve the quality of chronic illness care (Rothman and Wagner 2003), but models that adopt an explicit patient-oriented approach are likely to have the greatest effects on patient outcomes (Zwar et al. 2006). However, much of the research evidence is on the management of a few specific diseases, such as diabetes. There has been less focus on individuals with coexisting conditions or multiple health problems (Piette and Kerr 2006; Struijs et al. 2006), even though it is this rapidly increasing population, with multiple disease processes and with diverse and sometimes contradictory needs, who pose the greatest challenge to health systems (Chapter 2). Also, research has concentrated on immediate to short-term outcomes only; relatively little is known about the long-term impact of approaches to chronic disease management, particularly as it relates to clinical and patient outcomes (Bailie et al. 2006). Importantly, available evidence seems to suggest that the impact of chronic disease management interventions will depend, to considerable extent, on the specific features of the healthcare setting within which they are introduced, and this observation seems to hold both within and between care systems. This issue will be examined briefly in the following section.

The system context of chronic disease management

Much of the conceptual thinking and empirical evidence originates from the United States, which is characterized by a highly fragmented system of generalist and specialized care and where the baseline outcomes from common chronic diseases such as diabetes are worse than, for example, in Europe (Nolte et al. 2006). Perhaps in response to this situation, a wide range of innovative approaches to disease management have been developed to improve the quality of care for those with chronic illness (Rothman and Wagner 2003). However, given differences in health systems, in particular as they relate to coverage and access, findings originating from the United States may not easily be transferable to healthcare systems that are characterized by (almost) universal access to healthcare such as those in Europe.

For example, the application of the Evercare approach to case management described earlier has been associated with reduced costs of care for older people living in nursing care homes in the United States. This was achieved through the reduced use of health services such as hospitalizations and use of emergency services (Kane et al. 2004; UnitedHealth Europe 2005). This approach was later adopted in England, with policy makers envisaging Evercare's experience as a means to free up hospital resources through targeted case management of high-intensity users or people at high risk of hospitalization (Boaden et al.

2006). This move was guided by the observation of substantial resource use by patients with complex conditions; for example, approximately 15% of people with three or more chronic problems were found to account for almost 30% of inpatient days (Wilson et al. 2005). Starting with pilots of the Evercare model of case management of frail elderly people in nine primary care trusts in England from April 2003 (UnitedHealth Europe 2005), case management subsequently became part of the United Kingdom government's national policy for supporting people with chronic conditions. The 2004 *NHS Improvement Plan* stipulated the introduction of case management in all primary care trusts through the appointment of senior nurses (community matrons) by 2007 (Department of Health 2004; see also Chapter 7). The anticipated benefits included improved quality of care and, by preventing or delaying complications, reduced (emergency) admissions and long hospital stays.

Yet these expectations seem not to be justified. Two reviews found that the evidence that case management prevented admissions to acute care and use of emergency departments was weak (Hutt et al. 2004; Singh 2005a). In both cases, the authors argued that the findings from studies in one healthcare setting could not be generalized easily to others, and the effectiveness of complex approaches to case management is, therefore, likely to depend on the nature of the intervention and on the nature of the target population and the care system into which it is introduced. This conclusion is supported by the evaluation of the "Evercare pilot" in the NHS in England, which failed to find the gains in lower emergency admissions and bed-days that would be expected based on the potential cost savings suggested for the Evercare model in the United States (Gravelle et al. 2007) (Box 4.3).

Case management has now become a key component of the national community matron policy in England, whereby senior nurses (matrons) act as case managers. Yet, as indicated by the findings of Boaden et al. (2006), while community matrons may be popular with patients and increase access to care, the policy on its own is unlikely to reduce hospital admissions in the absence of a more radical system redesign.

Similar conclusions were drawn from a series of studies undertaken within in the Veterans Health Administration in the United States, which provides healthcare for military veterans in the United States and which, with its integrated structure, has many features in common with systems such as the United Kingdom NHS. These studies suggested that use of case management or coordination strategies alone did not lead to reductions in hospital (re-) admissions of patients with complex needs; only subsequent major system-wide changes incorporating a range of strategies that also encouraged greater use of primary care services were associated with reduced admission rates (Kizer et al. 2000).

A recent study by Schmittdiel et al. (2006) assessed the association between primary care orientation (see below) and implementation of the CCM in a cross-sectional sample of United States medical groups and independent practice associations that had more than 20 physicians treating patients with chronic disease. Measures of primary care orientation were adapted from the work by Barbara Starfield and colleagues (for an overview see Starfield et al. (2005)), who identified a series of core practice features of primary care, such as the

Box 4.3 Case management in England

Gravelle et al. (2007) analysed the impact on patient outcomes of the Ever-care pilot, which introduced case management for elderly people in England. This involved a before and after analysis of hospital admissions data in 62 general practices implementing the Evercare model (April 2004 to March 2005). A key feature of the approach is the use of specialist nurses (advanced practice nurses) who monitor and coordinate the care of patients at risk according to individual care plans designed to improve a patient's functional status and quality of life and avoid hospital admissions. In a linked qualitative study, Boaden et al. (2006) highlighted the improvements in quality of care, such as frequency of contact, regular monitoring, psychosocial support and a range of referral options, that had not previously been provided to frail elderly people, but Gravelle et al. (2007) were unable to demonstrate any significant effects of the intervention on rates of emergency admissions, emergency bed-days and mortality for a population aged over 65 years at high risk for hospitalization. Gravelle et al. (2007), therefore, concluded that the implementation of case management of frail elderly people in England introduced an additional range of services into primary care but did not lead to an associated reduction in hospital admissions. While this lack of an association might be attributable, in part, to additional cases being identified, the overall findings of this evaluation do not support the use of nurse practitioners as a means to reduce hospital admissions in patients who have had previous emergency admissions (Gravelle et al. 2007; Sargent et al. 2007).

extent of gatekeeping, continuity/longitudinality, comprehensiveness, degree of service coordination and accountability. Implementation of the CCM was measured in terms of five elements: community linkages, self-management support, delivery system design, decision support and clinical information systems. These were then subdivided into 11 dimensions. The study found that of the eight measures indicating primary care orientation, six (representing level of comprehensiveness, accountability and coordination) were significantly and positively associated with adoption of 11 dimensions of the CCM. Schmittdiel et al. (2006) concluded that organizations "that have adopted 6 core attributes of primary care . . . appear to use more chronic care management practices". The nature of the study, using a cross-sectional design, does not allow determination of the direction of causality (i.e. whether greater primary care organization facilitates implementation of CCM elements or vice versa). However, the findings suggest that a strong primary care orientation may positively impact on the adoption of elements of chronic disease management and, consequently, systems elsewhere that are characterized by strong primary care orientation are likely to find it easier to introduce practices that benefit those with chronic conditions.

This consideration is important because the nature of primary care varies considerably within Europe. At the risk of generalization, the model found in the United Kingdom also exists in the Netherlands and Scandinavian countries. Primary care is based largely on multiprofessional teams of physicians, nurses and other health professionals (Ettelt et al. 2006). Patients are registered with a particular primary care facility, which acts as a gatekeeper to secondary care. In many countries where strong primary care teams exist, there has been a progressive shift in the management of many chronic diseases to nurse-led clinics in primary care (Box 4.4). There is now considerable evidence from various countries and for different diseases that this approach yields better results than traditional physician-led care, and it may also reduce costs (Singh 2005b; Vrijhoef et al. 2001), although the model cannot be generalized universally (Smith et al. 2001; see also Chapter 7).

In contrast, in most of the countries in Europe where healthcare is funded through social insurance, there is free choice of family practitioners and specialists working in ambulatory care. In this model, physicians are much more likely to work as individual practitioners and, as in many systems in the United States, the ambulatory and hospital sector tend to be strictly separated. As a consequence, countries such as Germany have tended to follow the United States

Box 4.4 Nurse-led clinics in Sweden

Nurses play an increasingly prominent role in the Swedish healthcare system through advanced care of patients with chronic and complex conditions such as diabetes and asthma; they also have limited authority to prescribe (Buchan and Calman 2005). By the late 1990s, two-thirds of hospitals ran nurse-led heart failure clinics, based on clinical protocols and with nurses empowered to change medication regimens within those protocols (Stromberg et al. 2001).

Nurse-led clinics are now common at primary healthcare centres and in hospital polyclinics across Sweden, managing diabetes and hypertension and with some also managing allergy/asthma/chronic obstructive pulmonary disease, psychiatry and heart failure (Karlberg 2008). The total number of nurse-led clinics in Sweden is difficult to assess; however, such clinics are established in almost every medical department and primary healthcare centre. While there are no significant regional differences in the number and design of nurse-led clinics, their staffing depends on the catchment area; one or more diabetes nurses may work with, among others, dieticians, foot therapists, surgeons and diabetes physician/endocrinologists.

The main reasons behind the growth in nurse-led clinics are both economic and to create new career opportunities for nurses. One other aspect is the development of a more patient-centred system that facilitates access, through telephone consultations and support for elderly persons with communication difficulties.

approach by introducing structured disease management programmes for selected conditions. Preliminary evidence indicates some success in terms of uptake and patient outcomes (Nordrheinische Gemeinsame Einrichtung Disease Management Programme GbR 2004; Petro et al. 2005) and systematic evaluations are underway (e.g. Joos et al. 2005). However, these are additional services that have not altered the general structure of primary care in the country (Siering 2008) and currently focus on single conditions only. Consequently, the current approach does not seem sufficient to meet the needs of the majority of patients with chronic disease (Gensichen et al. 2006; Siering 2008).

Conclusions

There is now an emerging consensus that the effective management of complex chronic diseases represents one of the greatest challenges now facing health systems. There is also a substantial consensus that this will require new ways of delivering healthcare, involving integration of care providers or, at least, much closer coordination of their activities. Yet beyond these areas of agreement, there is much less consensus about how this should be achieved. In part, this is a result of the plethora of terminology involved, which tends to confuse rather than clarify. Frequently, the same words mean very different things to different people. However, it also reflects the reality that health systems exhibit the property of path dependency, whereby the options to go forward are constrained by what has happened in the past. Each health system is characterized by a particular set of relationships between the different professionals and institutions that deliver care, and change must take account of what is possible (although, where constraints created by the existing system are insurmountable, more radical approaches may be needed). For both of these reasons, it cannot be assumed that a model of care developed in one setting can be transplanted to another. The experience of implementing United States models in the United Kingdom demonstrates the pitfalls that may arise. It does, however, seem that innovative models of care can be more easily implemented in health systems where there is a strong orientation to primary care, with a single point of access to the health system providing continuity.

The decision on how to move forward must be made for each health system. It is appropriate to begin by determining the nature of the integration being pursued, including the type, breadth, degree and process of integration. It should also take account of the very diverse population of people with chronic disorders, some of whom will require only that the services they need communicate with each other while others will need carefully managed and tightly integrated services so that no-one falls through the gaps.

There are now a number of models that policy makers can learn from as they seek a solution that is appropriate to their needs. The CCM has the advantage of a sound theoretical underpinning, identifying key elements that should be considered in any strategy. However, the policy maker is handicapped, first, by the paucity of high-quality evidence available on the different elements of the CCM and similar approaches and, second, by the even more limited evidence on transferability of such models to different systems. Perhaps the only area where there is some degree of certainty is that innovative models of care cannot be relied on to yield cost savings. There is a clear need for many more evaluations of the innovations being introduced in Europe in order to expand this evidence base.

Notes

1. In the Bible this was a tower built in an attempt to reach heaven, which God frustrated by confusing the languages of its builders so that they could not understand one another (Genesis 11:1–9) (Soanes and Stevenson 2005).
2. Building on the same notion of a continuum, others have refined this approach further (Goodwin et al. 2004; Ahgren and Axelsson 2005). For example, Ahgren and Axelsson (2005) distinguished five levels: (i) full segregation, the complete absence of any form of integration between services; (ii) linkage; (iii) coordination in networks; (iv) cooperation, where organizations or organizational units are still separate but closely coordinated by appointed network managers; and (v) full integration, a "new" organization that pools funds from the various sources and is responsible for the entire spectrum of services.
3. Kaiser Permanente is a collaboration of three distinct legal entities: the Kaiser Foundation Health Plan (includes the insurance and financing activities), Kaiser Foundation Hospitals (owns large parts of the physical assets of the delivery system, including hospitals and clinics) and the Permanente Medical Groups (responsible for care delivery). The eight regionally based Permanente Medical Groups are organized and operated as autonomous multispecialty group practices; each has a medical services agreement with the payer (KHFP-H) and is responsible for the organization and provision of the necessary medical care for members in the given geographical region (Wallace 2005).

References

Adams, S., Smith, P., Allan, P. et al. (2007) Systematic review of the Chronic Care Model in chronic obstructive pulmonary disease prevention and management, *Arch Intern Med*, 167: 551–61.

Ahgren, B. and Axelsson, R. (2005) Evaluating integrated health care: a model for measurement, *Int J Integr Care*, 5: 1–9.

Axelsson, R. and Axelsson, S. (2006) Integration and collaboration in public health: a conceptual framework, *Int J Health Plann Manage*, 21: 75–88.

Bailie, R., Robinson, G., Kondalsamy-Chennakesavan, S., Halpin, S. and Wang, Z. (2006) Investigating the sustainability of outcomes in a chronic disease treatment programme, *Soc Sci Med*, 63: 1661–70.

Boaden, R., Dusheiko, M., Gravelle, H. et al. (2006) *Evercare Evaluation: Final Report*. Manchester: National Primary Care Research and Development Centre.

Bodenheimer, T. (1999) Disease management: promises and pitfalls, *N Engl J Med*, 340: 1202–5.

Bodenheimer, T. (2000) Disease management in the American market, *BMJ*, 320: 563–6.

Bodenheimer, T., Wagner, E. and Grumbach, K. (2002a) Improving primary care for patients with chronic illness, *JAMA*, 288: 1775–9.

Bodenheimer, T., Wagner, E. and Grumbach, K. (2002b) Improving primary care for patients with chronic illness: the chronic care model, Part 2, *JAMA*, 288: 1909–14.

Boston Consulting Group (2006) *Realizing the Promise of Disease Management*. Boston, MA: Boston Consulting Group.

Buchan, J. and Calman, L. (2005) *Skill-mix and Policy Change in the Health Workforce: Nurses in Advanced Roles*. Paris: OECD.

Cavanaugh, K., White, R. and Rothman, R. (2007) Exploring disease management programs for diabetes mellitus, *Dis Manage Health Outcomes*, 15: 73–81.

Congressional Budget Office (2004) *An analysis of the Literature on Disease Management Programs*. Washington, DC: Congressional Budget Office.

Conrad, D. and Shortell, S. (1996) Integrated health systems: promise and performance, *Front Health Serv Manage*, 13: 3–40.

Delnoij, D., Klazinga, N. and Glasgow, I. (2002) Integrated care in an international perspective, *Int J Integr Care*, 2: 1–4.

Department of Health (2004) *The NHS Improvement Plan. Putting People at the Heart of Public Services*. London: Department of Health.

Department of Health (2005) *Supporting People with Long Term Conditions. An NHS and Social Care Model to Support Local Innovation and Integration*. London: Department of Health.

Dowling, B., Powell, M. and Glendinning, C. (2004) Conceptualising successful partnerships, *Health Soc Care Commun*, 12: 309–17.

Ellrodt, G., Cook, D., Lee, J. et al. (1997) Evidence-based disease management, *JAMA*, 278: 1687–92.

Epping-Jordan, J., Pruitt, S., Bengoa, R. and Wagner, E. (2004) Improving the quality of care for chronic conditions, *Qual Saf Health Care*, 13: 299–305.

Epstein, R. and Sherwood, L. (1996) From outcomes research to disease management: a guide for the perplexed, *Ann Intern Med*, 124: 832–7.

Ettelt, S., Nolte, E., Mays, N. et al. (2006) *Health Care Outside Hospital. Accessing Generalist and Specialist Care in Eight Countries*. Copenhagen: World Health Organization on behalf of the European Observatory on Health Systems and Policies.

Fabbricotti, I. (2007) *Taking Care of Integrated Care: Integration and Fragmentation in the Development of Integrated Care Arrangements*. Rotterdam: Erasmus University.

Fireman, B., Bartlett, J. and Selby, J. (2004) Can disease management reduce health care costs by improving quality? *Health Aff*, 23: 63–75.

Gensichen, J., Muth, C., Butzlaff, M. et al. (2006) The future is chronic: German primary care and the Chronic Care Model, *Zaerztl Fortbild Qual Gesundheitswes*, 100: 365–74.

Geyman, J. (2007) Disease management: panacea, another false hope, or something in between? *Ann Fam Med*, 5: 257–60.

Gillespie, J. and Rossiter, L. (2003) Medicaid disease management programmes, *Dis Manage Health Outcomes*, 11: 345–61.

Glasgow, N., Zwar, N., Harris, M., Hasan, I. and Jowsey, T. (2008) Australia, in E. Nolte, C. Knai and M. McKee (eds) *Managing Chronic Conditions: Experience in Eight Countries*. Copenhagen: European Observatory on Health Systems and Policies.

Gonseth, J., Guallar-Castillon, P., Banegas, J. and Rodriguez-Artalejo, F. (2004) The effectiveness of disease management programmes in reducing hospital re-admission in older patients with heart failure: a systematic review and meta-analysis of published reports, *Eur Heart J*, 25: 1570–95.

Goodwin, N., Perri, 6, Peck, E., Freeman, T. and Posaner, R. (2004) *Managing Across Diverse Networks of Care: Lessons From Other Sectors*. London: National Co-ordinating Centre for NHS Service Delivery and Organisation R&D.

Gravelle, H., Dusheiko, M., Sheaff, R. et al. (2007) Impact of case management (Evercare) on frail elderly patients: controlled before and after analysis of quantitative outcome data, *BMJ*, 334: 31–4.

Groene, O. and Garcia-Barbero, M. (2001) Integrated care. A position paper of the WHO European office for integrated health care services, *Int J Integr Care*, 1: 1–16.

Hardy, B., Mur-Veemanu, I., Steenbergen, M. and Wistow, G. (1999) Inter-agency services in England and the Netherlands, *Health Policy*, 48: 87–105.

Howarth, M. and Haigh, C. (2007) The myth of patient centrality in integrated care: the case of back pain, *Int J Integr Care*, 7: e27.

Hroscikoski, M., Solberg, L., Sperl-Hillen, J. et al. (2006) Challenges of change: a qualitative study of chronic care model implementation, *Ann Fam Med*, 4: 317–26.

Hunter, D. and Fairfield, G. (1997) Managed care: disease management, *BMJ*, 315: 50–3.

Hutt, R., Rosen, R. and McCauley, J. (2004) *Case-managing Long-term Conditions. What Impact does it have in the Treatment of Older People?* London: King's Fund.

Jiwani, I. and Dubois, C. (2008) Canada, in E. Nolte, C. Knai and M. McKee (eds) *Managing Chronic Conditions: Experience in Eight Countries*. Copenhagen: European Observatory on Health Systems and Policies.

Joos, S., Rosemann, T., Heiderhoff, M. et al. (2005) ELSID-Diabetes study-evaluation of a large scale implementation of disease management programmes for patients with type 2 diabetes. Rationale, design and conduct: a study protocol, *BMC Public Health*, 5: 99.

Kane, R., Homyak, P., Bershadsky, B., Flood, S. and Zhang, H. (2004) Patterns of utilization for the Minnesota Senior Health Options Program, *J Am Geriatrics Soc*, 52: 2039–44.

Karlberg, I. (2008) Sweden, in E. Nolte, C. Knai and M. McKee (eds) *Managing Chronic Conditions: Experience in Eight Countries*. Copenhagen: European Observatory on Health Systems and Policies.

Kizer, K., Demakis, J. and Feussner, J. (2000) Reinventing VA health care: systematizing quality improvement and quality innovation, *Med Care*, 38(Suppl I): 7–16.

Knight, K., Badamgarav, E., Henning, J. et al. (2005) A systematic review of diabetes disease management programmes, *Am J Manag Care*, 11: 241–50.

Kodner, D. and Spreeuwenberg, C. (2002) Integrated care: meaning, logic, applications, and implications: a dicussion paper, *Int J Integr Care*, 2: e12.

Krumholz, H., Currie, P., Riegel, B. et al. (2006) A taxonomy for disease management: a scientific statement from the American Heart Association Disease Management Taxonomy Writing Group, *Circulation*, 114: 1432–45.

Leichsenring, K. (2004) Developing integrated health and social care services for older persons in Europe, *Int J Integr Care*, 4: e10.

Leutz, W. (1999) Five laws for integrating medical and social services: lessons from the United States and the United Kingdom, *Milbank Q*, 77: 77–110.

Leutz, W. (2005) Reflections on integrating medical and social care: five laws revisited, *J Integrated Care*, 13: 3–11.

Mattke, S., Seid, M. and Ma, S. (2007) Evidence for the effect of disease management: is $1 billion a year a good investment? *Am J Manag Care*, 13: 670–6.

Maynard, A. and Bloor, K. (1998) *Managed Care: Panacea or Palliation?* London: Nuffield Trust.

McCall, N., Cromwell, J. and Bernhard, S. (2007) *Evaluation of Phase 1 of Medicare Health Support (formerly Voluntary Chronic Care Improvement) Pilot Program under Traditonal Fee-for-service Medicare*. Baltimore, MD: Centers for Medicare and Medicaid Services.

Neumeyer-Gromen, S., Lampert, T., Stark, K. and Kalligschnigg, G. (2004) Disease management programs for depression. A systematic review and meta-analysis of randomized controlled trials, *Med Care*, 42: 1211–21.

Niskanen, J. (2002) Finnish care integrated? *Int J Integr Care*, 2: 1–10.

Nolte, E., Bain, C. and McKee, M. (2006) Diabetes as a tracer condition in international benchmarking of health systems, *Diabetes Care*, 29: 1007–11.

Nordrheinische Gemeinsame Einrichtung Disease Management Programme GbR

(2004) *Qualitätssicherungsbericht 2004. Disease-Management-Programme in Nordrhein.* Düsseldorf: Nordrheinische Gemeinsame Einrichtung Disease Management Programme GbR.

Norris, S., Nichols, P., Caspersen, C. et al. (2002) The effectiveness of disease and case management for people with diabetes. A systematic review, *Am J Prev Med*, 22: 15–38.

Norris, S., Glasgow, R., Engelgau, M., O'Connor, P. and McCulloch, D. (2003) Chronic disease management. A definition and systematic approach to component interventions, *Dis Manage Health Outcomes* 11: 477–88.

NSW Department of Health (2004) *NSW Chronic Care Program 2000–2003. Strengthening Capacity for Chronic Care in the NSW Health System.* Sydney: NSW Department of Health.

Ofman, J., Badamgarav, E., Henning, J. et al. (2004) Does disease management improve clinical and economic outcomes in patients with chronic diseases? A systematic review, *Am J Med*, 117: 182–92.

Ouwens, M., Wollersheim, H., Hermens, R., Hulscher, M. and Grol, R. (2005) Integrated care programmes for chronically ill patients: a review of systematic reviews, *Int J Qual Health Care* 17: 141–6.

Ovretveit, J. (1998) *Integrated Care: Models and Issues. A Nordic School of Public Health Briefing Paper.* Goteborg: Nordic School of Public Health.

Pearson, M., Wu, S., Schaefer, J. et al. (2005) Assessing the implementation of the chronic care model in quality improvement collaboratives, *Health Serv Res*, 40: 978–95.

Petro, W., Schulenburg, J., Greiner, W. et al. (2005) Effizienz eines Disease Management Programmes bei Asthma, *Pneumologie*, 59: 101–7.

Piatt, G., Orchard, T., Emerson, S. et al. (2006) Translating the Chronic Care Model into the community. Results from a randomized controlled trial of a multifacted diabetes care intervention, *Diabetes Care*, 29: 811–17.

Piette, J. and Kerr, E. (2006) The impact of comorbid chronic conditions on diabetes care, *Diabetes Care*, 29: 725–31.

Plochg, T. and Klazinga, N. (2002) Community-based integrated care: myth or must? *Int J Qual Health Care*, 14: 91–101.

Renders, C., Valk, G., Griffin, S. et al. (2000) Interventions to improve the management of diabetes mellitus in primary care, outpatient and community settings, *Cochrane Database Syst Rev* 4: CD000541.

Roberts, D. (2002) Reconceptualizing case management in theory and practice: a frontline perspective, *Health Serv Manage Res*, 15: 147–64.

Rothman, A. and Wagner, E. (2003) Chronic illness management: what is the role of primary care? *Ann Intern Med*, 138: 256–61.

Sargent, P., Pickard, S., Sheaff, R. and Boaden, R. (2007) Patient and carer perceptions of case management for long-term conditions, *Health Soc Care Commun*, 15: 511–19.

Schmittdiel, J., Shortell, S., Rundall, T., Bodenheimer, T. and Selby, J. (2006) Effect of primary health care orientation on chronic care management, *Ann Fam Med*, 4: 117–23.

Shortell, S., Gillies, R. and Anderson, D. (1994) The new world of managed care: creating organized delivery systems, *Health Aff*, 13: 46–4.

Shortell, S., Gillies, R., Anderson, D., Erickson, K. and Mitchell, J. (2000) *Remaking Health Care in America. The Evolution of Organized Delivery Systems*, 2nd edn. San Francisco, CA: Jossey-Bass.

Siering, U. (2008) Germany, in E. Nolte, C. Knai and M. McKee (eds) *Managing Chronic Conditions: Experience in Eight Countries.* Copenhagen: European Observatory on Health Systems and Policies.

Simoens, S. and Scott, A. (1999) *Towards a Definition and Taxonomy of Integration in Primary Care.* Aberdeen: University of Aderdeen.

Singh, D. (2005a) *Transforming Chronic Care. Evidence about Improving Care for People with Long-term Conditions.* Birmingham: University of Birmingham, Surrey and Sussex PCT Alliance.

Singh, D. (2005b) *Which Staff Improve Care for People with Long-term Conditions? A Rapid Review of the Literature.* Birmingham: University of Birmingham and NHS Modernisation Agency.

Singh, D. and Fahey, D. (2008) England, in E. Nolte, C. Knai and M. McKee (eds) *Managing Chronic Conditions: Experience in Eight Countries.* Copenhagen: European Observatory on Health Systems and Policies.

Singh, D. and Ham, C. (2006) *Improving Care for People with Long-term Conditions. A Review of UK and International Frameworks.* Birmingham: University of Birmingham, NHS Institute for Innovation and Improvement.

Smith, B., Appleton, S., Adams, R., Southcott, A. and Ruffin, R. (2001) Home care by outreach nursing for chronic obstructive pulmonary disease, *Cochrane Database Syst Rev*, 3: CD000994.

Smith, V., Gifford, K., Ellis, E. et al. (2006) *Low Medicaid Spending Growth amid Rebounding State Revenues. Results From a 50-state Medicaid Budget Survey, State Fiscal Years 2006 and 2007.* Washington: Kaiser Commission on Medicaid and the Uninsured.

Soanes, C. and Stevenson, A. (2005) *The Oxford Dictionary of English.* Oxford: Oxford University Press. http://www.oxfordreference.com/ (accessed 19 July 2007).

Solberg, L., Crain, A., Sperl-Hillen, J. et al. (2006) Care quality and implementation of the chronic care model: a quantitative study, *Ann Fam Med*, 4: 310–16.

Starfield, B., Shi, L. and Macinko, J. (2005) Contribution of primary care to health systems and health, *Milbank Q*, 83: 457–502.

Stromberg, A., Martensson, J., Fridlund, B. and Dahlstrom, U. (2001) Nurse-led heart failure clinics in Sweden, *Eur J Heart Fail*, 3: 139–44.

Struijs, J., Baan, C., Schellevis, F., Westert, G. and van den Bos, G. (2006) Comorbidity in patients with diabetes mellitus: impact on medical health care utilization, *BMC Health Serv Res*, 6: 84.

Tsai, A., Morton, S., Mangione, C. and Keeler, E. (2005) A meta-analysis of interventions to improve care for chronic illness, *Am J Manag Care*, 11: 478–88.

UnitedHealth Europe (2005) *Assessment of the Evercare Programme in England 2003–2004.* London: UnitedHealth.

Velasco-Garrido, M., Busse, R. and Hisashige, A. (2003) *Are Disease Management Programmes (DMPs) Effective in Improving Quality of Care for People with Chronic Conditions?* Copenhagen: WHO Regional Office for Europe. http://www.euro.who.int/document/e82974.pdf.

Vondeling, H. (2004) Economic evaluation of integrated care: an introduction, *Int J Integr Care*, 4: e20.

Vrijhoef, H., Spreeuwenberg, C., Eijkelberg, I., Wolffenbuttel, B. and van Merode, G. (2001) Adoption of disease management model for diabetes in region of Maastricht, *BMJ*, 323: 983–5.

Wagner, E. (1998) Chronic disease management: what will it take to improve care for chronic illness? *Eff Clin Pract*, 1: 2–4.

Wagner, E., Austin, B. and von Korff, M. (1996) Organizing care for patients with chronic illness, *Milbank Q*, 74: 511–14.

Wagner, E., Davis, C., Schaefer, J., Von Korff, M. and Austin, B. (1999) A survey of leading chronic disease management programs: are they consistent with the literature? *Manage Care Q*, 7: 56–66.

Wagner, E., Austin, B., Davis, C. et al. (2001) Improving chronic illness care: translating evidence into action, *Health Aff*, 20: 64–78.

Wallace, P. (2005) Physician involvement in disease management as part of the CCM, *Health Care Financ Rev*, 27: 19–31.

Weingarten, S., Henning, J., Badamgarav, E. et al. (2002) Interventions used in disease management programmes for patients with chronic illness: which ones work? Meta-analysis of published reports, *BMJ*, 325: 925–32.

WHO (2003) *Innovative Care for Chronic Conditions: Building Blocks for Action*. Geneva: World Health Organization.

Wilson, T., Buck, D. and Ham, C. (2005) Rising to the challenge: will the NHS support people with long-term conditions? *BMJ*, 330: 657–61.

Zwar, N., Harris, M., Griffiths, R. et al. (2006) *A Systematic Review of Chronic Disease Management*. Sydney: Australian Primary Health Care Institute.

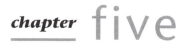
Preventing chronic disease: everybody's business

Thomas E. Novotny

Introduction

This chapter will address the prevention of chronic diseases, as the future burden of these diseases in Europe and globally will be determined in large part by the reduction in the major risk factors for such diseases, including tobacco use, obesity/diet, hypercholesterolaemia, hypertension, alcohol abuse, sedentary lifestyle and certain infectious diseases. Further, the chapter will consider the influences on these risk factors of distal factors, such as demographic changes, poverty and other social determinants, globalization and the environment. It will present examples of effective prevention efforts in both the individual and population-based context and it will conclude by outlining the specific role of health systems in preventing chronic disease.

Risk factors for chronic diseases in Europe

Trends in risk factors and in the burden of disease associated with specific risk factors have been evaluated thoroughly in recent scientific reports, including Ezzati et al. (2004) (*Comparative Quantification of Health Risks*) and Lopez et al. (2006) (*Global Burden of Disease and Risk Factors*). Quantifying these risk factors and the disease burden attributable to them is key to understanding how to prevent chronic diseases through appropriately targeted health policies. Since its publication in 1990, the approach outlined in the *Global Burden of Disease* has become the main method to assess the impact of disease on health systems and populations and to provide the basis for setting research priorities. It provides a common metric to describe disease burdens using diagnostic categories from the *International Classification of Diseases* and their major risk factors. Readers are referred to the online technical material in Lopez et al. (2006)

(http://www.dcp2.org/pubs/GBD) for detailed description of methodologies. The basic schema to understand the relationship between social and environmental determinants, risk factors, and health outcomes is shown in Figure 5.1.

To refresh the reader's memory on risk factors and how they can be considered causal for chronic diseases, it may be helpful to consider the following five causal criteria (Hill 1965):

- consistency of the association
- strength of the association
- specificity of the association
- temporal relationship of the association
- coherence of the association.

This chapter will mainly focus on an additional criterion for asserting causality, namely that the removal of the risk factor will be associated with a reduction in disease. Prevention can reduce the burden of chronic disease by reducing exposure to risk factors; the prevention framework should include primary, secondary or tertiary approaches. Briefly, primary prevention works before the onset of disease (e.g. preventing young people from becoming addicted to smoking to prevent lung cancer); secondary prevention works on those with early signs of or preconditions of chronic disease (e.g. hypertension screening in clinic patients to control this condition and prevent stroke); and tertiary prevention works on those with established disease to reduce disability and morbidity (e.g. taking low-dose aspirin after the first myocardial infarct to prevent recurrence).

The importance of distal risk factors such as socioeconomic status, demographic changes, globalization, environmental disadvantages and inadequate information on risk factors for chronic disease must be emphasized at the outset. Much evidence has been reported, especially since the 1960s, that the health of individuals and populations is fundamentally determined by their social and physical environments (Marmot and Wilkinson 2006). Those with the least knowledge about health risks suffer from an asymmetry of information: knowledge of risk associations and disease, the long-term health consequences of these risks, and the difficulty of abandoning such risks is much more difficult for those below the poverty line and for those with the least access to healthcare than for others. A thorough discussion of these determinants is beyond the scope of this chapter, but health systems interactions with them will be discussed.

In this chapter, risk factors and determinants for chronic disease (Table 5.1) will be disaggregated and individually addressed with respect to the European

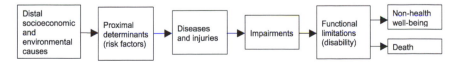

Figure 5.1   Overview of the burden of disease framework.

Source: Adapted from Mathers et al. (2002).

Table 5.1 Deaths and burden of disease attributable to common risk factors, 2001

Chronic disease risk factors	Low and middle income (No. (%))		High income (No. (%))		World (No. (%))	
	Deaths	DALY	Deaths	DALY	Deaths	DALY
Smoking	3340 (6.9)	54,019 (3.9)	1462 (18.5)	18,900 (12.7)	4802 (8.5)	72,919 (4.7)
High blood pressure	6223 (12.9)	78,063 (5.6)	1392 (17.6)	13,887 (9.3)	7615 (13.5)	91,950 (6.0)
High cholesterol	3038 (6.3)	42,815 (3.1)	842 (10.7)	9431 (6.3)	3880 (6.9)	52,246 (3.4)
Overweight and obesity	1747 (3.6)	31,515 (2.3)	614 (7.8)	10,733 (7.2)	2361 (4.2)	42,248 (2.8)
Low fruit and vegetable intake	2308 (4.8)	32,836 (2.4)	333 (4.2)	3982 (2.7)	2641 (4.7)	36,819 (2.4)
Physical inactivity	1559 (3.2)	22,679 (1.6)	376 (4.8)	4732 (3.2)	1935 (3.4)	27,411 (1.8)

DALY, disability adjusted life years.

Source: Lopez et al. (2006).

situation. The chapter will focus on tobacco use, obesity/diet, hypertension, alcohol abuse, sedentary lifestyle and infectious diseases. Influences on chronic disease to be discussed with regard to prevention include demographic changes, globalization, health systems, and the built environment.

Tobacco use

Tobacco use as a preventable risk factor for chronic disease has perhaps been studied more than any other. The main chronic diseases concerned are cancers, cardiovascular diseases and respiratory diseases, and there is no longer any doubt as to the role that tobacco use plays in their development (Department of Health and Human Services 2004). There is also substantial evidence on the causal relationship between several chronic diseases and exposure to passive smoking (Department of Health and Human Services 2006). Tobacco use acts in synergy with other risk factors to cause cardiovascular disease (hyper-cholesterolaemia, diabetes mellitus and hypertension), thus multiplying risk for cardiovascular disease as these various risk factors cluster.

There is now substantial evidence of the effectiveness of a number of prevent-ive efforts at both the population and individual level of intervention in differ-ent national settings (Jha and Chaloupka 2000; Department of Health and Human Services 2004). In California, where a comprehensive tobacco control programme has been in place since approximately 1990, adult smoking preva-lence declined at a faster pace than for all the other states (Siegel et al. 2000). During 1988–1997, age-adjusted incidence of lung cancer declined 14% in California compared with only 2.7% in other parts of the United States (Centers for Disease Control and Prevention 2000). One would also expect a rapid decline in heart disease mortality, and, in fact, Fichtenberg and Glantz (2000) reported 33,300 fewer deaths than expected compared with the rest of the United States.

In Finland, the European model for cardiovascular risk reduction is the North Karelia Project, wherein reductions in multiple cardiac risk factors have produced substantial falls in cardiovascular mortality since the early 1970s. In this community, where a comprehensive cardiovascular disease prevention programme was implemented in 1972, changes in mortality were significantly greater than in the rest of Finland between 1969 and 1982 (Figure 5.2).

The annual decline in mortality from ischaemic heart disease in men was 2.9%, whereas in the rest of Finland it was 2.0%. Among women the respective average annual declines in mortality were 4.9% and 3.0%. Smoking cessation was a major part of this programme (Sankila 2003).

Lung cancer mortality may be reduced by smoking cessation, both at the population level and at the individual level (Figure 5.3). Clearly, the benefits of quitting at an earlier age are far greater than those who wait until middle age or later to quit.

Lung cancer mortality rates among men have peaked or are decreasing in all European countries except for Hungary and Spain (Brennan and Bray 2002). These trends reinforce the evidence for the effectiveness of any tobacco control programmes that can reduce smoking prevalence on lung cancer mortality (as an indicator disease for all smoking-attributable chronic illnesses). The evidence from across Europe is that chronic diseases caused by tobacco use can be prevented if a large proportion of current smokers can quit and fewer new smokers are recruited. However, in central and eastern Europe, the actions of the tobacco industry, coupled with sociodemographic and economic stresses, bode ill for the future in tobacco control (Levintova and Novotny 2004; Bobak et al. 2006).

Tobacco interventions

There is clear evidence for the effectiveness of several specific prevention approaches in tobacco control, articulated by the World Bank (Jha and Chaloupka 2000) and reemphasized by the Disease Control Priorities Project (2007). Briefly, the effective interventions are as follows.

Higher prices for cigarettes. Evidence from many developed countries indicates that the price elasticity of cigarette demand ranges from –0.25 to –0.50, meaning that a 10% price increase for cigarettes will reduce cigarette smoking by 2.5 to 5.0% (Chaloupka et al. 2000). Importantly, this means that tax rises will both increase government revenues and reduce smoking prevalence.

Public smoking bans. Comprehensive restrictions on cigarette smoking in public places may reduce smoking prevalence rates by 5 to 15% (Woolery et al. 2000) and are important in changing social norms relating to smoking.

Public information. The "information shocks" provided by the 1962 United Kingdom Royal College of Physicians Report and the 1964 United States Surgeon General's Report on the Health Consequences of Smoking led to significant reductions in cigarette consumption, with initial declines of 4–9% and longer-term cumulative declines of 15–30% (Kenkel and Chen 2000).

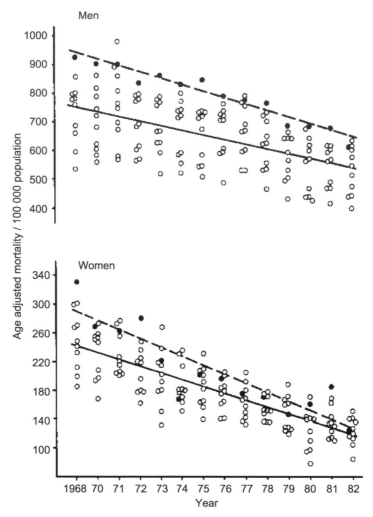

Figure 5.2 Age-standardized annual mortality from all cardiovascular diseases per 100,000 population in men and women aged 35 to 64 years in Finland, 1969–1982. North Karelia, filled circles and dashed fitted regression line; 10 other Finnish provinces, open circles and continuous fitted regression line.

Source: From Tuomilehto et al. (1986) *BMJ*, 293: 1068–71. Reproduced with permission from the BMJ Publishing Group.

Bans on advertising and promotion. Comprehensive bans may achieve up to 6% reduction in cigarette consumption if coupled with strong tobacco control programmes in other areas. Partial bans can be expected to have little effect owing to the proven capacity of the tobacco industry to subvert the intent of such restrictions (Saffer and Chaloupka 2000).

Smoking cessation. Reductions in smoking-attributable mortality will only be seen if cessation is more widely adopted by current smokers. Behavioural

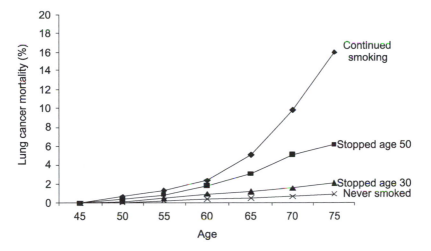

Figure 5.3   Cumulative risk of lung cancer mortality men in the United Kingdom, based on 1990 smoking rates.

Source: Adapted from Peto et al. (2000).

assistance includes self-help manuals, community-based programmes, and minimal or intensive clinical interventions, but there is significant evidence for the use of nicotine-replacement and/or pharmacological therapy with bupropion (Novotny et al. 2000), which can increase quit rates by a factor of two or three.

Controlling smuggling. This is really the only useful supply-side intervention according to World Bank research (Merriman et al. 2000). In effect, restricting the availability of cheap, smuggled cigarettes increases the price, thus making smuggling control a demand-side approach. Such controls depend on reducing corruption, establishing tracking mechanisms and monitoring the efforts of the tobacco industry in support of smuggling.

Other interventions. There is little evidence to support an effect with restrictions on sales to minors, prohibitions of cigarette sales in general or agricultural interventions such as crop substitution and diversification (Jacobs et al. 2000).

One particularly important multinational approach recently implemented is the Framework Convention on Tobacco Control (FCTC), which is the first-ever health treaty made by the WHO. This treaty calls for implementation of advertising bans, labelling restrictions, actions to tackle smuggling, higher prices, restrictions on smoking in public places, increased cessation services and other evidence-based approaches, enacted by means of domestic law but obligated under the international treaty. In the future, similar multinational agreements may be useful in terms of food policy, alcohol policy and harmonization of prevention practices.

Overweight and obesity

Energy balance is determined by caloric intake and physical activity, so consequently nutritional excess as well as socioenvironmental and demographic changes such as urbanization may lead to increased levels of overweight/obesity. As incomes increase, dietary changes may favour high-fat fast foods, influenced by the globalization of food markets. Although awareness of the problem is rising, the International Obesity Task Force (2003) showed that, excluding Portugal, over 50% of people living within each European Union Member State (EU before May 2004) were failing to meet at least three of the four dietary and health targets set by the WHO regarding healthy diets (WHO 2003). Almost a third of all people living in Europe are overweight, defined as a body mass index (kg/m²) of 25 or greater (30 or greater is considered to indicate obesity). Overweight varies significantly by age, with older age groups showing higher prevalence (up to 57% of men in western Europe at age 70–79 years) (James et al. 2004).

Childhood obesity is already considered an epidemic in Europe. According to a 2003 study by the London-based International Obesity Task Force, 14 million of the 77 million children living in the European Union are overweight (Figure 5.4). This number, given current trends, is predicted to rise by 400,000 each year.

Obesity negatively impacts on blood pressure, blood cholesterol and lipid levels, and the metabolic effects of insulin, leading to the onset of diabetes mellitus. In addition, respiratory diseases, chronic musculoskeletal problems, osteoporosis, gall bladder disease, infertility and adverse dermatological conditions are associated with obesity. The main issues are, however, cardiovascular disease, diabetes type 2 and some cancers, including breast cancer. Europe has a

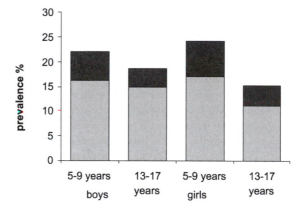

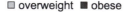

Figure 5.4   Overweight and obesity in the European region.

Source: Reprinted from International Obesity Task Force (2003). *Waiting for a green light for health? Europe at the crossroads for diet and disease.* IOTF Position Paper, September 2003. London: International Obesity Task Force, with permission from the International Obesity Task Force, the policy arm of the International Association for the Study of Obesity.

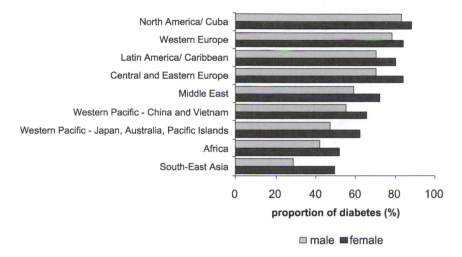

Figure 5.5 Proportion of diabetes attributable to weight gain by region for adults aged over 30 years.

Source: Adapted from James et al. (2004).

high burden of diabetes mellitus attributable to weight gain compared with other global regions (Figure 5.5).

The global epidemic of diabetes mellitus is of great concern to governments because of the secondary complications (visual, orthopaedic, renal, dermatological, etc.) that lead to premature mortality and disability and impose significant fiscal burdens on health systems and society.

Obesity and diabetes interventions

From the preceding discussion, it becomes clear that obesity is a vexing problem in a "globalized" world. There appears to be little new in the world of cost-effective interventions, but increasingly governments must consider a more paternalistic approach as a public good in the battle against the growing, and critically costly, epidemic of obesity and diabetes. The following policy actions may eventually have traction in preventing obesity in Europe (Gostin 2007).

Public information and disclosure. Inform consumers through easily understood labels on packaged foods, of the risks from added sodium, fat and sugar, such as the traffic-light schemes. Canada and the United States mandate labelling of *trans*-fatty acids on prepackaged foods. Informed consumers are essential if social norms are to change.

Targeting children and adolescents. Studies suggest that advertising can significantly shape the eating habits of children and youth and the purchasing patterns of their parents. Regulating the content of food advertising to prevent misleading messages directed toward young people may protect them from ill-advised lifelong eating patterns.

Taxation of unhealthy food. Some public-health advocates have proposed a "fat tax" as an economic disincentive on highly promoted unhealthy food products.

The WHO recognizes the influence of price on food choices and supports such a fiscal approach. In addition, subsidies or tax policies may be provided by governments to encourage healthy food choices at the agricultural level, institutional food programme level or at the trade level. In Poland and the Czech Republic, changes in food policies were associated, as they were in Finland, with marked reductions in body mass index and subsequent reduced cardiovascular disease burden (McKee and Zatonski 1998).

The built environment. The built environment in many poor communities does not support healthy living, including access to nutritional foods, recreational facilities and safe places for outdoor activity. Governments could use planning laws to limit the invasion of fast-food outlets and provide incentives to stores that sell nutritious and affordable foods.

Food prohibitions. Owing to the scientific evidence linking *trans*-fatty acids to cardiovascular disease, the United States Institute of Medicine concluded that there is no safe consumption level for this food element nor that it provides any benefit to human health (Instutute of Medicine 2005). Denmark was the first country to restrict the percentage of *trans*-fat in foods, and New York City recently restricted artificial *trans*-fat in all restaurants.

Primary prevention is the most important approach to obesity control. In 1998, the European Commission funded a major study, coordinated by the University of Crete, to gather existing evidence on health promotion programmes addressing nutrition, diet and lifestyles and to develop an action plan for European dietary guidelines (European Commission 2000). The study describes population goals for nutrients and lifestyle for the prevention of chronic diseases in Europe (Table 5.2).

This approach to multinational standard setting may have significant implications for health systems, national policy and, ultimately, individual human behaviour. In terms of nutrient intakes, for example, available data indicate that few European nations have diets containing less than 30% of dietary energy from fat, and that only three have intakes of less than 35% dietary energy from fat. Since 1960, cereal consumption has fallen by approximately 25%. Nutrient intakes may be addressed in school programmes, public information campaigns, direct counselling of patients in healthcare settings and other means.

Looking more specifically at the potential contribution of health services in preventing or reducing obesity, screening, counselling and chemoprevention are important, although the cost-effectiveness of these interventions is variable and difficult to determine. Using quality-adjusted life years saved as an endpoint, Cawley (2007) reported a range of costs for primary, secondary and tertiary preventions from US$4305 for school-based interventions to US$35,600 for bariatric surgery (Table 5.3).

Some researchers have pointed out that physical activity and diet are cost-effective for prevention of diabetes (Narayat et al. 2006), but the actual delivery of these types of intervention is highly context specific and requires intensive monitoring and policy backing to assure adherence.

The evidence presented here makes it clear that multiple interventions at the social, health system and individual levels will be necessary simultaneously if the looming obesity and consequent diabetes crises in Europe is to be addressed effectively.

Table 5.2 Population goals for nutrients and features of lifestyle consistent with the prevention of major public health problems in Europe

Component	Population goals	Levels of evidence
Physical activity levels	> 1.75	++
Body mass index	22–22	++
Dietary fat as percentage of energy intake	< 30	++
Fatty acids as percentage total energy		
Saturated	<10	++++
Trans	<2	++
Polyunsaturated fat intake		
n-6	4–8 g	+++
n-3	2 g linoleic acid + 200 mg very long chain acids	++
Carbohydrates as percentage total energy	> 55	+++
Sugary food consumption (occasions per day)	≤ 4	++
Fruit and vegetables (g/day)	> 400	++
Folate from food (µg/day)	> 400	+++
Dietary fibre	> 25 (or 3 g/MJ)	++
Sodium (expressed as sodium chloride) (g/day)	<6	+++
Iodine (µg/day)	150 (infants, 50; pregnancy, 200)	+++
Exclusive breast feeding	Approximately 6 months	+++

Levels of evidence: ++++, multiple double-blind placebo-controlled trials; +++, single study of double-blind analyses (breast feeding: series of non-double-blind analyses); ++, ecological analyses compatible with non-double-blind intervention and physiological studies; +, integration of multiple levels of evidence by expert groups.

Source: European Commission (2000).

Hypertension

Globally, approximately 14% of deaths and 6% of disability-adjusted life years (DALYs) are attributable to hypertension, with a higher proportion (17.6% of deaths and 9.3% of DALYs) in developed countries. Over the long term, damage to the heart and cardiovascular system resulting from uncontrolled hypertension represents a major cause of morbidity and mortality for ischaemic heart disease, stroke and end-stage renal disease. Underlying renal diseases also eventually produce hypertension, which then leads to ischaemic heart disease, the single largest cause of death in developed countries. Hypertension must be considered in the context of multiple cardiac and vascular risk factors, especially hypercholesterolaemia, obesity, smoking and sedentary lifestyle. Therefore, the approach to hypertension must not be singular but should be combined with reduction strategies for other ischaemic heart disease risk factors; this is most effectively addressed through comprehensive programmes at both the population and individual clinical levels. At the individual level, the predicted 10-year

Table 5.3 Cost per quality-adjusted-life-year saved by interventions to reduce or prevent obesity

Intervention	Target population	Estimated cost per QALY (US$)	Source
Planet health (a school-based intervention to improve nutrition and increase physical activity)	Middle-school children	In girls, 4305	Wang et al. (2003)
Orlistat	Overweight and obese patients with type 2 diabetes mellitus	8327	Maetzel et al. (2003)
Bariatric surgery	Middle-aged men and women who are morbidly obese	Women: 5400–16,100 Men: 10,000–35,600	Craig and Tseng (2002)
Diet, exercise, and behaviour modification	Adult women	12,640	Roux et al. (2006)

QALY, quality-adjusted-life-year.

Source: Cawley (2007).

cardiovascular disease risk for someone with blood pressure of 140/90 mmHg can vary from 5 to 50% depending on the number of concomitant risk factors (Jamison et al. 2006). At the population level, clinical trials indicate that a 10 mmHg reduction in systolic blood pressure would result in a 32% reduction in stroke risk and a 14% relative reduction in ischaemic heart disease risk in the general population.

Hypertension interventions

Continuous blood pressure reduction will slow the progression of ischaemic heart disease, stroke and many forms of renal disease in individual patients. The generally agreed threshold for treating hypertension is systolic blood pressure above 140 mmHg, and diastolic blood pressure above 90 mmHg. The distinction between primary and secondary prevention in hypertension is unnecessary from a population health perspective. Patients with a family history, multiple risk factors and no overt history of ischaemic heart disease require treatment, and those with a positive history of ischaemic heart disease, stroke or renal disease need careful attention to reduce their multiple risk factors.

Risk factor reduction programmes for multiple risks include weight loss, healthy diet (high in potassium and low in sodium, low fat, adequate fruit and vegetable consumption), physical activity and moderate alcohol consumption (Chobanian et al. 2003). Although there is clear evidence for the efficacy of antihypertensive (and anticholesterol) medications to reduce ischaemic heart disease outcomes, patient adherence is notoriously problematic. Combinations of education, attentive monitoring based on clinical practice guidelines, and easy-to-use fixed-dose therapies have been shown to improve adherence.

An intriguing pharmacological approach to multiple risk factor reduction proposes use of a "polypill" involving four medications (Wald and Law 2003). This includes a statin to reduce cholesterol, folic acid to reduce arterial plaque formation, low-dose aspirin to prevent platelet adhesiveness and an antihypertensive drug to lower blood pressure. The polypill strategy has been proposed as a population-based intervention to prevent ischaemic heart disease and stroke for all persons aged 55 and older or all those with existing cardiovascular disease. Estimates of ischaemic heart disease and stroke reduction are as high as 80%, and the benefits of a fixed-dose combination medication with proved component effectiveness has generated considerable discussion regarding costs, regulatory approaches and clinical effectiveness (Sleight et al. 2006).

Alcohol abuse

Alcohol-related diseases account for approximately 4% of global DALYs each year, while the figure for eastern Europe is 10.7%. Approximately 75% of this disease burden is chronic illness, including alcohol dependence, vascular disease such as hypertension, hepatic cirrhosis and various cancers. Injuries (particularly road traffic accidents) contribute a substantial portion of the DALYS (25%) (Jamison et al. 2006).

Policies to combat alcohol abuse

Policies on alcohol abuse are, in many cases, analogous to those on tobacco use. Taxing alcohol raises the price and thereby reduces consumption. Advertising bans may reduce the social acceptability of excess drinking. Sales of alcohol may be restricted to limited licensed retail outlets, minimum ages, or limited hours. Strictly enforced drunk-driving laws discourage excessive drinking and prevent traffic accidents. These measures require effective enforcement and laws, including policing, regulatory enforcement on licensing, and education of alcohol sellers to reduce illegal sales to minors or inebriated persons. In limited quantities, alcohol consumption may have some measurable effects on cardiac disease prevention among those with a preexisting risk (which excludes almost all people under the age of 40), but alcohol abuse is a tremendously costly and vexing public health problem.

Clinical treatment of alcoholism includes individual counselling, therapeutic support communities such as Alcoholics Anonymous and family therapy. Alcohol dependence is in part genetically determined but is also related to social factors, mental health, quantities and frequency of consumption, and marketing by the alcohol industry. Multiple policy approaches as well as integration of brief advice, screening and referral within clinical settings may reduce the disease burden caused by alcohol abuse. The clinician has a particular role to play in determining individual risk for alcohol-related medical and psychosocial problems. Non-directive interviewing and counselling have been shown to be effective in identifying and addressing problem drinking prior to the onset of chronic disease consequences (Burge and Schneider 1999).

Sedentary lifestyle

Regular physical activity is a key element in weight control and prevention of obesity (International Agency for Research on Cancer 2002). In addition, regular physical activity reduces the risk of coronary artery disease, stroke, type 2 diabetes, colon and breast cancer, osteoporotic fractures, osteoarthritis and depression. Important health benefits have been associated even with walking for half an hour each day, but greater reductions in risk are seen with longer durations of physical activity and more intense activity. Increasingly, there are less opportunities and motivations in developed nations to engage in sports, physical work or a physically active home life (Koplan and Dietz 1999). Dramatic reductions in physical activity also occur as a result of urbanization, with less access to walking and bicycle riding, and mechanization of labour. This is discussed further below in the section on the built environment.

Interventions promoting physical activity

Physical activity is especially important for the healthy development of children and young people, and physical activity will improve physical well-being and reduce the impact of chronic disease among older people, especially cardiovascular disease and diabetes. Specific advice by health providers on physical activity may improve self-care by providing manageable targets for patients. In Europe, targets for physical activity level (PAL; the ratio of total daily energy expenditure to estimated basal metabolic rate) have been developed as a sort of prescription that may be offered to patients by providers (the target of over 1.75 is 60–80 minutes walking daily to avoid weight gain and 30 minutes per day to prevent cardiovascular diseases and diabetes) (Table 5.2).

Weight-bearing exercises also reduce age-related bone loss and maintain muscular strength. These outcomes, in turn, prevent stumbling and reduce the risk of falls and fractures in the elderly. As noted above, socially disadvantaged populations tend to be less active in their leisure time because they are less able to access programmes and facilities, and they are more likely to live in neighbourhoods suffering from crime and traffic safety concerns, which both create barriers to physical activity.

Opportunities for physical activity need to be created close to where people live. Local governments have a crucial role to play in creating such environments and for programmes encouraging physical activity and active living.

Infectious diseases

Growing evidence is emerging for an aetiological role for several infectious agents, particularly viruses, in human cancer. Prominent among these is hepatitis B virus and human papilloma virus (HPV), offering the potential for prevention of hepatic carcinoma and cervical cancer, respectively, through targeted immunization. A bacterium, *Helicobacter pylori*, which is a cause of stomach cancer, can be easily treated with antibiotics. Other carcinogenic infectious agents include liver flukes, schistosomes, Epstein–Barr virus, herpes simplex, and T-lymphotrophic viruses. Infectious agents causing chronic disease include hepatitis C virus (causing an acute infection and chronic active hepatitis), human immunodeficiency virus (HIV, causing the acquired immunodeficiency syndrome (AIDS), which is now considered a chronic disease in countries where antiretroviral therapy has reduced mortality significantly). Overall, there would be 26.3% fewer cancers in developing countries (1.5 million cases per year) and 7.7% in developed countries (390,000 cases) if these infectious diseases were prevented. The fraction attributable to these infections varies among sites, from 100% of cervix cancers attributable to HPV to a tiny proportion (0.4%) of liver cancers (worldwide) caused by liver flukes (Parkin 2006).

Cervical cancer is the third commonest form of cancer globally. Approximately 45% of women diagnosed with cervical cancer in Europe die prematurely from this disease. Of several risk factors, HPV infection and subsequent failure to detect precancerous lesions by regular Papanicolau tests are the major cause of this disease. The development of an effective vaccine against HPV offers scope to prevent much of this disease in Europe and elsewhere (Arun 2007).

Infectious disease interventions

Current prevention efforts for hepatic cancer and chronic active hepatitis must focus on universal application of hepatitis B vaccine, given to children at birth, in an appropriate schedule during childhood and to household members of infected persons. Hepatitis B vaccine was the first vaccine to prevent a form of cancer.

HPV vaccine to prevent cervical cancer has been approved for use in the United States for girls prior to onset of sexual activity. Routine vaccination with three doses of quadrivalent HPV vaccine is recommended for females 11–12 years of age, but the vaccination series can be started in females as young as 9 years of age (Centers for Disease Control and Prevention 2006) and may be used to catch up until the age of 26. Curiously, the vaccine is not recommended for boys even though HPV is sexually transmitted and has been implicated in penile cancer and anal carcinoma in homosexually active men. Despite the potential to prevent a significant proportion of cervical cancer, there is no plan to reduce the screening regimens for cervical cancer using Papanicolau testing in the United States at least. The approval of the vaccine in Europe allowed it to be incorporated into several national immunization programmes. As of the end of March 2007, Austria, Germany, France and Italy have decided to include the HPV vaccination in their national programmes. Other countries that recommend the use of the vaccine are Belgium, Luxembourg, Norway, Sweden, Switzerland and the United Kingdom (Arun 2007).

Prevention of gastric cancer must focus on the clinical management of patients symptomatic with dyspepsia, stomach ulcer or gastritis. *H. pylori* may infect 50% of adults in developed countries and is a primary cause of gastric cancer. A test (serology for specific IgG using enzyme-linked immunosorbent assay) and treat strategy is recommended for patients with undifferentiated dyspepsia who have not undergone endoscopy. Endoscopy is reserved for use in patients with symptoms suggesting ulcer complications or cancer, or those who do not respond to treatment. Treatment involves a multidrug regimen including antibiotics and acid suppressants for 10–14 days plus education about avoidance of other ulcer-causing factors (such as smoking, acidic foods, stress) and close follow-up (Meurer and Bower 2002).

Distal influences on chronic disease risk factors

Poverty and social inequalities

Poverty and social inequalities may be the most important determinants of poor health worldwide, and poverty itself may also be an independent determinant of many risk factors for chronic disease. For example, tobacco use and alcohol abuse are much more common among persons of lower socioeconomic status. However, in the well-known Whitehall cohort studies of civil servants in the United Kingdom, confirmed by the Multiple Risk Factor Intervention Trial (MRFIT) study in the United States, only about one-quarter to one-third of the difference in mortality rates between rich and poor can be explained by differences in risk factors such as smoking, obesity, low physical activity, hypertension and high blood cholesterol (McCally et al. 1998).

Demographic changes

Demographic changes in Europe may have a considerable impact on current and future chronic disease burdens and subsequently on opportunities for prevention (Chapter 2). Primary demographic determinants include population ageing, reduced fertility, increasing urbanization and continued economic growth. Additionally, in the European region, the overall population is expected to decline over the next decade or so, owing to declines in fertility, unless there is a substantial increase in immigration. This has implications for dependency ratios as populations are also ageing, leading to increased requirements for chronic care resources, additional care needs of the elderly being provided by a dwindling younger population, and increased demands on health systems from chronic diseases.

Globalization

Globalization is a term with multiple meanings, but generally it encompasses the way nations, businesses and people are more interconnected and interdependent across national boundaries through increased economic integration, communication, travel and cultural diffusion (Labonte and Schrecker 2006). Globalization begets ethical concerns, given that there are information asymmetries between populations and that social justice issues arise in the provision of services and protection against harms (Novotny et al. 2006). As the spread of infectious diseases across borders has created awareness about some aspects of health security, there is need for sovereign nations to address other global health threats with equal consciousness. These include tobacco use, obesity, sedentary lifestyle and other risk factors for chronic disease that could be addressed through the beneficial aspects of globalization (i.e. multinational cooperation and standards, healthy trade policy and international communication systems).

The environment

Participation in physical activity is not only through sport or organized activity but is influenced by the built, natural and social environments in which people live. Urban design may permit access to environments that can be either an encouragement or a barrier to physical activity and active living. Collective social norms also influence greatly the participation in physical activity. In an analysis of built environment clusters, Nelson et al. (2006) found that aggregate indices of socioeconomic status are not the only issue of importance in explaining low levels of physical activity. They also found that race/ethnicity, crime, types of road, street walkability and the presence of recreational facilities were also important factors. There is no single approach that addresses these factors. Meaningful combinations of approaches, supported by urban planning theory and empirical evidence on the complexity and origins of neighbourhood, are needed.

Physical activity is an essential component of any strategy that aims to address the problems of sedentary living and obesity among children and adults. Active living contributes to individual physical and mental health but also to social cohesion and community well-being. People are more active when they can easily access key facilities such as parks, green spaces, workplaces and shops. Other barriers to active living include fears about crime and road safety, transport emissions and pollution, problems with access and/or a lack of recreational facilities, and negative attitudes to physical activity.

The role of the private sector in chronic disease prevention

The private sector should be a key partner in chronic disease prevention. For one thing, private employers suffer economically when employees experience prolonged absences or are limited in job performance by chronic illness (see also Chapter 3). Therefore, there is both a rationale for worksite-based health risk reduction and a larger responsibility for the private sector to contribute to population-based chronic disease prevention. The population from which the private sector derives both employees and customers would be better off without preventable disabilities caused by chronic disease. Prevention efforts by companies and industries could have a potentially far-reaching effect on consumers and communities (Oxford Health Alliance Newsletter 2006).

With respect to environmental design for prevention of ill health, designers, architects and urban planners can assist in creating an environment in which the healthy choices are the easy choices. Commercial design linked to the common good would make for good business practice and would show concern for public health.

Private–public partnerships, by virtue of their potential global reach, could be formed by a number of different partners from academia, government, the food industry, non-governmental organizations and the pharmaceutical industry. Such alliances might have a profound effect in mobilizing resources, getting the attention of policy makers and "branding" the prevention approach to chronic diseases. The private sector has the potential to expand the reach of prevention efforts through marketing and promotion; the Oxford Health Alliance (2006) is one current attempt to combine forces among disparate partners in the pursuit of chronic disease prevention.

The role of health services and health systems in preventing chronic disease

Interventions to combat the increase in the prevalence of chronic diseases, as well as the risk factors for these diseases, can occur at the individual, community and societal levels, supported by government policy and health system interventions. In most European nations, the budget for health promotion programmes is less than 1% of the total health budget (European Commission 2000), and yet there is ample evidence for the effectiveness of health promotion and education programmes (European Commission 1990), with many of these interacting with healthcare policies. Although the Disease Control Priorities Project (2007) identified several chronic disease interventions as cost-effective (see above), governments have, in general, not yet resonated with the need for prevention of chronic diseases on a programmatic level. The reasons for this relatively weak response are manifold.

- Many chronic conditions are related to lifestyle, and, consequently, there are residual public sentiments that these result from personal choices and are not under the influence of government.
- Prevention programmes need to be multisectoral and so require leadership at all levels of government to ensure policy integration of prevention programmes across various sectors. For this to occur, a broad vision of prevention needs to be adopted by unfamiliar government participants.
- Vested interests oppose many government prevention programmes. The tobacco industry is the strongest case in point. With responsibility to its shareholders to sell cigarettes, there is significant political interference and influence exercised against effective tobacco-control programmes at multiple governmental levels. In addition, fast-food and junk food enterprises often use similar tactics to support free choice by consumers to purchase unhealthy foods. These actions require advocacy groups to alert the public to their existence, support sensible prevention programmes within government and engage prevention within the private sector as well.
- It is difficult to assess the effectiveness of individual prevention programmes

as isolated initiatives. There is an understandable need for accountability in government public health programmes, but prevention is difficult to separate into measurable individual components. Often, a multiplicity of interventions is required to achieve results. Too often, prevention programmes are subjected to short-term, limited and segmented evaluations that may not show significant results. These programmes need to be evaluated in the context of comprehensive approaches involving multiple, integrated channels of action.

Programmes to prevent and manage chronic diseases in the United Kingdom, Canada and elsewhere emphasize integrated approaches, with clinical care systems being explicitly seen as an integral part of a broader systems approach to addressing chronic disease, involving public health and health promotion efforts that are linked to disease management and support for self-care. Health services form a key component of prevention, and various guidelines have been developed to assist health service providers in addressing prevention systematically.

Specific preventive activities taken by health service provider systems include screening, counselling, immunization and chemoprevention. Screening is the systematic application of a test to identify individuals at risk of a specific disease. The goal is for people who have or have not sought medical attention to benefit from further investigation or direct preventive action. Effectively implemented, medical screening can prevent disability and death and improve quality of life. Screening tests are available for some chronic diseases, including cardiovascular disease, diabetes and several site-specific cancers (Strong et al. 2005). The number of proven screening procedures for chronic diseases is limited (Chapter 2), although evidence for cost-effectiveness supports the following: screening for elevated risk of cardiovascular disease using an overall risk approach; screening for early detection of breast and cervical cancer where there are sufficient resources to provide appropriate treatment; and more targeted screening of persons with suggestive symptoms (e.g. screening for *H. pylori* among persons with dyspepsia).

In 2003, the *European Journal of Cardiovascular Prevention and Rehabilitation* published guidelines on cardiovascular disease prevention (De Backer et al. 2003) (Table 5.4). These are geared toward patients with established cardiovascular disease, asymptomatic individuals with multiple risk factors, individuals with markedly raised levels of single risk factors (elevated blood lipids, blood pressure greater than 180/110 mmHg, diabetes), individuals with close relatives with cardiovascular disease, smokers, and other individuals encountered in routine clinical practice through screening.

Clinicians must develop a therapeutic alliance with the patient to ensure that patients understand the relationship between behaviour, health and disease and can take action with assistance from the health system, whether through behavioural programmes, drug therapy or lifestyle change prescriptions.

Immunizations are critically important in the practice of prevention. These include the careful monitoring of vaccine schedules and indications (such as hepatitis B and HPV as discussed above). Proactive ascertainment of cervical cancer screening status among eligible women, and prevention of exposure to

Table 5.4 Key elements for prevention of chronic diseases in clinical settings

Intervention	Screening	Counselling	Specific interventions
Stop smoking	Ask if patient smokes	Advise to quit, provide behavioural counselling, follow-up	Assist with nicotine replacement or buproprion
Healthy foods	Food history	Fat no more than 30% of total calories	Omega-3 fatty acids, found in fish, low-fat foods, whole grains, fruits and vegetables
Physical activity	Comprehensive clinical judgement, especially for cardiovascular disease	Promote in all age groups;	30 minutes 5 days per week to 60–75% of maximum heart rate
Overweight	Body mass index $\geq 30\,kg/m^2$	Weight reduction through diet and physical activity	Consider chemotherapy and surgery only for morbid obesity
Blood pressure	$>140/90\,mmHg$	Ensuring adherence to therapy, physical exercise, diet, stop smoking	Antihypertensive drug therapy to achieve $<140/90\,mmHg$
Blood lipids	Assess total cardiovascular risk	Strict diet, physical activity, stopping smoking	Statin therapy to lower total cholesterol to $<175\,mg/dl$, and low density lipoprotein cholesterol to $<100\,mg/dl$
Diabetes	Fasting blood glucose $>110\,mg/dl$, haemoglobin A1c $>6.1\%$	Lifestyle: exercise, diet and blood glucose control	Insulin, oral hypoglycaemic drugs
Alcohol abuse	Drinking history, alcohol-related medical problems or alcohol-related family, legal or employment problems	Interventions based on the severity of the alcohol problem and the patient's readiness to change risk behaviour	Non-directive counselling, referral, laboratory testing, family therapy
Other prophylaxis?			The "polypill"?

Source: adapted from De Backer et al. (2003).

second-hand smoke by those sharing households with smokers, may be thought of as analogous to immunization in chronic disease.

However, the realm of health systems in preventing chronic disease goes far beyond the provision of selected clinical services. Clinicians have multiple opportunities for health education and prevention in the office setting, but they also have wider responsibilities for advocacy and support for policy changes that can prevent disease and disability. For example, each contact a smoker has with the health service provider should be a teaching opportunity and a channel through which cost-effective interventions may be applied. Health professionals can provide sustained messages to all smokers who are exposed to the system, through strict non-smoking policies in health facilities and consistent attention by all health providers to support smoking cessation among all patients who seek care. In addition, parents who bring in children for care should be counselled about the need to quit and, if not able to do so, at least not to smoke in the presence of children.

Health systems also have a crucial role in addressing more distal influences on chronic disease, such as social disadvantage, by reducing barriers to and providing incentives for healthier lifestyles; improving access to appropriate, effective preventive health and social services; and participating in population-based approaches to risk factor reduction that address the highest-risk groups (McKee 2002). Clinical preventive services incorporate behavioural, structural and communication functions to reduce risk factors, and in some countries, such as the United Kingdom, the work of primary care teams incorporates risk factor reduction into the health system. Health systems may directly support physical activity programmes in healthcare settings, workplaces, schools and transport systems, and they should participate in partnerships that enhance opportunities for active living.

Space does not permit a complete analysis of potential avenues for advocacy through the health system, but physicians and other health providers have been instrumental in advocating for sound food policy, the reduction of *trans*-fatty acids in commercial food products, the implementation of clean indoor air legislation to prevent exposure to tobacco smoke at the worksite, and improvements in school lunches to address the epidemic of childhood obesity. Much more can be done through partnerships at several levels, but governments are crucial in establishing preventive approaches as part of a state's responsibility. Further, international cooperation among governments is critical in controlling globalized health risks through multinational actions. Food policy, trade policy, advertising policy and information dissemination are all critical multinational approaches. Each nation has a responsibility to work on these issues for the greater global public good.

Conclusions

Prevention of chronic diseases is founded on an integrated approach involving government policy, healthcare systems and preventive practice standards, public information, and individual responsibility for self-care. In the case of tobacco use, substantial evidence is available on effective integrated interventions, but with obesity, the evidence for population or even clinically based approaches remains limited. With cardiovascular diseases occupying first place in the chronic disease burden, there is ample evidence for a multiple risk factor reduction approach at both the population and individual level. Hypertension, hypercholesterolaemia, smoking, obesity and physical inactivity require multiple channels of intervention for optimal effect. The healthcare system is critically important in this respect, as those patients with risks but without established cardiovascular disease, as well as those with early or subclinical chronic disease, can be effectively treated. This will reduce future burdens on the health system as well as on the patient. It is clear, however, that prevention is truly "everyone's business", with government, the private sector, the healthcare system and the individual all having substantial responsibilities to apply scientifically based prevention practices to the growing epidemic of chronic diseases.

References

Arun, A.K. (2007) *HPV Vaccination: Current Status in Europe*. Frost & Sullivan Market Insight. http://www.frost.com/prod/servlet/market-insight-print.pag?docid= 100775178 (accessed 6 July 2007).

Bobak, M., Gilmore, A. and McKee, M. (2006) Changes in smoking prevalence in Russia, 1996–2004, *Tob Control*, 15: 131–5.

Brennan, P. and Bray, I. (2002) Recent trends and future directions for lung cancer mortality in Europe, *Br J Cancer*, 87: 43–8.

Burge, S.K. and Schneider, F.D. (1999) Alcohol-related problems: recognition and intervention, *Am Fam Physician*, 59: 361–70.

Cawley, J. (2007) The cost-effectiveness of programs to prevent or reduce obesity: the state of the literature and a future research agenda, *Arch Pediatr Adolesc Med*, 161: 611–14.

Centers for Disease Control and Prevention (2000) Declines in lung cancer rates: California, 1988–1997, *MMWR*, 49: 1066–9.

Centers for Disease Control and Prevention (2006) General recommendations on immunization: Recommendations of the Advisory Committee on Immunization Practices (ACIP), *MMWR*, 55: 1–48.

Chaloupka, F., Hu, T.W. and Warner, K.E. (2000) The taxation of tobacco products, in P. Jha and F. Chaloupka (eds) *Tobacco Control in Developing Countries*. Oxford: Oxford University Press.

Chobanian, A.V., Bakris, G.L., Black, H.R. et al. (2003) The Seventh Report of the Joint National Committee on Prevention, Detection, Evaluation, and Treatment of High Blood Pressure: the JNC 7 report, *JAMA*, 289: 2560–72.

Craig, B.M. and Tseng, D.S. (2002) Cost-effectiveness of gastric bypass for severe obesity, *Am J Med*, 113: 491–8.

De Backer, G., Ambrosioni, E., Borch-Johnsen, K. et al. (2003) European guidelines on cardiovascular disease prevention in clinical practice: Third Joint Task Force of European and other societies on cardiovascular disease prevention in clinical practice (constituted by representatives of eight societies and by invited experts), *Eur J Cardiovasc Prev Rehabil*, 10: S1–S10.

Department of Health and Human Services (2004) *The Health Consequences of Smoking: A Report of the Surgeon General*. Atlanta, GA: US Department of Health and Human Services, Centers for Disease Control and Prevention, National Center for Chronic Disease Prevention and Health Promotion, Office on Smoking and Health.

Department of Health and Human Services (2006) *The Health Consequences of Involuntary*

Exposure to Tobacco Smoke: A report of the Surgeon General. Atlanta, GA: US Department of Health and Human Services, Centers for Disease Control and Prevention, National Center for Chronic Disease Prevention and Health Promotion, Office on Smoking and Health.

Disease Control Priorities Project (2007) *Cost-effective interventions*. Washington: Disease Control Priorities Project. http://www.dcp2.org/page/main/BrowseInterventions.html (accessed 3 September 2007).

European Commission (1990) *International Union for Health Promotion and Education. The Evidence of Health Promotion Effectiveness: Shaping Public Health in a New Europe*. Brussels: European Commission.

European Commission (2000) *EURODIET Core Report*. Heraklion, Crete: European Commission and the University of Crete School of Medicine.

Ezzati, M., Lopez, A.D., Rogers, A. and Murray, C.J. L. (2004) *Comparative Quantification of Health Risks*. Geneva: World Health Organization.

Fichtenberg, C.M. and Glantz, S.A. (2000) Association of the California tobacco control program with declines in cigarette consumption and mortality from heart disease, *N Engl J Med*, 343: 1772–7.

Gostin, L.O. (2007) Law as a tool to facilitate healthier lifestyles and prevent obesity, *JAMA*, 297: 87–90.

Hill, A.B. (1965) The environment and disease: association or causation? *Proc R Soc Med*, 58: 295–300.

Insitute of Medicine (2005) Dietary reference intakes for energy, carbohydrates, fiber, fat, fatty acids, cholesterol, protein and amino acids (micronutrients). Washington DC: The National Academies Press.

International Agency for Research on Cancer (2002) *Weight Control and Physical Activity*. Lyon, France: IARC Press.

International Obesity Task Force (2003) *Waiting for a Green Light for Health? Europe at the Crossroads for Diet and Disease. IOTF Position Paper*. London: International Obesity Task Force.

Jacobs, R., Gale, H.F. and Capehart, T.C. (2000) The supply-side effects of tobacco-control policies, in P. Jha and F. Chaloupka (eds) *Tobacco Control in Developing Countries*. Oxford: Oxford University Press.

James, W., Jackson-Leach, R., Mhurchu, C. et al. (2004) Overweight and obesity (high body mass index), in M. Ezzati, A.D. Lopez, A. Rogers and C.J. L. Murray (eds) *Comparative Quantification of Health Risks*. [CD] Geneva: World Health Organization.

Jamison, D.T., Breman, J.G., Measham, A.R. et al. (2006) *Disease Control Priorities in Developing Countries*. New York: Oxford University Press and World Bank.

Jha, P. and Chaloupka, F. (2000) *Tobacco Control in Developing Countries*. Oxford: Oxford University Press.

Kenkel, D. and Chen, L. (2000) Consumer information and tobacco use, in P. Jha and F.J. Chaloupka (eds) *Tobacco Control in Developing Countries*. Oxford: Oxford University Press.

Koplan, J.P. and Dietz, W.H. (1999) Caloric imbalance and public health policy, *JAMA*, 282: 1579–81.

Labonte, R. and Schrecker, T. (2006) *Globalization and Social Determinants of Health: Analytic and Strategic Review Paper*. Ottawa: University of Ottawa Institute of Population Health.

Levintova, M. and Novotny, T. (2004) Non-communicable disease mortality in the Russian Federation: from legislation to policy, *Bull WHO* 82: 875–80.

Lopez, A.D., Mathers, C.D., Ezzati, M., Jamison, D.T. and Murray, C., J L (2006) *Global Burden of Disease and Risk Factors*. New York: Oxford University Press and World Bank. Technical material at http://www.dcp2.org/pubs/GBD.

Maetzel, A., Ruof, J., Covington, M. and Wolf, A. (2003) Economic evaluation of orlistat in overweight and obese patients with type 2 diabetes mellitus, *Pharmacoeconomics*, 21: 501–12.

Marmot, M. and Wilkinson, R. (2006) *Social Determinants of Health*, 2nd edn, p. 376 Oxford: Oxford University Press.

Mathers, C.D., Stein, C., Ma Fat, M. et al. (2002) *The Global Burden of Disease 2000 Study*, Version 2: *Methods and Results. Discussion Paper* No. 50. Geneva: World Health Organization. http://www.who.int/healthinfo/discussionpapers/en/index.html (accessed 25 January 2007).

McCally, M., Haines, A. and Fein, O. (1998) Poverty and ill health: Physicians can, and should, make a difference, *Ann Int Med*, 129: 726–33.

McKee, M. (2002) What can health services contribute to the reduction of inequalities in health? *Scand J Publ Health*, 30: 54–8.

McKee, M. and Zatonski, W. (1998) How the cardiovascular burden of illness is changing in eastern Europe, *Evidence-based Cardiovasc Med*, June: 39–41.

Merriman, N.D., Yurekli, A. and Chaloupka, F. (2000) How big is the worldwide cigarette smuggling problem? in P. Jha and F.J. Chaloupka (eds) *Tobacco Control in Developing Countries*. Oxford: Oxford University Press.

Meurer, L.N. and Bower, D.J. (2002) Management of *Helicobacter pylori* infection, *Am Fam Physician*, 65: 1327–36.

Narayat, V.K. M., Zhang, P. and Kanaya, A.M. (2006) Diabetes: the pandemic and potential solutions, in D.T. Jamison, J.G. Breman, A.R. Measham et al. (eds) *Disease Control Priorities in Developing Countries*, 2nd edn, pp. 591–604. New York: Oxford University Press and World Bank.

Nelson, M.C., Gordon-Larsen, P., Song, Y. and Popkin, B.M. (2006) Built and social environments-Associations with adolescent overweight and activity, *Am J Prev Med*, 31: 109–17.

Novotny, T.E., Cohen, J. and Yurekli, A. (2000) Smoking cessation and nicotine-replacement therapies, in P. Jha and F. Chaloupka (eds) *Tobacco Control in Developing Countries*. Oxford: Oxford University Press.

Novotny, T.E., Mordini, E. and Chadwick, R. (2006) Bioethical implications of globalization: an international consortium project of the European Commission, *PLoS Med*, 3: e43.

Oxford Health Alliance (2006) *Oxford Health Alliance Newsletter*, Issue 1(April). Oxford: Oxford Health Alliance. www.oxha.org.

Parkin, D.M. (2006) The global health burden of infection-associated cancers in the year 2002, *Int J Cancer*, 118: 3030–44.

Peto, R., Darby, S., Deo, H. et al. (2000) Smoking, smoking cessation, and lung cancer in the UK since 1950: combination of national statistics with two case-control studies, *BMJ*, 321: 323–9.

Roux, L., Kuntz, K.M., Donaldson, C. and Goldie, S.J. (2006) Economic evaluation of weight loss interventions in overweight and obese women, *Obesity* (Silver Spring), 14: 1093–106.

Saffer, H. and Chaloupka, F. (2000) Tobacco advertising: economic theory and international evidence, *J Health Econ*, 19: 1117–37.

Sankila, R. (2003) Epidemiology of tobacco related cancers in Finland, *Finn Med J* 58: 2965–7.

Siegel, M., Mowery, P.D., Pechacek, T.P. et al. (2000) Trends in adult cigarette smoking in California compared with the rest of the United States, 1978–1994, *Am J Public Health*, 90: 372–9.

Sleight, P., Pouleur, H. and Zannad, F. (2006) Benefits, challenges, and registerability of the polypill, *Eur Heart J*, 27: 1651–6.

Strong, K., Wald, N., Miller, A. and Alwan, A. (2005) Current concepts in screening for noncommunicable disease: World Health Organization Consultation Group Report on methodology of noncommunicable disease screening, *J Med Screen*, 12: 12–19.

Tuomilehto, J., Geboers, J., Salonen, J.T. et al. (1986) Decline in cardiovascular mortality in North Karelia and other parts of Finland, *BMJ*, 293: 1068–71.

Wald, N.J. and Law, M.R. (2003) A strategy to reduce cardiovascular disease by more than 80%, *BMJ*, 326: 1419.

Wang, L.Y., Yang, Q., Lowry, R. and Wechsler, H. (2003) Economic analysis of a school-based obesity prevention program, *Obes Res*, 11: 1313–24.

WHO (2003) *Obesity and Overweight*. Geneva: World Health Organization.

Woolery, T.S., Asma, S. and Sharp, D. (2000) Clean indoor-air laws and youth access, in P. Jha and F. Chaloupka (eds) *Tobacco Control in Developing Countries*. Oxford: Oxford University Press.

chapter SİX

Supporting self-management

Mieke Rijken, Martyn Jones, Monique Heijmans and Anna Dixon

Introduction

Chronic conditions, such as diabetes mellitus, stroke and cardiovascular disease, have a significant impact on both the mental and the physical health of individuals (Mackay and Mensah 2004). The increase in the prevalence of chronic conditions represents a growing challenge to healthcare systems worldwide (Singh 2005). Some health systems have adopted a system-wide approach based on a framework such as the Chronic Care Model (Wagner et al. 2001) (Chapter 4) while others focus on specific elements of care or target people who are intensive users of services or at greatest risk of hospitalization (Singh 2005). Given the long-term nature of these conditions, governments and health service providers are engaged in initiatives to develop new ways of supporting people living with chronic conditions to manage their own health. There is increasing recognition that reduced risk and improved outcomes cannot depend solely on the actions of health professionals but are also contingent on the individual's own actions. Support for people to self-care is, therefore, a vital element of any policy to tackle the rising tide of chronic disease.

This chapter will clarify the definitions of terms such as self-care, self-management and self-management support and will detail the theoretical approaches that underpin many self-management support interventions. The nature and effectiveness of self-management support in chronic disease will be analysed critically, highlighting the challenges of providing such support to people with multiple conditions, or who experience social deprivation. This analysis will be illustrated with examples from selected countries. Finally, we will identify health system facilitators that are necessary for the implementation of self-management support. As such, this chapter will be of interest to policy makers and providers engaged in the redesign of services to improve the quality of chronic disease management.

Defining self-care, self-management and self-management support

The concept of self-care features prominently in policy documents in many countries, for example the United Kingdom *NHS Plan* (Department of Health 2005) and the Danish strategy for the management of chronic conditions (National Board of Health 2005a, 2005b). Similar policy initiatives in Australia refer to self-management (Walker et al. 2003). The concept of self-management support is also used in most countries (Glasgow et al. 2003). There is a lack of clarity and some overlap in the way these terms have been defined and used in current policy and research since the early 1990s (Bentzen et al. 1989; Dean 1989; Haugh et al. 1991; Meetoo and Temple 2003) (Table 6.1).

Self-care

The WHO defines self-care as, "the activities individuals, families, and communities undertake with the intention of enhancing health, preventing disease, limiting illness, and restoring health" (WHO 1983). The Department of Health (2005) uses a similar but slightly elaborated definition of self-care: "the actions people take for themselves, their children and their families to stay fit and maintain good physical and mental health; meet social and psychological needs; prevent illness or accidents; care for minor ailments and long-term conditions; and maintain health and well-being after an acute illness or discharge from hospital".

These definitions reflect the fact that self-care skills and knowledge stem from lay experience and suggest that self-care is a part of daily living. Some definitions emphasize that self-care involves a partnership between health service users, their carers and health professionals (NHS Scotland 2005), others suggest self-care activities may exclude healthcare professionals (Eales and Stewart 2001). Self-care can include a broad range of activities ranging from doing nothing in a particular situation (Haugh et al. 1991), or taking painkillers for a headache, to a patient developing expertise in managing a long-term condition (NHS Scotland 2005). Self-care may include behaviour and actions taken by those who are healthy, at risk of ill health, experiencing symptoms, diagnosed with an illness or receiving treatment. Thus, it encompasses specific types of self-care such as self-diagnosis, self-management, self-medication and self-monitoring.

Self-management

The term self-management was first used by Creer in the mid 1960s to denote the active participation of patients in their treatment (Koch et al. 2004). The aim of self-management is to minimize the impact of chronic disease on physical health status and functioning, and to enable people to cope with the psychological effects of the illness (Lorig and Holman 1993). Self-management is described as a collaborative activity between patient and healthcare practitioner

Table 6.1 Key characteristics of self-care, self-management and self-management support for chronic conditions

	Who is involved	Goals or targets	What is involved
Self-care	Broad spectrum: Ranges from the individual person or patient to families and communities in collaboration with healthcare professionals and healthcare systems; Healthcare professionals need not be involved	Optional Prevention of disease and accidents, limitation of illness and restoration of health Improvement in the existing state of health, which may be associated with a chronic condition Changes in lifestyle, maintenance of optimal levels of health Recovery from minor ailments and following discharge from hospital	May include doing nothing Taking responsibility for health for self, children, family and helping others Asserting control Managing emotion Goal attainment and behavioural change (Hobbs et al. 1999)
Self-management	More focused networks Patients, peers, healthcare practitioners and support networks Includes healthcare professional as collaborator with the person with the chronic condition	Desirable prerequisite Minimization of the impact of chronic disease on physical health status and functioning; coping with the psychological effect of the illness Minimization of pain; patient participating in decision making about treatment, gaining a sense of control over their lives Initiation or maintenance of access to health services and practitioners Targeting change in behaviour, existing and new	Active participation by person/patient Symptom management (Barlow et al. 2002) Generic versus illness-specific behavioural tasks Individual versus group tasks Medical and role management Self-regulation/self-monitoring Lifestyle change and education

Self-management support	More focused and complex networks: patients, practitioners and the healthcare system	Essential prerequisite	Emphasizes collaboration between patient, healthcare practitioner and healthcare system, in standardized, programmatic interventions to improve self-management behaviour
	May require a refocus of health practitioner activity	Service development and chronic disease management improvement, including the provision of self-management support, decision support, delivery system redesign, and clinical information systems	Generic programmes, include the Chronic Disease Self Management Program Chronic Care Model; Expert Patient Programme
		Development of new skills in practitioners (e.g. problem solving and goal setting), with the patient as a key resource	Disease-specific applications are seen in e.g. diabetes and heart failure
		Patient empowerment, activation and education	
		Increasing self-management skills	
		Cognitive symptom management, positive changes in health behaviour, self-efficacy, health status, and number of hospitalizations	

(Lorig 1993). Self-management activities are usually undertaken by the patient between planned contacts with healthcare practitioners and services. These activities involve managing symptoms, treating the condition, coping with the physical and psychosocial consequences inherent in living with a chronic condition and making lifestyle changes (Glasgow et al. 2003). At-home management tasks and strategies are undertaken with the collaboration and guidance of the individual's physician and other healthcare providers (Clark et al. 1991). As such, self-management is not regarded as an option but rather as an inevitable series of activities that should be an integral part of primary care (Glasgow et al. 2003).

Self-management support

Self-management support involves a patient-centred collaborative approach to care to promote patient activation, education and empowerment (Goldstein 2004). Self-management support expands the role of healthcare professionals from delivering information and traditional patient education to include helping patients build confidence and make choices that lead to improved self-management and better outcomes (Coleman and Newton 2005). Self-management support is a key feature of the Chronic Care Model, which emphasizes the centrality of an informed, activated patient to productive patient–provider interactions (Glasgow et al. 2002).

Self-management support includes patient education, the collaborative use of a wide range of behavioural-change techniques to foster lifestyle change, the adoption of health-promoting behaviours and skill development across a range of chronic conditions (Farrell et al. 2004). Patients are trained in problem solving, goal setting, and the use of evidence-based standardized interventions in chronic conditions such as diabetes (Coster et al. 2000; Balas et al. 2004), heart failure (Ara 2004), hypertension (Khan et al. 2005) and angina (McGillion et al. 2004). Collaborative care planning is an important way in which individual providers can support self-management. A collaborative care plan not only focuses on the medical management of the condition but also facilitates role management, negotiation of behaviour change necessitated by the chronic disease, and management of the emotional impact of living with a chronic disease (Fuller et al. 2004).

Self-management support may be delivered through standardized, programmatic interventions. Programmes generally target the way the person with the chronic condition thinks or represents his or her illness. They include a range of cognitive–behavioural interventions, with the goals of such programmes directed at self-efficacy beliefs, health behaviour, health status and reducing the number of unplanned hospitalizations (Dongbo et al. 2003). The aim of self-management support programmes is to prepare patients to engage with medical management, to maintain life roles and to manage negative emotions such as fear and depression by offering patients the opportunity to acquire the necessary knowledge, skills and confidence (self-efficacy) to deal with disease-related problems. In this way they seek to improve the quality of chronic disease management (Goldberg et al. 2003, 2004).

The theoretical basis of self-management support

Most self-management support provided to people with chronic conditions aims to influence their behaviour in some way. People living with one or more chronic diseases are expected to undertake a variety of activities to manage their condition and may need to modify their behaviour in order to minimize the impact of the illness and to prevent further deterioration. For example, they may need new skills or knowledge to use aids and devices, to manage symptoms and pain, to take medications as directed or to cope with the limitations of their illness. They may be advised to take more regular exercise, control their weight, modify their diet, give up smoking or reduce their alcohol intake. Many self-management support interventions are based on one or more theories of human behaviour. For example, techniques such as motivational interviewing and brief negotiation explicitly claim to draw on theories such as self-perception theory (people are more powerfully influenced by what they hear themselves say than by what others say) and decisional balance theory (decision making can be facilitated by weighing the advantages and disadvantages of a certain issue) (Kaiser Permanente 2005).

Table 6.2 summarizes some of the key behavioural theories and gives examples of relevant self-management support interventions. These theories are not mutually exclusive and many theories adopted and adapted earlier ideas. They provide different ways of thinking about what motivates behaviour change. An appreciation of the basic ideas behind theories of human behaviour is useful to understand both the appropriateness and the likely effectiveness of self-management support.

Rational choice theory

Theories of decision making that derive from utility theories date back to the work of Jeremy Bentham (1748–1832) and John Stuart Mill (1806–1876), and are used widely in economics and political science. They assume that individuals seek to maximize their welfare when taking action or making decisions. Rational decision making assumes that, when faced with a number of alternatives, people choose an action in line with stable preferences by weighing the expected costs and benefits. In the case of health behaviours, rational choice suggests individuals will only change their behaviour or adopt new behaviours where they perceive that the value of doing so outweighs the costs. If people are not fully informed about the outcomes of a particular behaviour or action, this might present a significant barrier to effective self-management. Therefore, educational interventions that seek to increase knowledge about a person's condition, available treatment options and preventive and management strategies are an important element of self-management support. Nevertheless, knowledge about the impact of behaviours does not necessarily lead to behaviour change. Strategies such as increasing the costs of risky behaviours, for example by taxing cigarettes, or subsidizing the costs of beneficial behaviours, as with vouchers for gym membership, are also used to modify behaviour. Evidence suggests that economic incentives are effective

Table 6.2 Overview of behavioural theories and related self-management support interventions

Behavioural theory	Underlying concept	Related self-management support interventions	Key texts
Rational choice theory	Humans seek to maximize their welfare within constraints and make decisions in line with stable preferences after weighing the expected costs and benefits of an action.	Information leaflets, educational interventions, financial incentives, patient decision aids	Mill and Bentham (1987); Hargreaves et al. (1992)
Theory of reasoned action, theory of planned behaviour attitude/social influence/self-efficacy model (ASE model)	Behavioural intention is the main determinant of human behaviour	Peer modelling, peer support	Fishbein and Aizen (1975); Aizen and Fishbein (1980); De Vries et al. (1988)
Self-regulation	The beliefs of individuals are important factors in how different people respond to their health and illness	Symptom awareness, self-monitoring, diaries	Leventhal et al. (1980, 1984)
Trans-theoretical model of change	Motivation and attitudes are important factors in behaviour change	Stages of change, social marketing	Prochaska and DiClemente (1983)
Social cognitive or social learning theory	Behaviour is influenced by outcome expectations, observational learning and self-efficacy expectations	Social marketing, peer modelling, goal setting and planning, self-belief/confidence building	Bandura (1977, 1997)
Stress-coping framework	People develop coping mechanisms in response to recurrent stressful situations that pose serious challenges to adaptation	Teach adaptive coping strategies, support groups, cognitive–behavioural therapy, education groups	Lazarus and Folkman (1984)
Self-determination theory	Three psychological needs must be met in order to motivate people to reach a particular health behaviour goal: autonomy, competence and relatedness to others	Collaborative care planning, personal goal setting, skill training	Deci and Ryan (1985)

in simple preventive care and for distinct, well-defined behavioural goals. There is less evidence that financial incentives can sustain long-term lifestyle changes (Kane et al. 2004). The rational approach to decision making has been criticized from a number of perspectives: there are limits on our ability to appraise all options rationally (Simon 1957), people use mental shortcuts to make decisions (Tversky and Kahneman 1974) and preferences are often unstable and can be shaped by the way in which information is presented (Lichtenstein and Slovic 2006).

Theory of planned behaviour

According to the theory of planned behaviour, behavioural intentions are determined largely by attitude (beliefs and evaluation of the outcomes), subjective norms (i.e. perceived social pressure) (Fishbein and Ajzen 1975; Ajzen and Fishbein 1980). A similar model, referred to as the attitude/social influence/self-efficacy (ASE) model, is an extension of the original theory but includes self-efficacy as a third component (De Vries et al. 1988). Interventions built on this model focus not only on influencing people's attitudes to the behaviour and their perception of the outcomes (i.e. is it worth it?) but also on external influences on behaviour (i.e. is this the right or acceptable thing to do?) and whether people are confident to take action (i.e. can I do it?).

Self-regulation model

An individual's beliefs about symptoms, the causes and prognosis of the illness and the possibilities for control are known as illness representations. Research since the 1970s has demonstrated the importance of illness representations to patient behaviour (Petrie and Weinman 1997). They have been linked to health-related outcomes such as depression and quality of life (Leventhal et al. 1980, 1984). Situational stimuli (such as symptoms) generate both cognitive and emotional representations of the illness; people adopt behaviours to cope with them and then appraise the efficacy of these behaviours. Changing patients' illness representations has been shown to improve recovery following myocardial infarction (Petrie et al. 2002) and patient outcomes for conditions as diverse as diabetes and the acquired immunodeficiency syndrome (AIDS) (Petrie and Broadbent 2003).

Trans-theoretical model of change

The trans-theoretical or transactional model focuses on the motivation or intention to change (Prochaska and DiClemente 1983). It identifies a series of motivational steps that have to be taken in order to change behaviour: precontemplation, contemplation, action, maintenance and relapse. The "stages of change" theory of human behaviour has been applied widely in health education and promotion, for example smoking cessation, condom use, weight loss, alcohol abuse, drug abuse and stress management.

The stages of change have also been applied to self-management and in this context "refer to a fixed sequence of psychological and behavioural states that patients move through from lacking the motivation to adopt new self-management behaviours in the beginning to having integrated the new behaviour in their life at the end" (Dijkstra 2005). Researchers have tried to classify people with chronic conditions according to the stages of change. The idea is that patients in different stages benefit from different types of self-management support. Such an approach to classifying theoretically derived stages may, however, oversimplify the reality.

Social cognitive or social learning theory

Bandura's (1977, 1997) social learning theory postulates that behaviour is influenced by outcome expectations (beliefs about the effectiveness of the behaviour, for example the advantages and disadvantages of an action), observational learning (social influences including social norms, social support or pressure, and the behaviours of others, also called modelling) and self-efficacy expectations (beliefs about the individual's ability to perform a particular behaviour or to change a specific cognitive state successfully regardless of circumstances or contexts). Improving the self-efficacy beliefs of patients is a key element of many self-management support interventions (Lorig et al. 2001). Use of peer modelling (i.e. using other patients as role models) and peer support are approaches grounded in this theory.

There is considerable evidence that self-efficacy plays an important role in the likelihood of adopting and maintaining health behaviour changes and is associated with improved affect, heightened motivation, better function, treatment adherence and improved clinical and social outcomes (Marks et al. 2005a, 2005b).

Stress-coping model

A chronic illness is seen as a major life event, characterized by a number of recurrent stressful situations that pose serious challenges to adaptation (Moos and Schaeffer 1984; Zautra 1996). People with chronic conditions face a range of stressors. For example, those with diabetes might have to adhere to a complex dietary regimen and perform self-management tasks on a daily basis. Patients with arthritis have to deal with pain, disfigurement, loss of functional ability and periods of remission. Their ability to cope with these stressors influences how well they can maintain adequate levels of physical, social and emotional functioning. Interventions based on the stress-coping model emphasize coping strategies and teach patients adaptive coping strategies. Many interventions try to improve coping by enhancing social support and personal coping resources, such as feelings of mastery, self-esteem or self-efficacy. Interventions ranging from cognitive–behavioural therapy and psychotherapy to education and support groups are linked with this theory.

Self-determination theory

Self-determination theory (Deci and Ryan 1985) emphasizes the importance of autonomy. According to this theory, healthcare practitioners must maximize the natural motivation of patients. "Motivation refers to the psychological forces or energies that impel a person towards a specific goal" (Sheldon et al. 2003). A patient's motivation to participate in self-management is predicted by the extent to which healthcare practitioners support autonomy and the extent to which an individual feels him- or herself responsible for initiating and maintaining that behaviour.

Summary of behavioural theories

In summary, understanding the theories that underpin human behaviour is important in order to design and assess interventions that support individuals in managing their condition. Self-management usually requires people to adopt new behaviours. The theories reviewed here suggest that interventions to support people in taking action to improve their health and manage their condition require a range of strategies depending on each person's level of knowledge, his or her illness and health beliefs, his or her attitudes towards the behaviour, the level of confidence, strength of social networks and the level of motivation. The support that is needed will vary for people in different social circumstances (as we shall see below), at different stages in their disease and with different skill levels (e.g. literacy). A wide range of interventions have been developed based on these theories, including those that involve the provision of educational support, financial incentives, peer support groups, motivational interviewing, problem solving, goal setting, action planning and strengthening coping skills. The next section will describe these interventions and summarize the evidence for their effectiveness.

Self-management support programmes: scope and effectiveness

Self-care interventions have been systematically reviewed elsewhere (Coulter and Ellins 2006). Here we provide an overview of self-management support programmes, by which we mean standardized interventions developed for specific target groups (e.g. elderly people, patients with diabetes, parents of children with asthma). As we have seen, self-management requires people with chronic conditions to undertake a variety of demanding tasks. It is, therefore, not surprising that many people with chronic conditions find it difficult to self-manage successfully, and patients may benefit from participating in self-management support programmes that aim to develop the attitudes and skills necessary for successful self-management. Since the early 1990s, there has been a substantial increase in the number of self-management support programmes used internationally, although the approaches vary. Box 6.1 provides selected examples of self-management support programmes.

Box 6.1 Examples of self-management support programmes

Chronic Disease Self-Management Program

The Chronic Disease Self-Management Program (CDSMP) was developed at Stanford University (Lorig et al. 1999, 2001) and comprises a six-week session of workshops, with weekly sessions of two and a half hours that usually take place in community settings such as senior centres, churches, libraries and hospitals. People with different chronic conditions attend together. Workshops are facilitated by two trained leaders, one or both of whom are non-health professionals with a chronic illness themselves.

Subjects covered in the workshop include (1) techniques to deal with generic problems of chronic illness such as frustration, fatigue, pain and isolation; (2) appropriate exercise for maintaining and improving strength, flexibility and endurance; (3) appropriate use of medication; (4) communicating effectively with family, friends and health professionals; (5) nutrition; and (6) ways to evaluate new treatments. Each participant in the workshop receives a copy of the companion book, *Living a Healthy Life with Chronic Conditions*, and an audio relaxation tape, *Time for Healing*.

It has been claimed that the format in which the programme is taught accounts for its effectiveness. Classes are highly participative, where mutual support and success are used to build up the participants' confidence in their abilities to manage their health and maintain activities. CDSMP does not conflict with other interventions or medical treatment of patients. It is designed to enhance regular treatment and disease-specific education. It is especially helpful for patients with multiple chronic conditions and disability, as the programme focuses on the development of skills to coordinate the different tasks necessary to manage health and to keep an active life.

Comprehensive Health Enhancement Support System

The Comprehensive Health Enhancement Support System (CHESS) is an interactive, computer-based system to support people with managing chronic conditions or other health-related crises or concerns (Gustafson et al. 2001). CHESS provides information, referral to service providers, support in making tough decisions and networking with experts and others facing the same concerns. CHESS is designed to improve access to health and human services for people who would otherwise face psychological, social, economic or geographic barriers to receiving services.

The system is accessed from a patient's home via the Internet or software installed on a personal computer. People participating in the CHESS project who do not have a computer are loaned one for up to a year. CHESS has also been installed in community centres, health centres, college dormitories and in the workplace. CHESS is currently being used by several major health organizations in the United States and Canada. CHESS has been successfully trialled with different target groups including the elderly, people with low education and people from minority populations. People have used the facility equally although in different ways.

Target population

The majority of self-management support programmes focus on people with a single disease. Barlow et al. (2002) showed that most interventions are designed to address either asthma or diabetes, or more rarely arthritis and heart disease. A respiratory rehabilitation programme for people with chronic obstructive pulmonary disease developed in Canada aimed to support patients to maintain optimal physical, psychosocial and mental functioning levels (Bourbeau et al. 2003). The programme was shown to reduce the number of admissions to hospitals and visits to the emergency department. It also showed an enhanced use of primary health services and improvement in the patients' quality of life.

Some support programmes are not disease specific but generic in design. These generic programmes address the needs of people with multiple comorbidities or those with chronic disability, often older patients. The Chronic Disease Self Management Program (CDSMP) (Lorig et al. 2001) is probably the best example of such a generic programme (Box 6.1).

Most support programmes target the person with the chronic condition. Carers and family members may accompany the person to one of the sessions but self-management support programmes exclusively designed for carers or family members are rare. Where they do exist, they mainly focus on carers of chronically ill patients who are dependent on intensive home care, for instance those with stroke, dementia or in a terminal phase of their illness. In these programmes, most attention is paid to helping the carer to deal with the emotional aspects of living with and caring for a person in need of intensive care. Few are designed specifically to help partners and other family members to provide positive self-management support to the patient (Clark and Dunbar 2003). The Family Partnership Intervention is an example of a support programme that focuses on developing supportive skills among family members of patients with heart failure (Clark and Dunbar 2003). A major part of this support programme aims to teach family members to use behaviours supportive of autonomy, such as expressing empathy and concern, providing a rationale for self-management, emphasizing the choice a patient has, reducing critical or guilt-provoking language, and helping the patient with problem-solving behaviours. However, further research is needed on the value of support programmes for partners or family members.

The majority of self-management support programmes target adults; few focus on children. There are exceptions, especially in the field of asthma, where several programmes are designed for both children and adults. Many programmes that are offered to children were originally developed for adults and insufficiently account for the developmental stage of the child (Mokkink et al. 2007). Most support programmes are only used in the country where they have been developed and few have been adapted for use in different countries or cultures. An exception is the Arthritis Self Management Program (ASMP), which was developed at Stanford University but has been delivered in a number of countries outside the United States including Denmark, the United Kingdom, the Nether-lands, Australia and Canada (Barlow et al. 2002). The CDSMP has also been adapted for use in the UK (known as the Expert Patient Programme) and Canada (British Columbia and Alberta; known as Live Better Everyday), and the National Board of Health in Denmark has recommended that it should be implemented nationwide following a successful trial (see accompanying volume).

Content

Lorig and Holman (2003) reported that most interventions address medical or behavioural management tasks, whereas a minority also pay attention to role management and/or emotional management. This, however, depends on the disease process involved: support programmes for patients with cancer are more likely to address the emotional aspects of the disease than programmes for patients with asthma, where correct use of medication comes first. Interventions that focus primarily on medication and symptom management are necessarily disease specific. Interventions that include management of psychological con-sequences (e.g. depressed mood), lifestyle (e.g. exercise), social support and communication are usually generic but can also be designed for individual diseases.

Early self-management programmes often lacked a sound theoretical basis or the theoretical principles were not explicit. As noted above, many of the current programmes are based on social learning theory developed by Bandura (1977, 1997) and focus on building self-efficacy or use self-regulation principles. It has been noted that support programmes for patients with diabetes and arthritis are generally more theory based than programmes for patients with asthma, for which interventions are mainly information based and instructional, with only a few incorporating techniques to address barriers to self-management (Newman et al. 2004).

Other characteristics of self-management programmes

Self-management programmes can be group based, developed for the individual or a combination of both. Groups typically have between 6 and 12 participants and often use written materials. Programmes for an individual can range from provision of a manual that participants work through at home to sessions with a health professional on a one-to-one basis in a clinical setting.

Most interventions are administered by health professionals such as medical doctors, psychologists and nurses. For example, in Australia, diabetes self-management education is provided largely by specialist nurses and dieticians through diabetes centres. In Sweden, the majority of self-management support for diabetics is given in nurse-led clinics. The CDSMP in the United States and the Expert Patient Programme in the United Kingdom use lay tutors with chronic conditions who are trained to deliver the intervention. An evaluation of Expert Patient Programme found that the perceived success of the group depended on the facilitation skills of the lay leader (National Primary Care Research and Development Centre 2007).

Most self-management programmes are offered within a clinical setting, such as a hospital or a rehabilitation centre. In some countries, the voluntary sector or patient organizations have traditionally run self-management programmes. For example, in France, diabetes networks have developed patients' guides and newsletters with instructions on foot care, insulin injections, fat intake reduction and exercise (REVESDIAB). In Canada, the provincial health systems are beginning to take a more active role in investing in self-management support programmes, having previously relied on diabetes and cancer associations. Increasingly self-management support programmes are funded as part of the public health system.

Effectiveness

For policy makers and providers, the main question is whether people with chronic conditions benefit from self-management support programmes. The answer is not straightforward. Systematic reviews and meta-analyses suggest that most programmes show positive results, but rarely on all outcome indicators that were measured.

Chodosh et al. (2005) carried out a meta-analysis of 53 randomized controlled trials on self-management interventions focusing on elderly patients with diabetes, hypertension or osteoarthritis and concluded that mostly beneficial effects were found on clinical outcomes such as blood glucose level (diabetic patients) and blood pressure (patients with hypertension), but not on outcomes such as pain and functional status (patients with osteoarthritis) and weight (diabetic patients). An explanation suggested by the authors is that programmes that address medication adherence may be particularly effective.

Two Cochrane reviews have examined the effectiveness of self-management support programmes. The first concerned self-management programmes for adults with asthma (Gibson et al. 2002). The interventions studied provided self-monitoring of symptoms and regular review by clinicians as well as use of written action plans. The authors found evidence that participation in these programmes had beneficial effects on the course of the disease: patients who had joined a self-management support programme had fewer hospital admissions and emergency department or unscheduled medical office visits; they reported fewer night time symptoms and less sickness absence from work or school. The second Cochrane review (Riemsma et al. 2002) focused on the effects of self-management support programmes for patients with rheumatoid arthritis. The interventions consisted of patient education combined with several other approaches, such as psychobehavioural methods, exercise, biofeedback and psychosocial support. There was evidence that the programmes had beneficial effects on functional status, the number of affected joints, self-reported health and overall psychological status, but not on the level of pain, anxiety and depression. The positive effects were found shortly after attending the support programmes; long-term benefits could not be established.

Lorig and Holman (2003) described the results of randomized trials conducted by the Stanford Patient Education Research Center of their own self-management programmes (e.g. CDSMP, ASMP). In general, they found positive effects on the frequency of behaviours such as exercising and symptom management. In all studies on patients with arthritis and back pain, patients experienced a reduction of pain; in most of these studies they also found disability to be reduced. Furthermore, participants reported improved communication with their physicians. In two studies, one with the English version of the ASMP and one with the generic CDSMP, significant reductions in healthcare utilization were also found. A randomized trial to assess effectiveness of the Expert Patient Programme in the United Kingdom found improvements in self-efficacy and energy levels among patients with chronic conditions, with some evidence of a (small) reduction in associated costs (Kennedy et al. 2007).

Barlow et al. (2002) conclude from several randomized clinical trials that self-management support programmes are effective in increasing knowledge, symptom management, use of self-management behaviours and self-efficacy, and promote beneficial medical outcomes.

Based on a systematic review, Coulter and Ellins (2006) concluded that educational programmes that teach practical self-management skills appear to be more effective than information-only patient education. Findings from studies evaluating self-management education were mixed, however, as there was a general association with improvements in knowledge, coping behaviour, adherence, self-efficacy and symptom management. The review found limited evidence for reductions in health service utilization, cost and enhanced quality of life but identified the following factors as being associated with larger effect sizes: longer and higher intensity interventions, regular review with health professionals, focus on specific rather than general educational topics, participative rather than didactic teaching methods, multicomponent approaches and involvement of informal carer or family members.

Methodological considerations

These studies have a number of limitations that need to be acknowledged. First, the follow-up period of the evaluation studies described above is seldom longer than 12 months and mostly shorter than six months, which makes it difficult to draw conclusions about the long-term effects of self-management support programmes. Second, although most support programmes show beneficial results, at least in the short term, none of the above-mentioned studies linked specific components of the programmes to outcomes. Most programmes are multicomponent, but the studies often fail to describe interventions in sufficient detail to allow a thorough understanding of them. This means that we still do not know which approaches, techniques or elements of self-management pro-grammes are most successful and should, therefore, be developed in future. Lorig and Holman (2003) observed that enhanced self-efficacy is one key mech-anism responsible for improvements in health status among those attending self-management programmes. They concluded that self-efficacy should form a key component in future self-management support programmes. Further research on this question is needed in order to prevent programmes being offered that include unnecessary components and so waste time and money.

The comparative effectiveness of generic and disease-specific programmes also needs further evaluation. Clark and Dunbar (2003) contended that support programmes that teach basic problem-solving and self-regulatory skills may be successful for many people irrespective of their specific chronic condition. Such programmes may be promising for people with rare diseases and the many people who have multiple chronic conditions for whom disease-specific support programmes are either not available or are inadequate. Coulter and Ellins (2006) found different results of self-management education with different diseases. Education for people with asthma was found to reduce health service utiliza-tion, with improvements in quality of life and self-efficacy, while education for people with arthritis had only a small and short-term impact on pain and functional disability (Coulter and Ellins 2006).

Only a few studies have analysed the cost-effectiveness of programmes (e.g. Kennedy et al. 2007). Those that have, mostly focused exclusively on the direct costs of the self-management programme, rarely considering the indirect costs to the participant (e.g. time off work or for substitute care, travel expenses etc.). It seems plausible that some interventions will be cheaper than others: peer-led programmes will probably be less expensive than programmes provided by medical personnel, group-based approaches less expensive than providing indi-vidual support, and offering the programme in community buildings less expensive than programmes provided in a clinical setting. These potential dif-ferences in costs have not, however, been systematically assessed.

Responding to the support needs of different patients

Despite the variety of self-management support programmes available, they may not be appropriate for everyone with a chronic condition. Here we identify at least three groups where greater (or different) self-management support may be needed: those with complex needs, those with limited resources and those who are not motivated.

Complex needs

Some groups of patients have particularly complex self-management tasks, such as those with multiple chronic conditions, the frail elderly and patients with severe or various impairments and disabilities (Bayliss et al. 2003; Young 2003; Levine et al. 2006; Suhl and Bonsignore 2006). Such people are usually excluded from participation in standardized interventions that are evaluated by random-ized clinical trials. Moreover, the existing support programmes – especially those that are disease specific – may not be relevant to the specific self-management support needs of patients with multiple comorbidities or chronic disability. Bayliss et al. (2003) reported that patients with multimorbidity often experience "competing demands" arising from their chronic conditions. Fur-thermore, engaging in activities to promote physical or psychological health may be hindered by comorbid conditions. For example, a person who is obese and has diabetes and who is advised to exercise may feel constrained from doing so because of coexisting arthritis. Also, depression or other mental disorders, which are concomitant conditions in many chronically ill people (Verhaak et al. 2005), have been found to impact adversely on self-management performance (e.g. Ciechanowski et al. 2000). Data from the Dutch National Panel of the Chronically Ill and Disabled shows that, in 2005, levels of self-reported inactiv-ity were significantly higher among patients with severe disability compared with people with no/mild disabilities (Table 6.3) (Rijken et al. 2005).

Tailoring of self-management support is in its infancy and so there is no evidence to guide policy makers as to the best approach. However, some inter-ventions appear promising in this respect. Generic self-management support programmes that focus on the development of self-efficacy and problem solving and how to integrate self-management behaviours in daily life may be effec-tive for patients with multiple morbidities or chronic disability. A disability approach (Heijmans et al. 2004), in which the generic disabilities of people with different chronic diseases in the social, emotional or physical area are taken as a starting point for intervention, may also appeal to patients with complex needs. Computer-based decision support tools have been developed that enable

Table 6.3 Level of inactivity among patients with at least one chronic disease by level of physical disability and income, 2005

	No.	*Inactive (%)*
Disability		
None/mild	1102	9
Moderate	450	20
Severe	167	52
Total	1719	
Income (€)		
<850	139	32
850–1450	775	29
1450–1900	435	18
1900–2300	296	18
2300–2700	176	14
2700–3300	184	14
>3300	126	8
Total	2131	

Source: Data of the National Panel of the Chronically ill and Disabled (NPCG, NIVEL), the Netherlands.

telephone-based nursing staff to counsel patients with multiple comorbidities to help them to focus on those self-management activities that evidence suggests will be most effective in bringing their condition under control. For example, a patient with diabetes and ischaemic heart disease will have to combine activities aimed at lipid lowering and glucose control (Mulley 2006). Other work is needed to establish meta-guidelines and information resources that recognize the interdependencies experienced by people with multiple comorbidities. Most existing information and decision support tools are disease specific. Finally, supporting people to manage mental as well as physical conditions will be important. Some providers are considering routine screening for depression and its treatment before embarking on self-management programmes for chronic physical conditions.

Levine et al. (2006) have warned that frailty "is not just the sum of several disease conditions": many frail elderly people do not only suffer from multiple diseases; cognitive impairments and poor mental health often also coexist. They argued that more research is needed to find out which disease management approach best meets the needs of the frail elderly. They predicted that approaches which respond to both the social and medical needs of frail elderly people and their caregivers will be most effective.

Lack of resources

Some people with chronic conditions may have inadequate access to resources to perform successful self-management or to attend support programmes. Although self-management support programmes are designed to develop resources such as knowledge, communication skills, effective coping strategies, social support and self-efficacy, a basic level of these resources is needed to be able to benefit from self-management support: patients need to be informed about the existence of such programmes; they need to speak the same language as the programme leader and other group members; they need to be sufficiently literate to be able to read and understand the accompanying written materials; and they must be able to reach the location and to afford the costs of participation or know how to get reimbursed where relevant. Reaching diverse and disadvantaged groups has been a challenge for CDSMP courses (National Primary Care Research and Development Centre 2007). Patients tend to be especially disadvantaged if they are older, are less educated, are on low incomes or do not have health insurance, have cognitive or intellectual impairments, or belong to an ethnic minority (Glasgow et al. 1997; Becker et al. 2004; Rothman et al. 2004; Suhl and Bonsignore 2006).

A 2005 study from the Netherlands of patients with chronic conditions found that those on lower incomes were significantly more likely to be inactive than those in high-income groups (Table 6.3). Understanding of medication was lower among those with less educational attainment (Table 6.4; Heijmans 2006). Similar examples can be found elsewhere. For instance, Becker et al. (2004), in a qualitative study among African-Americans suffering from chronic illness, found that regular exercise was reported less often by respondents who were uninsured. Those who had some form of health insurance had many more

Table 6.4 Knowledge about medication use in 440 patients with chronic obstructive pulmonary disease by educational level, 2006

Educational level	Mean score (out of 11)	Standard deviation
No education/primary school	3.3	2.6
Lower vocational	4.1	3.2
Intermediate vocational	4.2	2.9
Higher vocational/university	4.6	3.0

P for trend < 0.05.
Source: Data of the National Panel of the Chronically ill and Did (NPCG, NIVEL), the Netherlands.

opportunities to discuss their illness and self-management problems with physicians and other health professionals.

Disadvantaged groups will benefit from basic patient education ("what to do and why") before addressing their skills and confidence to carry out these self-management tasks ("how to do things"). Individual support from a clinician involved in their care could be appropriate, or a group consultation with other patients with the same condition, preferably complemented with written or audiovisual education material in the patient's native language. In some countries, patients are simply not getting access to basic education about their condition. For example only 28% of people with diabetes in Ontario had access to structured education (see accompanying volume).

Once basic patient education and counselling has been provided, ongoing support, involving goal setting and action planning, with regular review and problem solving can help these patients to gain the skills and confidence they need to take on self-management tasks. This could either be provided by a health professional from their care team or health coaches accessed by telephone. Referral to financially and physically accessible community self-management programmes can be considered once the patient feels confident and motivated to attend a support programme (Coleman and Newton 2005).

Lack of motivation

The third group of chronically ill patients who appear not to be served well by existing support programmes are those who lack motivation. Barlow et al. (2002) referred to this group as patients who "may not feel able to embrace the concept of self-management". Since attendance at self-management support programmes is voluntary, participants must be willing to improve their self-management, or at least to think about it seriously (Dijkstra 2005). Patients who are not motivated to adopt healthy behaviours are unlikely to benefit from support programmes that focus on enhancing self-efficacy and formulating personal action plans. These patients generally know "what to do", but not "why". In terms of the trans-theoretical model, these patients find themselves in the precontemplation phase. Barlow et al. (2002) noted that patients "may need support in making the transition from precontemplation to contemplation of making self-management a part of their lives". The patient activation model, developed and validated in the United States, sees such patients as having the lowest level of knowledge, skills and confidence and consequently failing to recognize that they have an active role to play in their health (Hibbard et al. 2005). By identifying which behaviours are realistic for patients at different stages of activation, it is possible to encourage them to take appropriate "next steps" suited to their level of knowledge and skill (Hibbard and Tusler 2007).

Unfortunately, very little is known about how to support patients in making this step. Further research is needed to understand why these patients lack motivation to self-manage and to explore their illness representations, as described earlier in this chapter. When patients consider their condition to be not very serious or do not experience any symptoms, they will feel less motivated to self-manage. Patients may also not believe that they can influence their health or control their disease, either by following medical advice or by self-care. False beliefs about the causes of their illness, its course and consequences, as well as the benefits of adequate self-management may be corrected by interventions that aim to develop autonomous behaviours. This may be by providing information relevant to the patient's personal goals, use of role models appealing to the patient, monitoring and feedback on progress, or creating peer support through "buddying". In addition, healthcare providers may wish to involve partners or other important members of the social network in the self-management process. This can be helpful for all patients but may be essential for patients who lack intrinsic motivation.

While there are many benefits from systematizing the care of people with chronic conditions (Chapter 4), self-management support must be tailored to the needs of the individual. Self-management support interventions need to be developed and evaluated with this in mind. However, further research is needed to understand the barriers to self-management that different patients experience.

In summary, proactive teams will make use of standardized assessments of patients' levels of self-management in different areas, including skills to manage their illness and confidence in minimizing barriers to self-management and gaining access to support. We have suggested that the support people will need might depend on the nature and number of their chronic conditions or their level of disability; their education, age, ethnicity, language, culture and income; their skills, knowledge and confidence to self-manage; and their beliefs, attitudes, readiness to change and motivation. Tools are needed that can be used easily in clinical practice to explore the kinds of self-management problem faced by patients so that appropriate self-management support can be provided.

Building a health system that supports self-management

It is only in recent years that healthcare providers and health insurers have recognized how crucial self-management support is to the achievement of better outcomes. If self-management is critical to good outcomes for patients and there is evidence that interventions can improve patients' ability to self-manage, what does it take to build a system that supports self-management?

Self-management requires a whole system approach. Glasgow et al. (2003) defined self-management support as a "process of making and refining multi-level changes in healthcare systems and the community to facilitate self-management". The healthcare system must give providers incentives to promote self-management (Chapter 9). In a system where providers are rewarded for more activity, they will be keen to see patients frequently, even if this brings little benefit to the patient, and even if it disadvantages them given the cost of travel and lost work. Patients can be trained to undertake much routine monitoring, such as blood pressure, blood glucose levels and peak respiratory flow. Capitation payments covering at least a year of care or outcome-related payments offer incentives to promote self-management. Financial incentives, in particular clinician rewards, are being used in a number of countries to drive changes in how patients with chronic diseases are supported (e.g. contracts for general practitioners in the United Kingdom and the Netherlands, and Pay for Performance within Medicare in the United States). Providers must also be given resources to support self-management. For example, in Ontario there is a commitment in the Physician's Service Agreement 2004 that the Ontario Health Ministry will identify and distribute appropriate self-care material to patients enrolled with a Family Health Team (see accompanying volume).

Physicians require training in how to support patients most effectively. Tattersall (2002) contended that many healthcare professionals feel uncomfortable with the idea of empowering their patients. Active participation of chronically ill patients in the management of their disease depends not only on the willingness and ability of the patients but also on positive attitudes and appropriate skills in their healthcare professionals. Support for self-management requires a fundamental shift in the patient–provider relationship. Encounters may require more time, they may be more educational in content and they will demand new skills from health professionals (Chapter 7). In Australia, following a series of 12 demonstration projects, the government is investing AU$515 million (316 million) over five years in self-management. The majority of resources are going into education about self-management for health professionals, in particular general practitioners (see accompanying volume). In France, in contrast, the legal framework makes substitution and delegation of tasks by doctors difficult and does not encourage educational approaches to self-management support.

Doctors who wish to maintain their professional authority and expect patients to comply with medical advice may undermine other efforts to support patients to self-manage. Endorsement for self-management activities and active referral to self-management programmes by doctors are rare in many countries. The national evaluation of the Expert Patients Programme in the United Kingdom found that professionals had not engaged in the process and few referred people to courses or knew about their content or rationale (National Primary Care Research and Development Centre 2005).

Self-management support should not be confined to efforts of individual healthcare providers. Support for self-management requires extensive coordination. This includes scheduling group visits for patients with comparable chronic conditions, using disease management guidelines as prompts to structure consultations, providing systematic support by regular phone calls (especially by nurses), and generating feedback or reminders by email or text messaging (short message system; Coleman and Newton 2005). Other changes might include giving patients access to non-physician members of the care team, providing alternative contact methods (e.g. telephone, email or drop-in visits (either individual or group)), giving patients access to electronic medical records, preparing patients for the consultation using agenda-setting tools, engaging patients in their care using goal setting and action planning tools, offering opportunities for peer-to-peer mentorship, and designating a care coordinator or advocate (Bergeson and Dean 2006).Where possible, self-management support also should be accessible via the Internet and call centres. An example of this approach is the Internet-based Australian government initiative "HealthInsite", which provides quality information on a range of health topics. Call centres extend this concept. Health First in the Australian Capital Territory provides a comprehensive health website on health and related services, easy access to health information and telephone contact with registered nurses giving health advice 24 hours a day, seven days a week (ACT Government 2007).

Group and community interventions such as weight-loss programmes and walking buddies require little direct support from the health system. However, schemes such as "exercise on prescription", which provide professional endorsement or financial subsidies, may increase take up, particularly among patients who are less engaged or from poorer backgrounds. Providers and insurers may need to promote awareness of community resources and their benefits to both the public and clinicians. More-advanced self-management tasks, for example when a patient monitors and reports clinical indicators associated with his or her condition, may require access to telecare and home monitoring devices. Results can be recorded automatically in the patient's electronic medical record and be available to view via a secure Internet connection, so enabling patients to track their progress over time. This requires investment in information technology and assistive technologies (Chapter 8).

The Chronic Care Model recognizes that self-management and the active relationship between a patient and the provider are embedded within the health system and the wider social environment. Policy makers should ensure that systems, organizations, individual professionals and the community all facilitate the patient to self-manage successfully.

Conclusions

In this chapter, we have focused on self-management as we view this as the most important element of self-care that applies to people with chronic conditions. Self-management requires individuals to take action to change their behaviour. Most individuals will need support in order to be successful in this role. In designing and evaluating self-management support, it is important to draw on our understanding of human behaviour. This brief review shows that there is some evidence that self-management support programmes improve outcomes, but more research is needed to understand which components impact on which outcomes and whether improvements are sustained over the long term. Support programmes vary in their design and content. More tailoring of self-management support is needed to ensure that it meets the needs of different people.

Although self-management support is recognized as an important element of chronic care, few countries seem to be developing or implementing systematic strategies to support this process. Data from a cross-national survey of "sicker adults" in five countries in 2004 found that significantly fewer respondents in the United Kingdom and United States reported that their doctor had given them clear advice on what to do and what symptoms to watch for compared with those in Australia, Canada and New Zealand (Coulter 2006; Davis et al. 2006). Fewer than two out of three respondents in all of these countries reported that the doctor gave them a plan for managing care at home, with as few as 37% reporting this in Germany (Coulter 2006). It is vital that health policy makers, insurers and providers create systems that enable all patients to self-manage effectively.

References

ACT Government (2007) *Welcome to Health First*. Canberra: ACT Government. http://www.healthfirst.net.au/providersearch.ser (accessed 5 January 2007).

Ajzen, I. and Fishbein, M. (1980) *Understanding Attitudes and Predicting Social Behaviour*. Englewood Cliffs, NJ: Prentice Hall.

Ara, S. (2004) A literature review of cardiovascular disease management programs in managed care populations, *J Manag Care Pharm*, 10: 326–44.

Balas, E.A., Krishna, S., Kretschmer, R.A. et al. (2004) Computerized knowledge management in diabetes care, *Med Care*, 42: 610–21.

Bandura, A. (1977) *Social Learning Theory*. Englewood Cliffs, NJ: Prentice Hall.

Bandura, A. (1997) *Self-efficacy: the Exercise of Control*. New York: W.H. Freeman.

Barlow, J., Wright, C., Sheasby, J., Turner, A. and Hainsworth, J. (2002) Self-management approaches for people with chronic conditions: a review, *Patient Educ Couns*, 48: 177–87.

Bayliss, E.A., Steiner, J.F., Fernald, D.H., Crane, L.A. and Main, D.S. (2003) Descriptions of barriers to self-care by persons with comorbid chronic diseases, *Ann Fam Med*, 1: 15–21.

Becker, G., Gates, R.J. and Newsom, E. (2004) Self-care among chronically ill African Americans: culture, health disparities, and health insurance status, *Am J Public Health*, 94: 2066–73.

Bentzen, N., Christiansen, T. and Pedersen, K.M. (1989) Self-care within a model for demand for medical care, *Soc Sci Med*, 29: 185–93.

Bergeson, S.C. and Dean, J.D. (2006) A systems approach to patient-centered care, *JAMA*, 20: 2848–51.

Bourbeau, J., Julien, M., Maltais, F. et al. (2003) Reduction of hospital utilization in patients with chronic obstructive pulmonary disease: a disease-specific self-management intervention, *Arch Intern Med*, 163: 585–91.

Chodosh, J., Morton, S.C., Mojica, W. et al. (2005) Meta-analysis: chronic disease self-management programs for older adults, *Ann Intern Med*, 143: 427–38.

Ciechanowski, P.S., Katon, W.J. and Russo, J.E. (2000) Depression and diabetes: impact of depressive symptoms on adherence, function, and costs, *Arch Intern Med*, 160: 3278–85.

Clark, N.M., Becker, M.H., Janz, N.K. et al. (1991) Self-management of chronic disease by older adults, *J Aging Health* 3: 3–27.

Clark, P.C. and Dunbar, S.B. (2003) Family partnership intervention: a guide for a family approach to care of patients with heart failure, *AACN Clin Issues*, 14: 467–76.

Coleman, M.T. and Newton, K.S. (2005) Supporting self-management in patients with chronic illness, *Am Fam Physician*, 72: 1503–10.

Coster, S., Gulliford, M.C., Seed, P.T., Powrie, J.K. and Swaminathan, R. (2000) Monitoring blood glucose control in diabetes mellitus: a systematic review, *Health Technol Assess*, 4: i–iv, 1–93.

Coulter, A. (2006) *Engaging Patients in Their Healthcare: How is the UK Doing Relative to Other Countries?* Oxford: Picker Institute.

Coulter, A. and Ellins, J. (2006) *Quest for Quality and Improved Performance. Patient-focused Interventions. A Review of the Evidence*. Oxford: The Health Foundation, Picker Institute Europe.

Davis, K., Schoen, C. and Schoenbaum, S.C. (2006) *Mirror, Mirror on the Wall: An Update on the Quality of American Health Care Through the Patient's Lens*. New York: Commonwealth Fund.

De Vries, H., Dijkstra, M. and Kuhlman, P. (1988) Self-efficacy: the third factor beside attitude and subjective norm as a predictor of behavioural intentions, *Health Educ Res*, 3: 273–82.

Dean, K. (1989) Conceptual, theoretical and methodological issues in self-care research, *Soc Sci Med*, 29: 117–23.

Deci, E. and Ryan, R. (1985) *Intrinsic Motivation and Self Determination in Human Behaviour*. New York: Plenum.

Department of Health (2005) *Self Care: A Real Choice*. London: Department of Health.

Dijkstra, A. (2005) The validity of the stages of change model in the adoption of the self-management approach in chronic pain, *Clin J Pain*, 21: 27–37; discussion 69–72.

Dongbo, F., Hua, F., McGowan, P. et al. (2003) Implementation and quantitative evaluation of chronic disease self-management programme in Shanghai, China: randomized controlled trial, *Bull World Health Organ*, 81: 174–81.

Eales, C.J. and Stewart, A.V. (2001) Health and responsibility: self-efficacy, self-care and self-responsibility, *S Afr J Physiother*, 57: 20–5.

Farrell, K., Wicks, M.N. and Martin, J.C. (2004) Chronic disease self-management improved with enhanced self-efficacy, *Clin Nurs Res*, 13: 289–308.

Fishbein, M. and Ajzen, I. (1975) *Belief, Attitude, Intention and Behaviour: An Introduction to Theory and Research*. Reading MA: Addison-Wesley.

Fuller, J., Harvey, P. and Misan, G. (2004) Is client-centred care planning for chronic disease sustainable? Experience from rural South Australia, *Health Soc Care Community*, 12: 318–26.

Gibson, P.G., Powell, H., Coughlan, J. et al. (2002) Limited (information only) patient education programs for adults with asthma, *Cochrane Database Syst Rev*, 2: CD001005.

Glasgow, R.E., Hampson, S.E., Strycker, L.A. and Ruggiero, L. (1997) Personal-model beliefs and social–environmental barriers related to diabetes self-management, *Diabetes Care*, 20: 556–61.

Glasgow, R.E., Toobert, D.J., Hampson, S.E. and Strycker, L.A. (2002) Implementation, generalization and long-term results of the "choosing well" diabetes self-management intervention, *Patient Educ Couns*, 48: 115–22.

Glasgow, R.E., Davis, C.L., Funnell, M.M. and Beck, A. (2003) Implementing practical interventions to support chronic illness self-management, *Jt Comm J Qual Saf*, 29: 563–74.

Goldberg, H.I., Ralston, J.D., Hirsch, I.B., Hoath, J.I. and Ahmed, K.I. (2003) Using an Internet comanagement module to improve the quality of chronic disease care, *Jt Comm J Qual Saf*, 29: 443–51.

Goldberg, H.I., Lessler, D.S., Mertens, K., Eytan, T.A. and Cheadle, A.D. (2004) Self-management support in a web-based medical record: a pilot randomized controlled trial, *Jt Comm J Qual Saf*, 30: 629–35, 589.

Goldstein, M.S. (2004) The persistence and resurgence of medical pluralism, *J Health Polit Policy Law*, 29: 925–45; discussion 1005–19.

Gustafson, D.H., Hawkins, R.P., Boberg, E.W. et al. (2001) CHESS: ten years of research and development in consumer health informatics for broad populations, including the underserved, *Medinfo*, 10: 1459–563.

Hargreaves Heap, S., Hollis, M. et al. (1992) *The Theory of Choice. A Critical Guide*. Cambridge: Blackwell.

Haugh, M.R., Akiyama, H., Tryban, G., Sonoda, K. and Wykle, M. (1991) Self care: Japan and the US compared, *Soc Sci Med*, 33: 1011–22.

Heijmans, M. (2006) *COPD Patients with Low SES: An Outline*. Utrecht:: NIVEL.

Heijmans, M., Rijken, M., Foets, M. et al. (2004) The stress of being chronically ill: from disease-specific to task-specific aspects, *J Behav Med*, 27: 255–71.

Hibbard, J.H. and Tusler, M. (2007) Assessing activation stage and employing a "next steps" approach to supporting patient self-management, *J Ambul Care Manage*, 30: 2–8.

Hibbard, J.H., Mahoney, E.R., Stockard, J. and Tusler, M. (2005) Development and testing of a short form of the patient activation measure, *Health Serv Res*, 40: 1918–30.

Hobbs, H., Wilson, J.H. and Archie, S. (1999) The Alumni program: redefining continuity of care in psychiatry, *J Psychosoc Nurs Ment Health Serv*, 37: 23–9.

Kaiser Permanente (2005) *Behavior Change Counseling Using the Brief Negotiation Method*. Oakland, CA: Regional Health Education, Northern California Region.

Kane, R.L., Johnson, P.E., Town, R.J. and Butler, M. (2004) Economic incentives for preventive care, *Evid Rep Technol Assess*, Summer: 1–7.

Kennedy, A., Reeves, D., Bower, P. et al. (2007) The effectiveness and cost effectiveness of a national lay-led self care support programme for patients with long-term conditions: a pragmatic randomised controlled trial, *J Epidemiol Community Health*, 61: 254–61.

Khan, N.A., McAlister, F.A., Lewanczuk, R.Z. et al. (2005) The 2005 Canadian Hypertension Education Program recommendations for the management of hypertension: part II: therapy, *Can J Cardiol*, 21: 657–72.

Koch, T., Jenkin, P. and Kralik, D. (2004) Chronic illness self-management: locating the "self", *J Adv Nurs*, 48: 484–92.

Lazarus, R.S. and Folkman, S. (1984) *Stress, Appraisal and Coping*. New York: Springer.

Leventhal, H., Meyer, D. and Nerenz, D. (1980) The common-sense representations of illness danger, in S. Rachman (eds) *Medical Psychology*, Vol. 2, pp 7–30. New York: Pergamon.

Leventhal, H., Nerenz, D.R. and Steele, D.S. (1984) Illness representations and coping with health threats, in A. Baum, S.E. Taylor and J.E. Singer (eds) *Handbook of Psychology and Health*, pp 219–52. Hillsdale,NJ: Erlbaum.

Levine, S., Reyes, J.Y., Schwartz, R. et al. (2006) Disease management of the frail elderly population, *Dis Manag Health Outcomes*, 14: 235–43.

Lichtenstein, S. and Slovic, P. (2006) The construction of preference: an overview, in S. Lichtenstein and P. Slovic (eds) *The Construction of Preference*, pp. 1–40. Cambridge: Cambridge University Press.

Lorig, K. (1993) Self-management of chronic illness: a model for the future, *Generations*, 17: 11–14.

Lorig, K. and Holman, H. (1993) Arthritis self-management studies: a twelve-year review, *Health Educ Q*, 20: 17–28.

Lorig, K.R. and Holman, H. (2003) Self-management education: history, definition, outcomes, and mechanisms, *Ann Behav Med*, 26: 1–7.

Lorig, K.R., Sobel, D.S. and Stewart, A.L. (1999) Evidence suggesting that a chronic disease self-management program can improve health status while reducing utilization and costs: A randomized trial, *Med Care*, 37: 5–14.

Lorig, K.R., Sobel, D.S., Ritter, P.L., Laurent, D. and Hobbs, M. (2001) Effect of a self-management program on patients with chronic disease, *Eff Clin Pract*, 4: 256–62.

Mackay, J. and Mensah, G. (2004) *Atlas of Heart Disease and Stroke*. Geneva: World Health Organisation, in collaboration with the Centre for Disease Control and Prevention.

Marks, R., Allegrante, J.P. and Lorig, K. (2005a) A review and synthesis of research evidence for self-efficacy-enhancing interventions for reducing chronic disability: implications for health education practice, part I, *Health Promot Pract*, 6: 37–43.

Marks, R., Allegrante, J.P. and Lorig, K. (2005b) A review and synthesis of research evidence for self-efficacy-enhancing interventions for reducing chronic disability: implications for health education practice, part II, *Health Promot Pract*, 6: 148–56.

McGillion, M., Watt-Watson, J., Kim, J. and Yamada, J. (2004) A systematic review of psychoeducational intervention trials for the management of chronic stable angina, *J Nurs Manag*, 12: 174–82.

Meetoo, D. and Temple, B. (2003) Issues in multi-method research: constructing self-care, *Int J Qualit Meth*, 2: article 1.

Mill, J.S. and Bentham, J. (1987) *Utilitarianism and Other Essays* (ed. by A. Ryan). Harmondsworth: Penguin.

Mokkink, L.B., van der Lee, J.H., Grootenhuis, M.A. et al. (2007) *Prevalence and Consequences of Chronic Conditions in Children*. Amsterdam: Academic Medical Centre.

Moos, R.H. and Schaeffer, J.A. (1984) The crisis of physical illness. An overview and conceptual approach, in R.M. Moss (eds) *Coping with Physical Illness*, Vol. 2: *New Perspectives*, pp. 3–39. New York: Plenum.

Mulley, A. (2006) *Personal Communication*. Boston, MA: Foundation for Informed Decision Making.

National Board of Health (2005a) *Patientskoler og gruppebaseret patientundervisning: en litteraturgennemgang med fokus på metoder og effekter*. Copenhagen: Danish National Board of Health.

National Board of Health (2005b) *Patient uddannelsesprogrammet: Lær at leve med Kronisk Sygdom*. Copenhagen: Danish National Board of Health.

Newman, S., Steed, L. and Mulligan, K. (2004) Self-management interventions for chronic illness, *Lancet*, 364: 1523–37.

National Primary Care Research and Development Centre (2005) *How has the Expert Patients Programme been Delivered and Accepted in the NHS During the Pilot Phase?* Manchester: National Primary Care Research and Development Centre. http://www.npcrdc.ac.uk/Publications/EPP_briefing_paper.pdf (accessed 28 May 2007).

National Primary Care Research and Development Centre (2007) *Spotlight on Support for Self Care in the NHS*. Manchester: National Primary Care Research and Development Centre.

NHS Scotland (2005) *National Framework for Service Change in NHS Scotland. Self Care, Carers, Volunteering and the Voluntary Sector: Towards a more Collaborative Approach*. Edinburgh: Scottish Executive Publications.

Petrie, K.J. and Broadbent, E. (2003) Assessing illness behaviour: what condition is my condition in? *J Psychosom Res*, 54: 415–16.

Petrie, K.J. and Weinman, J.A. (1997) *Perceptions of Health and Illness*. Amsterdam: Harwood Academic.

Petrie, K.J., Cameron, L.D., Ellis, C.J., Buick, D. and Weinman, J. (2002) Changing illness perceptions after myocardial infarction: an early intervention randomized controlled trial, *Psychosom Med*, 64: 580–6.

Prochaska, J.O. and DiClemente, C.C. (1983) Stages and processes of self-change of smoking: toward an integrative model of change, *J Consult Clin Psychol*, 51: 390–5.

REVESDIAB (2006) http://www.revediab.asso.fr/ (accessed 17 March 2006).

Riemsma, R.P., Kirwan, J.R., Taal, E. and Rasker, J.J. (2002) Patient education for adults with rheumatoid arthritis, *Cochrane Database Syst Rev*, 3: CD003688.

Rijken, M., van Kerkhof, M., Dekker, J. and Schellevis, F. (2005) Comorbidity of chronic disease, *Qual Life Res*, 14: 45–55.

Rothman, R.L., DeWalt, D.A., Malone, R. et al. (2004) Influence of patient literacy on the effectiveness of a primary care-based diabetes disease management program, *JAMA*, 292: 1711–16.

Sheldon, K.M., Arndt, J. and Houser-Marko, L. (2003) In search of the organismic valuing process: the human tendency to move towards beneficial goal choices, *J Pers*, 71: 835–69.

Simon, H. (1957) A behavioral model of rational choice, in (eds) *Models of Man, Social and Rational: Mathematical Essays on Rational Human Behavior in a Social Setting*. New York: Wiley.

Singh, D. (2005) *Transforming Chronic Care*. Birmingham: University of Birmingham and Surrey and Sussex PCT Alliance.

Suhl, E. and Bonsignore, P. (2006) Diabetes self-management education for older adults: general principles and practical application, *Diabetes Spectrum* 19: 234–40.

Tattersall, R.L. (2002) The expert patient: a new approach to chronic disease management for the twenty-first century, *Clin Med*, 2: 227–9.

Tversky, A. and Kahneman, D. (1974) Judgment under uncertainty: heuristics and biases, *Science*, 185: 1124–31.

Verhaak, P.F., Heijmans, M.J., Peters, L. and Rijken, M. (2005) Chronic disease and mental disorder, *Soc Sci Med*, 60: 789–97.

Wagner, E.H., Glasgow, R.E., Davis, C. et al. (2001) Quality improvement in chronic illness care: a collaborative approach, *Jt Comm J Qual Improv*, 27: 63–80.

Walker, C., Swerissen, H. and Belfrage, J. (2003) Self-management: its place in the management of chronic illness, *Aust Health Rev*, 26: 34–42.

WHO (1983) *Health Education in Self-care: Possibilities and Limitations. Report of a Scientific Consultation*. Geneva: World Health Organization.

Young, H.M. (2003) Challenges and solutions for care of frail older adults, *Online J Issues Nurs*, 8: 5.

Zautra, A.J. (1996) Investigations of the ongoing stressful situations among those with chronic illness, *Am J Community Psychol*, 24: 697–717.

seven

The human resource challenge in chronic care

Carl-Ardy Dubois, Debbie Singh and Izzat Jiwani

Why are workforce issues important?

Changing patterns of illness, ageing populations, changing expectations, technological developments and new patterns of practice and funding techniques are all altering the way healthcare is delivered by providers and accessed by service users.

The systems most successfully responding to the needs of people with long-term conditions build on continuum-based approaches that proactively identify populations with, or at risk of, chronic conditions and translate these into specific programmes of care tailored to individual needs, while taking a holistic perspective (Kodner 1993; Epstein and Sherwood 1996; Ouwens et al. 2005). Changes in staffing and human resources are critical elements of successful chronic care.

Workforces in the health, social care and voluntary sectors are under pressure from the increasing demands posed by the epidemic of chronic diseases, yet they are constrained by a lack of capacity and capabilities (Pruitt and Epping-Jordan 2005). In labour-intensive areas such as healthcare, the provision of essential services to people with long-term conditions depends largely on the availability of an appropriately organized and skilled workforce. Integrated systems aim to involve many different professionals working as teams to ensure that the right people get the right type of care at the right time (Norris et al. 2003; Singh 2005a).

Other chapters in this book describe how it is important to change approaches to chronic disease management, to support self-care, to use evidence-based approaches and decision support tools, and to finance changes appropriately. To achieve these changes, the right people must be in place to provide and manage services. Human resources are thus central to every component of the emerging models of chronic care.

Methods

Although much attention has been paid to devising new delivery structures for chronic care in recent years, the crucial role of workforce development has sometimes been overlooked. Yet improvements in the quality of health and social services are predicated on both the redesign of organizational systems *and* a workforce that is prepared and organized to work in these new systems. Furthermore, while redesigning chronic care may have significant benefits for service users, it is less clear how restructuring delivery systems impacts on those providing care. Therefore, this chapter explores the implications for the workforce of new models of chronic care. Drawing on case studies from different countries and published literature, we explore how the changes associated with emerging systems of chronic care delivery impact on the paid workforce, particularly in healthcare. In addition, we discuss how proactive changes to the workforce may be a lever that can be used to improve chronic care.

The information on which this chapter is based was derived from systematic review of the literature, sourcing more than 30,000 relevant studies from electronic databases. We also contacted experts in the field and drew on case studies of chronic care in different countries. The review methods and country case studies have been described in other publications (Singh 2005b), including the accompanying volume (Nolte et al. 2008).

In this chapter, the term "workforce" refers to the entire range of practitioners or caregivers relied upon to deliver healthcare, including formal and paid caregivers, informal carers and self-caregivers. The main focus of this chapter is on how nurses, family doctors, hospital specialists, home helpers, social workers, social care practitioners and service managers might be experiencing change at individual, organizational and system levels. However, our analysis also shows that these changes need to be reflected in work with service users, their family members and informal carers, who make up an important part of the human resources available in healthcare. Chapter 6 provides a more detailed focus on these aspects of self-care.

How does the workforce need to change?

Since the late 1980s, many countries and regions have developed explicit policies and frameworks to guide the redesign of chronic care and to improve responsiveness to the needs of people with long-term conditions (Sperl-Hillen et al. 2000; Barr et al. 2003; Ministry of Health Planning 2003). Most of the frameworks adopted in developed countries draw, to some extent, on the Chronic Care Model originally developed in the United States (Wagner 1998). As outlined in Chapter 4, delivery system design is one of the six key components of the Chronic Care Model. Human resources are an important part of such delivery systems.

There are at least four distinctive components of new models of chronic care that have significant implications for human resources:

- increased integration and multidisciplinary approaches
- person-centred care: focusing on service users' perspectives
- population-based approaches
- focusing on quality improvement.

This section discusses why these changing characteristics of chronic disease management models have important implications for the workforce. The next section outlines some of the impacts of these key changes on workforce composition, roles, skill requirements and practice environments.

Change 1: increased integration

Changing models of chronic disease management impact on integration in relation to individual professionals, teams and organizational structures.

Historically, healthcare workforces have been structured to provide services based largely on an acute medical model focused on the treatment of discrete episodes of disease. Within this perspective, care was conceptualized as a discrete event occurring in a single location and often involving a single provider (WHO 2002a). Chronic conditions provide a fundamentally different picture because they are permanent, non-reversible conditions that are in essence gradual and long term, and that may be expected to require an extended period of supervision, observation and some degree of support across settings and providers (Nodhturft et al. 2000). For example, a person with hypertension diagnosed with severe stroke may receive acute care in hospital, attend a separate residential facility for rehabilitation and visit a community-based organization or care home for long-term therapy. Furthermore, they may receive practical support from social services and the voluntary sector, and ongoing support from community nurses and their family doctor. They will benefit from a diverse array of services provided over a sustained period by different types of provider.

There is a large body of evidence to suggest that the most effective care pathways for people with long-term conditions involve integrated approaches (Wagner et al. 2001; Bodenheimer et al. 2002; McDonald et al. 2002; Neumeyer-Gromen et al. 2004). A key challenge for the workforce involved in chronic care is to manage the transitions of service users between and within services (Challis et al. 1995).

The comprehensive and systematic process of assessing, planning, arranging and monitoring numerous services to meet each person's multiple and complex needs involves some form of individual management and coordination of cases (Kodner 1993). This involves a shift from a task-oriented approach towards integrated provision. This means that workers must possess a broader range of skills and be able to demonstrate a more reflexive attitude in their work. Individual management does not solely involve formal "case management" staff. Being able to draw linkages and take a whole systems approach is increasingly important for many members of the chronic care workforce, whether or not they have a formal "case management" role.

Case-level coordination is closely intertwined with interprofessional coordination. Because people often have more than one long-term condition, and because chronic illness has many facets, care must be coordinated among different practitioners. Care is often provided by a team of caregivers from different disciplines with varying skills, knowledge and experience. In terms of workforce development, this moves the focus from single professionals to multiprofessionalism and it means that workers need to be able to work in teams and communicate with the other providers who have roles in managing coexisting conditions.

Effective interprofessional coordination relies, in many respects, on effective interagency coordination. Caring for people with multiple chronic conditions shifts provision from a hospital-centred paradigm to one that values a continuum of care by multiple organizations, including formal health and social care groups and community resources. Enhanced communication between these different groups has the potential to develop more effective referral pathways, facilitate navigation between services and link practitioners operating at different levels (Von Korff et al. 1997). The chronic care workforce can be instrumental in these processes and has a fundamental role in stimulating and maintaining the partnerships needed between different components of the system. A key challenge for workers is to accommodate a practice environment where traditional boundaries between organizations or occupational groups are blurred, leading to new forms of working and delivering services.

This trend toward increased integration is reflected by the creation in some countries of intermediary vertically integrated organizations that are responsible for a wide continuum of health services. Box 7.1 provides some examples.

The introduction of organizations with responsibility for the planning, management and funding (through direct provision or purchase) of the full continuum of health services for a defined population is linked to several major developments in workforce organization, including a shift from predominantly solo practices towards team-based practices, role expansion for nurses, a search for more flexibility in using the workforce and the emergence of new channels

Box 7.1 Developing integrated organizations

In Sweden, chronic care services are organized predominantly in county-owned health centres that are managed with interdisciplinary teams of physicians, nurses and other providers at multiple sites. District nurses with limited prescription rights play a crucial role, as they are responsible for many first contacts with the healthcare system. In many cases, they make a first assessment of service users and direct them to the most appropriate resource (Glenngård 2005).

In England, primary care trusts and practice-based commissioning groups aim to bring together local providers of primary and community services under a board representing general practitioners, nurses and other community staff. Primary care trusts are also responsible for commissioning acute hospital services.

of accountability for professionals (Bindman et al. 2001; Gillam and Schamroth 2002). These changes mean that new approaches to chronic care may challenge traditional professional boundaries, conventional team structures and job skills (McKee et al. 2006). There are few empirical studies of the impact of role redefinition on the workforce, but the existing evidence suggests that there is a need to consider the feelings and needs of the workforce as a priority. For example, one study of nurses' education and preparation for working with people with chronic conditions at home suggested that nurses were well informed and adapting to the core values and practices of case management but expressed immense insecurity about changes in their roles (Pratt 2006).

Traditionally, the clinical roles of medical professionals have been specialized, with little room for delegating tasks to those outside a particular profession. Yet research suggests that many medical professionals, such as doctors, nurses and allied health professionals, spend a large proportion of their time performing tasks that do not necessarily require their particular professional expertise (Richardson et al. 1998). Given the shortage of medical professionals in many countries, the emerging policy focus involves shifting some tasks from more specialized highly skilled professionals to less-qualified, lower-cost workers. This vertical delegation is resulting in blurring of role boundaries and professional values (Brown et al. 2000). For example, in some countries, a social worker may take over some functions of nurses (e.g. counselling) as an integral part of a chronic care team.

Role overlap can also occur horizontally between disciplines, such as physio-therapists and occupational therapists (Booth and Hewiston 2002). Some suggest that role overlap could threaten professional identity (Brown et al. 2000; Booth and Hewiston 2002). However, other research suggests that services such as "intermediate care" do not threaten role boundaries or professional identity (Nancarrow 2004). The key implication is that we need to acknowledge that the workforce is changing and allow for role delegation, flexibility and appropriate training. Central to this is taking the time to find out what individual workers think, and putting strategies in place to alleviate any fears they may have.

Another impact of integration is on education and training. Achieving the kind of flexibility needed for interdisciplinary working may require professionals to develop new skills. While numerous strategies have been trialled for increasing skills of professionals, including audit and feedback, reminder systems and individual and group education, the overall conclusion is that changing professional skills takes time and effort – and there is no single strategy for success (Munro et al. 2002; Smits et al. 2002; Robertson et al. 2003; Lewin et al. 2004; Jamtvedt et al. 2004). In driving forward change, we must consider ways to acknowledge and modify the attitudes of the workforce, because only by addressing attitudes and values will we be able to encourage the sustainable behavioural changes needed to transform chronic care.

Change 2: focusing on service users' perspectives

In the paternalistic model that has prevailed in the management of acute illness, the provider is often depicted as the guardian of the service user's best interests and is given the role of determining the approach to treatment (Szasz and Hollender 1956; Emanuel and Emanuel 1992). However, redesigning models of chronic care requires a new focus to involve service users fully. Service users must engage in their ongoing treatment, make behavioural changes and adjust to the consequences of their conditions on a long-term basis; consequently, service users inevitably become a major caretaker and a crucial part of the human resources or "workforce" in chronic care.

As well as having implications for the role of service users themselves (Chapter 6), this focus on service users' perspectives also has implications for the paid workforce. New models of chronic disease management shift decision making from paternalistic patient–physician relationships towards an ideal of a deliberative and partnering model that is more responsive to individual needs, embodies a central role for the service user and their families, incorporates their perspectives and preferences in the care process and offers them the educational and psychosocial supports needed for an effective care partnership (Clark et al. 1995; Laine and Davidoff 1996; Quill and Brody 1996). The role of practitioners thus broadens to include advising service users about recommended approaches to disease management, teaching healthcare skills, providing emotional and psychological support, assisting in access to health and social care resources and promoting healthy behaviours (Stubblefield and Mutha 2002).

The person-centred approach moves staff away from a provider-driven health and social care system towards a system that incorporates service users' perspectives and focuses on providing tailor-made support to individuals. This applies in primary, secondary and tertiary care. Box 7.2 contains an example of this approach.

Box 7.2   Changes to provide a person-centred service

In Quebec, the "Live well with COPD" programme provides a person-centred approach for people with chronic obstructive pulmonary disease. The programme is designed to help people to take more responsibility for their illness and maintain optimal physical, psychosocial and mental functioning. It builds on the capacity of individuals to assess their own needs, determine how and by whom these needs should be met, and adopt behaviours that are likely to influence the course of their disease. As part of this programme, specialized centres run by multidisciplinary teams offer a package of interventions including courses about the disease, its symptoms and management; telephone follow-up; and individual counselling. A randomized trial found that the programme helped to reduce hospital admissions and visits to the emergency department and to foster more appropriate use of primary health services (Bourbeau et al. 2003). This is one of many similar examples, backed up by research evidence, of the benefits of seeing service users as an integral part of the chronic care workforce (Lorig et al. 1999; Osman et al. 2002; Bourbeau et al. 2003; Chiang et al. 2004).

Change 3: population-based approaches

The new generation of chronic care models such as the Expanded Chronic Care Model and the Innovative Care for Chronic Conditions frameworks feature an approach to care that departs from a sole focus on disease management for individuals and instead adds a focus on broad determinants of health (Glasgow et al. 2001; WHO 2002a; Barr et al. 2003). These newer models involve building a comprehensive system of coordinated interventions that cuts across the primary, secondary and tertiary levels of care and extends beyond the boundaries of the healthcare system to cover issues such as population health promotion, prevention, screening and early detection, diagnosis, management of diagnosed cases, rehabilitation and palliative care.

Such population-based perspectives do not detract from individual needs and are, in fact, complementary to person-centred approaches. A person-centred perspective emphasizes the responsiveness of treatment decisions to the specific needs and preferences of individuals. A population-based approach builds on this to take account of the entire continuum of services and the broad set of interrelated factors (socioeconomic status, housing, physical environment, lifestyles) that impact on health.

This component of chronic disease management also has implications for the workforce. Population-based approaches move the workforce from caring for a single unit (one person seeking care) towards planning and delivering care to defined populations and ensuring that effective interventions reach all people who need them within a given population. To meet this challenge, practitioners have to assume new roles and demonstrate the ability to manage populations, assess the health needs of wider groups and plan and implement appropriate levels of health and social care interventions.

There are also implications for the deployment of workers beyond the traditional boundaries of formal health or social care institutions. For example, population-based care may mean that a worker previously located in "primary" or "secondary" care must be able to work in community settings or in the social care or voluntary sector environments in order to reach the communities of their defined populations. Such a perspective also implies that the community-based organizations need to be staffed and skilled adequately so as to fill the gaps in services that are not provided in formal organizations and to enable them to play a full role in the prevention and management of chronic conditions.

The shift towards a population-based approach has motivated the development of a number of new roles in different countries (Box 7.3).

Change 4: focusing on quality improvement

The increased focus on quality improvement within new models of chronic care also has implications for the workforce. Continuous quality improvement, with a focus on patient safety, is particularly salient in the context of chronic care. Medical errors and other lapses in safety are particularly likely to harm people with serious and progressive chronic conditions. Chronically ill people, as

Box 7.3   The development of new roles for chronic disease management

Community matrons are nurses in England who use population risk assessment strategies to target those with complicated needs or most at risk of hospital admission. Community matrons provide advice, coaching and an extensive range of nursing services and support in community settings and in people's own homes. This new role is central to the government's policy for supporting people with long-term conditions, with 3000 community matrons to be in post by March 2007. Although community matrons are working in different ways in different areas, there are some commonalities. They tend to be nurses based in primary care and to aim to coordinate primary and secondary care and social services. In large part, community matrons have been recruited from existing pools of primary care nurses, so there has been little shift of skills from secondary care. Most community matrons take part in advanced clinical and case management training offered through universities or private providers. National competency frameworks and training commissioning guidance have been developed. Community matrons use standardized risk assessment tools to identify people who may benefit from support and to undertake detailed initial and ongoing assessments. Increasingly community matrons are working alongside pharmacists to review medication. The key components of this model are:

- segmentation of people at high risk of admission or frequent service users
- use of clinical information systems to identify people at high risk, simplification of care pathways (by having one person coordinating other services)
- supporting self-management and individualized care planning, ongoing case management, often for an extended period.

Local areas have also been assessing the impacts of community matrons on hospital admissions. Early evidence is mixed. In some areas, community matrons have had little impact on overall admission rates whereas other areas report avoided admissions. Areas where community matrons have most success appear to be those where the role is implemented as one part of a broader chronic disease management programme, working in an integrated way with other services.

Similar approaches have occurred in other countries, such as Canada, where incentives have been introduced to encourage family physicians and family practice groups to enlarge the scope of their interventions and to provide a comprehensive package of care to defined populations with chronic conditions. In many cases, this has included more funding for activities related to preventive care, early diagnosis and effective management of people with chronic conditions (College of Family Physicians of Canada 2004).

intensive users of healthcare services and medications, have more interactions with the health system and consequently have a greater risk of exposure to potential failures in the system or medical errors (Corcoran 1997; Kohn et al. 2000). Chronically ill people with poor health status, comorbid conditions and multiple functional and physical limitations may be more severely impacted by errors because they often cannot protect themselves from risks and have fewer reserves with which to overcome adverse effects (Lynn and Schuster 2000). The complexity of care and collaboration required to respond to the needs of the chronically ill also means that there may be more scope for flawed system designs and consequent errors (Institute of Medicine 2001; Wunderlich and Kohler 2001).

Safety and quality improvement are embedded in recent efforts to foster optimal management of care for people with chronic conditions and to ensure that these people receive treatment consistent with evidence-based practice. Yet achieving such objectives depends on an ability to modify the practice environment in which professionals work in order to promote a culture of safety, to encourage open and systematic handling of errors and to reward individual and organizational behaviour directed at quality improvement. Historically, professionals may not have been rewarded for identifying gaps or suggesting improvements. Therefore, this focus on whole systems learning, creating an opportunity to develop and share learning in order to benefit both individuals and the wider system, may require significant shifts in organizational and professional culture – as well as shifts in individual practice.

Much current debate about preparing the workforce to embrace new models of care delivery is focused on the clinical skills and abilities of professionals to engage in new forms of relationships with their clients. Yet while the need to develop new competencies and skills is undoubtedly important, the need to develop organizational competencies is often overlooked. It is important to develop governance and change management capabilities at all levels of the health and social care system in order to implement new models of care. For decades, innovative clinicians and researchers have been developing and testing new ways to care for people with chronic conditions, and there is much evidence about how services can be better organized to improve the quality of care and service users' experiences (Bodenheimer et al. 2002; Zwar et al. 2006). However, these changes involve significant organizational and system improvements and achieving these requires full commitment of the workforce. Motivated personnel are a key tool for facilitating changes in the system and tailoring changes to individual contexts. This underlines the importance of developing a flexible, innovative and adaptive workforce that will be not only capable of accepting change but also prepared to lead it, manage it and capitalize on it in their day-to-day practice. The best strategies for encouraging such a transformed and motivated workforce remain uncertain.

What are the impacts on human resources?

This outline of the four key ways that new chronic care models necessitate workforce change indicates that major human resource challenges pervade the overall process. Human resources are a crucial link in chronic care policies and need to be addressed adequately if successful implementation of changes in chronic care delivery systems is to be achieved. Yet few studies have devoted attention to the impact on the workforce of new models of organizing and delivering chronic care or to the vast set of workforce changes needed to keep pace with emerging processes of care. In this section, we examine selected policy levers that may help to optimize the workforce's contribution to chronic care, and the potential impact of these levers on the workforce. The areas considered include conceptualizing a human resource continuum, reconfiguring roles, developing generic competences and reconfiguring the practice environment.

Impact 1: conceptualizing a human resource continuum

Although the number of health and social care occupations has increased in recent years, the formal health and social care system has traditionally recognized only a small segment of the potential human resources available. Often informal and lay caregivers and self-care providers have been overlooked. Such a narrow focus is in sharp contrast with the context of chronic care.

The needs of people with chronic conditions range from minimal personal assistance to virtually total everyday care. Interventions to meet these needs are offered in a variety of settings (hospitals, rehabilitation centres, nursing homes, residential care facilities, family practices, people's own homes) and extend to a vast range of activities, including health promotion, acute care, rehabilitation and psychosocial support. If the management of services for people with chronic conditions must be person centred, population based and integrated, workforce policies cannot be restricted to formal caregivers. Instead, a broader understanding of human resources is required that takes into consideration the whole spectrum of caregivers, ranging from those who strive to keep themselves healthy to those who look after chronically ill and disabled relatives and those who provide institutionalized or professional services (Pong et al. 1995; WHO 2006). The concept of a human resources continuum is also congruent with the objective of continuity of care, which implies the ability to mobilize a diverse range of caregivers providing services or assistance at different times.

While the workforce involved in providing chronic care can be divided into professionals and paraprofessionals, employees and independent contractors, paid workers and volunteers, and into a myriad of different professional or sectoral groups, it may be more useful to consider personnel in three main categories: formal caregivers, informal caregivers and self-care providers.

Formal caregivers are workers who are paid to provide their services, including nurses, physicians, social workers, pharmacists, therapists and dieticians. Many of these occupations are subject to legal sanction through licensure, certification and registration. However, within this formal caregiver category, providers range from highly qualified specialists to workers who have received minimal training. Non-professionals who provide the majority of personal care services, such as assistance with eating or bathing and other forms of support, make a significant contribution to service delivery and have a major impact on the quality of life of people with long-term conditions. Service providers for public and private home care also employ workers who are an important human resource in chronic care. These home-care workers could be health professionals, such as nurses, social workers or personal care workers, or "less trained" support workers. In addition to these direct care providers, the formal caregiver category also includes administrative workers, food service workers and housekeeping staff, who play essential support roles in chronic care. Grouping all these providers into a similar category may help to override professional territories and divisions that do not further the development of high quality support. This will span the boundaries between primary and secondary care and emphasizes that change is important in all contexts and not solely in one sphere of care.

While discussions about chronic care sometimes emphasize the role of formal caregivers, there is evidence that most care provided to people with long-term conditions is delivered by unpaid, informal caregivers, including family members, neighbours, friends and volunteers from religious and community organizations (Wunderlich and Kohler 2001; Hussein and Manthorpe 2005). The sustainability of the formal health and social care system depends to some extent on the contribution of these informal caregivers because, without them, there would not be sufficient resources to meet all health and social care needs.

The importance of self-care providers is also increasingly recognized (Lorig and Holman 1989; Barlow et al. 1999; Chapter 6). Individual behaviours (diet, exercise, smoking cessation and alcohol consumption) play a key role in the progression of many chronic conditions such as cardiovascular disease, cancer and diabetes. Service users, therefore, have a significant role to play in managing their own health. A growing body of literature suggests that, with appropriate training and support, most people with conditions such as diabetes, hypertension, asthma and arthritis can perform many tasks that were previously the preserve of formal caregivers in intuitional settings (Pong et al. 1995; Lorig et al. 1999; Astin et al. 2002; Gibson et al. 2003; Coulter and Ellins 2006). Many types of treatment and monitoring, such as self-assessment (taking blood pressure, blood glucose monitoring for diabetes), physical therapy for arthritis, self-administration of factor VIII for haemophilia and continuous ambulatory peritoneal dialysis, have been delivered safely and effectively by service users themselves (Kobayashi et al. 1990; McDonald et al. 1995).

In addition to providing self-care, people with long-term conditions can also provide peer support or act as lay workers to help others with chronic illnesses. There is empirical evidence that lay workers can play a vital role in supporting people with chronic disease or those in need of palliative care (Department of Health 2001; Barlow et al. 2005). There is also growing evidence of the valuable contribution lay workers can play as part of a care team for low-income communities (Whitmer et al. 1995; Corkery et al. 1997).

There is a lack of information available about whether using lay workers or community workers impacts on the views and responsibilities of professionals. It is conceivable that professionals may feel "challenged" by informal or self-caregivers or be concerned about the quality of care provided.

There is also only a little evidence in the literature on how people with long-term conditions feel about their role as part of the care team. There is evidence that self-management and peer support can be valuable and that people with long-term conditions are sometimes eager to take on these roles (Hainsworth and Barlow 2001; Struthers et al. 2003). However, less is known about how service users view their position in relation to other professionals, or any challenges and barriers that they face.

Recognizing the critical importance of informal caregivers and self-caregivers raises the question of how they can be supported to optimize their contribution. Of particular importance are the knowledge and skills of community members and the tools and support available to individuals to manage their health needs. A related question is how formal, informal and self-caregivers can best complement each other. In order to encourage integrated provision of chronic care, more attention needs to be given to coordinating all these formal, informal and unofficial resources and promoting communication and collaboration between them. Formal caregivers that are mostly trained to work in institutions will need to develop a broader understanding of health and social care services, familiarize themselves with community-based and voluntary services and be prepared to work in a greater variety of settings, including the community sector.

Conceptualizing the workforce as a continuum of human resources has several implications for workforce policy development. Efforts to improve chronic care would benefit from effective mobilization of all sectors in human resources. By looking outside the traditional boundaries and taking account of the entire continuum of resources, the health and social care system can enhance care for chronically ill people, fill gaps and avoid duplication.

Finally, while shortages in the formal health workforce have attracted the attention of policy makers and planners, any sustainable framework for chronic care needs to consider the socioeconomic changes that are likely to pose a threat to the informal caregiving workforce. Changes in family structure, increases in the contribution of women to the labour force and an increasingly unfavourable dependency ratio created by declining birth rates and longer lifespan are among the factors that could limit the availability of informal care in the future (Brodsky et al. 2000; WHO 2002b).

Impact 2: reconfiguring roles

WHO has documented the global shortage of human resources in health, in particular physicians and nurses. While this shortage is more evident in poorer countries, developed countries such as Australia, Canada and the United States are also experiencing shortages. This shortage of human resources impacts on how long-term conditions can be managed (Australian Medical Workforce Advisory Committee 2005; Productivity Commission 2005). One study found that 3.5 hours out of every family physician's day was spent managing people with the 10 leading chronic illnesses, even assuming the conditions were stable and under control. The estimated time required was multiplied three times for uncontrolled chronic diseases (Ostbye et al. 2005). A range of strategies have been developed to respond to the limited availability of staff, including reconfiguring roles. This process of reconfiguration can be grouped into two dominant patterns: redefining existing roles and creating new types of provider.

Redefining existing roles

Governments and professional governing bodies specify the scope of practice for most clinical professionals. Sometimes regulatory boundaries may act as obstacles to positive change, innovation and effective use of professionals. In France, each health professional's role is defined by law enacted by Parliament. In the Netherlands, a regulatory body (the MOBG) is in charge of the qualifications for (new) disciplines and educational programmes. Professional interest groups may also try to protect their position by influencing outcomes and decisions related to disciplines.

However, redefining roles, or the scope of practice in particular roles, is a strategy that can be used to make better use of an increasingly diversified workforce and ensure adequate supplies of the right type and mix of workers. These changes in professional boundaries fall into four categories: enhancement, substitution, delegation and innovation (Sibbald et al. 2004; McKee et al. 2006).

Nurses have been particularly targeted by these changes. A number of countries have provided nurses with opportunities to work in a much wider range of clinical roles and to assume functions previously restricted to physicians (Frich 2003; Loveman et al. 2003). The most commonly researched strategies for expanding the role of nurses include support from specialist nurses in primary or secondary care, nurse-led clinics in primary or secondary care and nurse-led outpatient follow-up by primary or secondary care nurses (Singh 2005a). For example, in the United Kingdom, nurses specializing in helping people with a particular type of condition (such as diabetes nurses or asthma nurses) substitute for general practitioners in routine appointments, running clinics to monitor and inform patients or undertaking outreach and educational work to increase the skills of other health and social care professionals (Griffiths et al. 2004). In Scandinavia, nurse anaesthetists have an important role in assessing chronic pain and managing postoperative pain (Moote 1993; Stromberg et al. 2001). Box 7.4 contains another example, from Canada.

A growing body of evidence suggests that these processes of redefinition can

Box 7.4   Primary care networks in Canada

With funding from the federal government, many primary care networks (PCN) in the Capital Health region of Edmonton, Canada have hired allied health professionals. The composition of allied health professionals varies with the needs of the particular region and may include such professionals as nurse practitioners, dieticians, mental health navigators, pharmacists and occupational therapists. Physicians in many PCNs work on a core set of practices and transfer some clinical roles to allied health professionals who can cover that area of practice. For example, an allied health professional may work with a person with diabetes to provide education, care planning, follow-up care and checking that foot and eye examinations and referrals have been provided. All allied health professionals receive necessary training to upgrade their skills.

improve outcomes for service users. Several systematic reviews have found that primary care nurses with expanded roles can provide care equivalent to that traditionally provided by family doctors, with the caveat that most studies reviewed included small numbers of clinicians and few examined long-term outcomes (Brown and Grimes 1995; Horrocks et al. 2002). There is good evidence that nurses who specialize in a particular long-term condition, either in hospital or in the community, can help to improve the health of patients and reduce their use of health services (Griffiths et al. 2004; Smith et al. 2004; Singh 2005b). Clinics run by specialist nurses have also been associated with improved patient satisfaction and clinical outcomes (Vrijhoef et al. 2000; Connor et al. 2002; Stromberg et al. 2003; Singh 2005a). Box 7.5 provides an example from Sweden (see also Chapter 4).

This process of role expansion is not confined to nurses. Changes associated with chronic care have also created opportunities for many other groups, such as pharmacists and social workers, to assume new roles in care delivery. For instance, a new pharmacists' contract adopted in England and Wales in 2004 gave pharmacists opportunities to expand their role into chronic disease management by providing repeat prescriptions, reviewing medication and compliance and providing smoking cessation services. However, few studies have investigated what these changes mean for professionals themselves – either the professionals with redefined roles or the colleagues working alongside them.

There is a further challenge in that alongside the move towards greater flexibility in roles is an equal and opposite pressure towards specialization, as reflected in the organization of integrated care pathways around diagnostic groups. The stated justification is that people with specialized skills may provide better treatment than generalists. Yet, while specialized services may increase the coherence of care for some types of service user, it presents a major challenge for managing the larger volume of demands in chronic care because so many

---

Box 7.5 Redefinition of the role of nurses in Sweden

Sweden is one of the leading countries in Europe in the area of nurse-led patient education and follow-up. Between 1990 and 1998, nurse-led heart failure clinics opened in two-thirds of all Swedish hospitals (Stromberg et al. 2001). Follow-up at these clinics with education, optimized treatment and social support has been found to improve survival and self-care behaviour and to reduce the need for hospital care (Cline 2002; Stromberg et al. 2003). However, these changes in the scope of practice are part of an overall process of reorganizing care delivery. They are not simply about substituting one staff group for another. While there is evidence to support this way of working, there are also studies suggesting that increased use of less-qualified staff is not effective in all situations, so caution is necessary to ensure that these changes reflect patient needs rather than short-term cost-reduction strategies.

people (particularly the elderly) have multiple conditions. Many people with multiple diagnoses will not easily fit into the integrated pathways set up around specific diagnoses and could be better served by generalists. This tension between specialization and generalists is an area in need of further exploration when developing and implementing new chronic care services.

Creating new types of provider

Diversification differs from merely redefining existing roles because it calls for the development of providers with new skill sets. Traditional professional roles do not necessarily fit the requirements of people with chronic conditions. Therefore, the field of chronic care has been a site of experimentation for a range of new types of care provider. Liaison nurses have been created in a number of countries to support activities such as post-hospital discharge follow-up, pulmonary rehabilitation for people with chronic obstructive pulmonary disease, supervision of medication and compliance, patient education and service navigation. As part of chronic care initiatives, case managers have been introduced in many jurisdictions as a way of a way of coordinating services for people with long-term conditions or complex social and medical needs. Such case managers assume a range of functions, including assessing people's needs, developing care plans, helping people to access appropriate care, monitoring the quality of care and maintaining contact with the person and their family.

Earlier legislation has sometimes focused on exclusive areas of practice for individual disciplines. New initiatives to reconfigure the workforce are building on new types of worker, who have multiple competencies or skills and who are trained to perform procedures and functions that overlap several disciplines. For example, in 2005, the Department of Health in England consulted about the possibility of a medical care practitioner, or physician's assistant, defined as a new healthcare professional who, while not a doctor, would work within the medical model, with the attitudes, skills and knowledge base to deliver holistic care and treatment within the general medical and/or general practice team.

In chronic care, there is an opportunity to promote generic professionals with a defined range of allied skills (nursing, physiotherapy, limited prescribing) working closely with other members of health and social care teams (Brooks 2003). The use of new technologies, such as telemedicine, also calls for more flexibility in roles and potentially more roles involving multiple skills (Piette et al. 1999; Montani et al. 2001; Montori et al. 2004).

To date, the quality of care provided by multi-skilled workers has not been researched extensively or systematically. Nor has the impact of such changes been assessed on practitioners themselves. Even assuming that "multi-skilling" is compatible with other models of care, there are a number of implementation issues that need to be addressed. Various impediments have been identified, such as resistance and fear of encroachment by practitioners in affected disciplines, practice restrictions arising from licensure and liability implications.

Of particular importance are debates about the risk of "deprofessionalization". Despite evidence that nurses achieve as good health outcomes as doctors in some circumstances, and that patient satisfaction with nurse-led care is generally high (Kinnersley et al. 2000; Horrocks et al. 2002), some physicians are reluctant to delegate or devolve their traditional responsibilities to nurses or other professionals as they see this as "deprofessionalization" or "deskilling" their profession.

Research in Canada found that fee-for-service physicians thought that collaborating with nurse practitioners was time consuming and perceived this as deskilling their profession (Centre for Nursing Studies and Institute for the Advancement of Public Policy 2001). One collaborative project ended when doctors refused to work with nurse practitioners. In this instance, the medical society and doctors who opposed the nurse practitioner programme said nurse practitioner duties intruded on the traditional role of the physicians (Canadian Health Services Research Foundation 2001). Similarly, in British Columbia, physicians surveyed felt they would be in competition with nurse practitioners (Schreiber et al. 2003).

Another type of "deskilling" is sometimes thought to occur as a result of striving for economic efficiency. In this context, deskilling refers to using fewer trained personnel to provide care (Baumann and Silverman 1998) or using non-regulated healthcare workers to do skilled professional jobs (WHO 2002c; Enhancing Interdisciplinary Collaboration in Primary Healthcare Initiative 2005). Using unqualified staff to replace qualified nurses became common in the 1990s, particularly in North America, for cost-containment purposes. In areas such as long-term care, unqualified nurse aides, assistants or support workers often carry out tasks previously completed by qualified medical workers, such as nurses. Sometimes nurses in this situation feel their skills are being devalued (Edwards 1997). Others have argued that unqualified workers add to indirect costs through skill dilution, absenteeism and high rates of turnover (Orne et al. 1998). There is conflicting evidence about the impact of greater numbers of qualified staff on the quality of care and efficiency (owing to reduced absenteeism or error) in the management of chronic disorders (Sibbald et al. 2004), although there is now clear evidence that lower numbers of registered nurses impacts adversely on quality of care in the acute sector (Aiken et al. 2002).

Impact 3: developing generic competencies

New strategies for chronic disease management signal a changing emphasis in user–provider relationships and in the settings where services are provided, the types of carer involved and the focus on change management. Such changes necessitate a new set of staff competences to sustain these shifts. Although existing competencies remain essential, the transition from acute to chronic health problems places a new set of demands on the health and social care workforce. In addition to skills that facilitate the diagnosis and treatment of acute illness and injury, new models for chronic disease management require the workforce to have an additional set of core competencies.

WHO suggests that core generic skills for delivering care to people with long-term conditions include skills and knowledge that transcend the boundaries of specific disciplines and are necessary for all professionals (WHO 2005). The following are seen as important.

- Delivering patient-centred care requires all workers to acquire communication skills, see things from the perspective of service users, provide education and information, involve service users in all aspects of decision making and motivate and train people in self-management.
- Managing the diverse transitions in chronic care means that the workforce must be capable of creating and maintaining effective partnerships with all caregivers who operate at different levels of the system: patients and their relatives, informal providers and other formal providers and the community. Of critical importance is the ability to collaborate with others and work in a variety of settings. Communication skills are necessary to negotiate, share decisions and collectively solve problems. The ability to use information technology is essential to support care, monitor people's navigation across different settings at different time points, exchange information with other providers and monitor response to treatments.
- Chronic care initiatives involve significant organizational and system changes to establish new ways of working and delivering care. Implementation of these changes requires a workforce skilled at managing the change process.
- Ensuring patient safety means that workers must possess basic knowledge about quality management and be able to make use of measurement and improvement tools in their practice. Clinicians need to be skilled at accessing the current knowledge base, gathering evidence about the best standards of care and integrating them into their practice. There is some evidence that identifying good practice and evaluating the success of services are gaps in the current competencies of many service managers and providers (Ham et al. 2007).
- Population-based care requires the workforce to engage in health promotion and prevention activities and to provide treatment and services across the entire continuum of care. This broadening of functions will likely require the development of public health capabilities, including reinforcing staffs members' understanding of their responsibility to broader populations as well as individuals.

Implications for training

Complementing the technical competencies of workers with this new core set of generic competencies has several implications for educational programmes. Although there is not a single educational model that would foster improved chronic care, existing approaches are flawed in a number of ways.

Recently, several promising didactic and experiential interdisciplinary initiatives have been set up in Canada to build a workforce that is multicompetent and skilled in working effectively in teams (Health Council of Canada 2005). The Interprofessional Education for Collaborative Patient-Centred Practice Initiative (IECPCP), led by Health Canada, aims to promote and demonstrate the benefits of interprofessional education in a wide range of settings and types of care delivery. Toronto Rehabilitation, a specialized teaching hospital, has initiated a new approach to clinical placements in rehabilitation and complex continuing care. Students are given an opportunity to see interprofessional care in action and to understand the roles of other professions. For eight weeks, a team of students from several faculties (medicine, nursing, social work and rehabilitation sciences) are placed with a clinical service that has demonstrated exceptional teamwork under the supervision of an interprofessional education leader. Such collaborative training is increasingly recognized as key in sharing responsibilities for patient care and making healthcare delivery more responsive to population health needs.

Two universities in Canada have established interprofessional programmes for health sciences education. At Memorial University of Newfoundland, the Centre for Collaborative Health Professional Education brings together five disciplines (medicine, nursing, pharmacy, social work and education) to deliver and evaluate interprofessional education for future health professionals. Similarly, the College of Health Disciplines at the University of British Columbia leads 15 health and human service programmes in interprofessional education and research. The task is summarized as follows (Pruitt and Epping-Jordan 2005):

> Common approaches to care are needed across different chronic conditions. Patients do better if they receive effective treatment within an integrated system, with multidisciplinary teams, support for self-management and regular follow-up. Enabling this requires a paradigm shift from a medical, curative model of healthcare towards a coordinated, comprehensive system . . . Healthcare teams need to be organized to coordinate care across providers and settings. Equipping physicians, nurses and other professionals with the necessary training and skills has implications for undergraduate curricula, specialist training and continuing education.

Some have argued that education programmes in health systems using the Chronic Care Model or similar need to encompass all aspects of the model, so that information technology, self-management support and teamwork are as important as clinical or managerial skills. Munro et al. (2002) commented: "What should medical schools be doing? For a start, they should create ambulatory care programs, such as the Chronic Care Model – which includes a practice team, information system, decision supports for practice, and patient self-management supports – to be the sites for new types of learning."

Training for managers is just as important as training for practitioners. When thinking about revising training programmes, it may be important to build in time to raise awareness among health and social care practitioners and managers about both substantive content and new ways of working, including:

- substantive content
  - the prevention, diagnosis, and treatment of long-term conditions
  - the psychological and social aspects of living with long-term conditions
- patient-centred care
  - the role of service users and carers, including how to support self-management
  - the needs of caregivers
  - how to work in different locations, including homes and community facilities
- team work
  - the roles of different professionals and service providers

- relationship building and listening skills
- teamwork and shared care, including how to work across organizations and specialities
- using technology
  - how to support service users by telephone, email, or video links
  - using integrated medical records to store and share information
- quality improvement
  - risk stratification and taking a public health perspective
  - project management, quality assessment and data analysis skills.

It is necessary, however, to sound a note of caution. Overall, the evidence available suggests that existing approaches to continuing professional development do not always improve skills or change behaviours (Oxman et al. 1995; Bero et al. 1998). It is, therefore, important that these skills are built into standard medical and management training, not solely as an "add on" after practitioners or managers are in post. Regular updating of skills, including how to work effectively across organizational structures and how to support self-care, should supplement this focus on enhanced generic competencies as part of routine training.

Another issue of concern is that training of health workers is still mostly confined to institutional settings. Yet, with new models of chronic care, more services are shifting to community-based settings. Educational programmes may, therefore, need to extend beyond the walls of teaching hospitals in order to give medical trainees educational experience that provides them with a broader understanding of healthcare issues, familiarizing them with community-based care and preparing them to work in a variety of settings.

A closely related issue is the lack of emphasis on primary healthcare. Many of the needs of people with chronic disease relate to primary care and require skills that are not acquired in current training programmes that focus on inpatient care (WHO 2002a, 2005; Institute of Medicine 2003, 2004). Preparing the workforce for the challenges of chronic care requires a shift from a curative orientation of healthcare education towards a more balanced curriculum that addresses health promotion functions and socio-psychological aspects of healthcare delivery as well as providing treatment and supporting services.

It is clear that changes to the conceptualization and roles of the chronic care workforce necessitate changes in how people are trained. Policy attention is most often focused on the competencies of formal caregivers. Yet, as pointed out above, informal caregivers and self-care providers are equally important. If they are to make an active contribution to delivery of chronic care, they must be given the opportunity to enhance their caring capabilities. Interventions to improve health literacy have proven to be of particular importance in improving the abilities of service users to read and understand health information, calculate the timing and dose of medication, evaluate and make decisions about treatment options and engage actively in the management of their conditions (Wakefield 2004).

Impact 4: reconfiguring the practice environment

The implementation of changes to service delivery depends not only on the composition of the workforce and practitioners' skills and roles but also on creating a practice environment that is likely to retain current workers and ensure each practitioner is able to contribute fully. Three key policy levers may be used by decision makers to improve the practice environment and sustain changes in chronic care: organizational arrangements, technology and organizational culture.

Organizational arrangements

Organizational arrangements refer to formal structures, administrative policies and rewards, including wages and benefits, non-financial incentives and career development opportunities. The challenge is to ensure that supportive systems are developed to foster the changes initiated.

Traditional arrangements for providing health and social services have focused largely on the individual practitioner. In the chronic care environment, many people require a complex array of services, which, in turn, are dependent on the knowledge and competencies of a multi-skilled team. Numerous studies have linked this multidisciplinary team model with care processes, clinical outcomes and service use that are superior to those achieved by traditional care arrangements, with many of these studies evaluating the addition of nurses, social workers, psychologists and clinical pharmacists to teams (Halstead 1976; Wells et al. 2000). For instance, in general practices in England, improved teamwork is associated with better processes of care, continuity of care, access to care and satisfaction (Campbell et al. 2001; Stevenson et al. 2001). However, the extent to which practitioners can work in teams depends on prevailing organizational arrangements.

The way resources are allocated and the systems for paying providers have long been identified as bottlenecks that may compromise the effective delivery of chronic care and that play a major role in whether healthcare providers embrace or resist changes in the mix of skills and responsibilities. Payment mechanisms that are based on individual reward (such as fee for service) and focus on face-to-face visits or specific procedures discourage team-based practices and do not account for many aspects of chronic care, including record keeping and office work, travel time, counselling and communication with other team members and professionals. Practice settings where *teams* are funded, rather than individual providers, appear to generate a workforce more willing to organize care to best suit the needs of the populations they serve and to optimize the skill mix of their staff. To remove financial disincentives to interprofessional practice, flexible compensation schemes such as capitation and full or partial salary have been used in many countries (Box 7.6; see also Chapter 9).

In transforming chronic care, it is important to consider the impacts of the organizational arrangements upon staff and to think about incentives to encourage change. Gaps in clinical support systems, unreasonable administrative burdens for clinicians and limitations in information systems are all

Box 7.6 Different payment models

In Canada, blended models of payment instituted through use of the intergovernmental Primary Healthcare Transition Fund have provided the opportunity and incentive to increase the time that various members of healthcare teams spend on health promotion, disease prevention and management of chronic diseases. In Ontario and Quebec, family practice physicians have been encouraged to shift to group practice structures through a variety of alternative payment schemes that reward the achievement of targets for health promotion and disease prevention or the use of certain procedures in chronic disease management.

In England, the general practitioner contract does not directly threaten the income of general practitioners if other skill groups are used. This allows use of nurses rather than doctors to provide services such as immunization, cervical screening and health promotion. In addition, the Quality Improvement and Outcomes Framework provides incentives through a system of points for general practitioners who use best practices to work with people with long-term conditions.

In Australia, incentives for care planning and case conferencing for people with chronic disease and complex care needs were introduced in the 1999 EPC package. To qualify for a Medicare benefit, a care plan must involve at least two care providers other than the general practitioner.

examples of organizational problems that can create barriers to developing more efficient and effective approaches to chronic care. All of these factors impact on the workforce and the extent to which team members are able to adapt to service delivery changes. For instance, a lack of resources may be a key barrier for physicians to work in a multidisciplinary team environment. In one study, general practitioners identified the main barriers as time, organization, communication, education and resources (Blakeman et al. 2001). Providing adequate resources can act as a catalyst to encourage general practitioners and others to join or expand teams.

Technology

Another key lever is technology. Technology is not restricted to machines and devices but encompasses a wide range of tools such as job and role design, clinical protocols and information systems. In chronic care, information technologies provide a powerful tool to facilitate transfer of information, eliminate redundant paperwork and monitor progress (Biermann et al. 2000; Kruger et al. 2003). Decision-support and clinical information systems, such as computer systems that provide prompt feedback on performance, can improve health professionals' adherence to guidelines for a range of chronic diseases (Zwar et al. 2006; Chapter 8).

Implementation of electronic health records has often proved difficult.

However, the burgeoning volume of clinical information confronting providers of chronic care makes technology an essential tool to facilitate communication between team members and to prevent errors. Robotics, monitoring technologies and telecommunications devices are other examples of tools that have many potential applications in chronic care and could improve both service delivery and the conditions of workers' practice. However, workers may need training and support to adopt new technologies, as well as the time and capacity to reap the rewards.

Organizational culture

A less tangible but no less important, lever in improving chronic care is professional and organizational culture (Stott and Walker 1965). This includes organizational philosophy and values, management styles and the patterns of behaviour and attitudes among an organization's members. Working in an interdisciplinary team environment means that professionals have to negotiate their own value system with those of other professionals while they also deal with the overriding organizational culture. Even if there are shared values, professionals may assume that they hold substantially different values and practices to others, and these perceptions may influence relationships with other professionals and organizations.

The magnitude of change involved in transforming chronic care means that the process cannot be approached as a one-off event or a discrete organizational intervention. Rather, changing chronic care is a long evolutionary process that necessitates forging a shared vision about what the system should be, identifying the direction in which the efforts should be focused and implementing strategic actions to deliver this vision. Such evolving and complex change may profit from building an organizational culture deliberately orientated towards innovation, negotiation, experimentation, critical appraisal and continuous learning. This too has implications for the workforce: people must be given the time, skills and scope for innovation, and perhaps be rewarded for making change.

Conclusions

This chapter has outlined why workforce issues are central to the development and implementation of new ways to manage chronic care. New models of conceptualizing and delivering chronic care involve at least four factors that herald the need for significant workforce changes: integration at an individual, team and organizational level; person-centred care; population-based focus; and increased focus on quality improvement.

Improving chronic care offers many clinical and quality benefits for service users, but it also impacts on staff. These impacts, while positive in the longer term, may be seen as challenges in the short term. Investing in staff, in terms of time, training and resources, will be crucial to the success of any system or programme-level changes in chronic care.

Yet, the country case studies reviewed for this chapter (Nolte et al. 2008) suggest that, while some targeted work is being undertaken to develop new staff roles and competency frameworks, less thought may have been put into tackling the more complex aspects of workforce and organizational development. Just how can we ensure that health and social care staff work together? What will motivate a hospital consultant to point out potential gaps in the system? What needs to happen to ensure a nurse is motivated to take on and develop the ideas of service managers and planners in day-to-day practice? We do not yet know the answers to these types of question – but we need to think about the answers if we are serious about transforming chronic care.

We know that audit and feedback, practitioner education sessions, shared learning approaches and clinical guidelines have mixed success in changing behaviours. We know that competency frameworks only go some way in addressing the new skills and roles needed. And we know that we must focus on changing more than the attitudes and behaviours of individual staff or groups of professionals; for change to be implemented in whole systems, there needs to be change at structural and organizational levels.

This chapter has illustrated that there are some key levers that can motivate change and enable the successful and sustainable implementation of chronic care models from a workforce perspective. These include conceptualizing a human resources continuum with service users taking a key role, redefining professional roles, developing generic competencies and reconfiguring the practice environment. However, perhaps the most important lesson from this chapter is that *someone* must make and sustain those changes in order to change chronic care. The workforce is that "someone" – so we may need to put more effort into considering the needs, perceptions and motivators of workforces in order to facilitate sustainable change.

References

Aiken, L.H., Clarke, S.P., Sloane, D.M., Sochalski, J. and Silber, J.H. (2002) Hospital nurse staffing and patient mortality, nurse burnout, and job dissatisfaction, *JAMA*, 288: 1987–93.

Astin, J.A., Beckner, W., Soeken, K., Hochberg, M.C. and Berman, B. (2002) Psychological interventions for rheumatoid arthritis: a meta-analysis of randomized controlled trials, *Arthritis Rheum*, 47: 291–302.

Australian Medical Workforce Advisory Committee (2005) *The General Practice Workforce in Australia: Supply and Requirements to 2013*. Sydney: Australian Medical Workforce Advisory Committee.

Barlow, J.H., Williams, B. and Wright, C.C. (1999) "Instilling the strength to fight the pain and get on with life": learning to become an arthritis self-manager through an adult education programme, *Health Educ Res*, 14: 533–44.

Barlow, J.H., Bancroft, G.V. and Turner, A.P. (2005) Volunteer, lay tutors' experiences of the chronic disease self-management course: being valued and adding value, *Health Educ Res*, 20: 128–36.

Barr, V.J., Robinson, S., Marin-Link, B. et al. (2003) The expanded Chronic Care Model: an integration of concepts and strategies from population health promotion and the Chronic Care Model, *Hosp Q*, 7: 73–82.

Baumann, A. and Silverman, B. (1998) De-professionalization in health care: flattening the hierarchy, in L. Groake (eds) *The Ethics of the New Economy: Restructuring and Beyond*, pp. 203–11. Ontario: Wilfred Laurier University Press.

Bero, L.A., Grilli, R., Grimshaw, J.M. et al. (1998) Closing the gap between research and practice: an overview of systematic reviews of interventions to promote the implementation of research findings, *BMJ*, 317: 465–8.

Biermann, E., Dietrich, W. and Standl, E. (2000) Telecare of diabetic patients with intensified insulin therapy. A randomized clinical trial, *Stud Health Technol Inform*, 77: 327–32.

Bindman, A.B., Weiner, J.P. and Majeed, A. (2001) Primary care groups in the United Kingdom: quality and accountability, *Health Aff* 20: 132–45.

Blakeman, T.M., Harris, M.F., Comino, E.J. and Zwar, N.A. (2001) Evaluating general practitioners' views about the implementation of the Enhanced Primary Care Medicare items, *Med J Aust*, 175: 95–8.

Bodenheimer, T., Wagner, E.H. and Grumbach, K. (2002) Improving primary care for patients with chronic illness: the chronic care model, Part 2, *JAMA* 288: 1909–14.

Booth, J. and Hewiston, A. (2002) Role overlap between occupational therapy and physiotherapy during in-patient stroke rehabilitation: an exploratory study, *J Interprofess Care*, 16: 31–40.

Bourbeau, J., Julien, M., Maltais, F. et al. (2003) Reduction of hospital utilization in patients with chronic obstructive pulmonary disease: a disease-specific self-management intervention, *Arch Intern Med*, 163: 585–91.

Brodsky, J., Habib, J. and Mizrahi, I. (2000) *Long-term Care Laws in Five Developed Countries: A Review*. Geneva: World Health Organization.

Brooks, P. (2003) The impact of chronic illness: partnerships with other healthcare professionals, *Med J Aust*, 179: 260–62.

Brown, B., Crawford, P. and Darongkamas, J. (2000) Blurred roles and permeable boundaries: the experience of multidisciplinary working in community mental health, *Health Soc Care Community*, 8: 425–35.

Brown, S.A. and Grimes, D.E. (1995) A meta-analysis of nurse practitioners and nurse midwives in primary care, *Nurs Res*, 44: 332–9.

Campbell, S.M., Hann, M., Hacker, J. et al. (2001) Identifying predictors of high quality care in English general practice: observational study, *BMJ*, 323: 784–7.

Canadian Health Services Research Foundation (2001) *Commitment and Care: The Benefits of a Healthy Workplace for Nurses, their Patients, and the System*. Ottawa: Canadian Health Services Research Foundation.

Centre for Nursing Studies and Institute for the Advancement of Public Policy (2001) *Final Report: The Nature of the Extended/Expanded Nursing Role in Canada*. St John's, Newfoundland: Centre for Nursing Studies. http://www.cns.nf.ca/research/finalreport.htm.

Challis, D., Darton, R., Johnson, L., Stone, M. and Traske, K. (1995) *Care Management and Health Care of Older People*. Aldershot, UK: Darlington Community Care Project.

Chiang, L.C., Huang, J.L., Yeh, K.W. and Lu, C.M. (2004) Effects of a self-management asthma educational program in Taiwan based on PRECEDE–PROCEED model for parents with asthmatic children, *J Asthma*, 41: 205–15.

Clark, N.M., Nothwehr, F., Gong, M. et al. (1995) Physician–patient partnership in managing chronic illness, *Acad Med*, 70: 957–9.

Cline, C. (2002) Nurse-led clinics for heart failure in Sweden: doing the right thing? *Eur J Heart Fail*, 4: 393–4.

College of Family Physicians of Canada (2004) *Family Medicine in Canada: Vision for the Future*. Mississauga, Canada: College of Family Physicians of Canada.

Connor, C.A., Wright, C.C. and Fegan, C.D. (2002) The safety and effectiveness of a nurse-led anticoagulant service, *J Adv Nurs*, 38: 407–15.

Corcoran, M. (1997) Polypharmacy in the older patient with cancer, *Cancer Control*, 4: 419–28.

Corkery, E., Palmer, C., Foley, M.E. et al. (1997) Effects of a biocultural community health worker on diabetes education in a Hispanic population. *Diabetes Care*, 20: 254–7.

Coulter, A. and Ellins, J. (2006) *Patient-focused Interventions: A Review of the Evidence.* Oxford: Picker Institute Europe.

Department of Health (2001) *The Expert Patient: A New Approach to Chronic Disease Management for the 21st Century.* London: Department of Health.

Edwards, M. (1997) The health care assistant: usurper of nursing? *Br J Community Health Nurs*, 10: 490–4.

Emanuel, E.J. and Emanuel, L.L. (1992) Four models of the physician-patient relationship, *JAMA*, 267: 2221–6.

Enhancing Interdisciplinary Collaboration in Primary Health Care Initiative (2005) *Barriers and Facilitators to Enhancing Interdisciplinary Collaboration in Primary Health Care.* http://www.eicp.ca/en/default.asp.

Epstein, R.S. and Sherwood, L.M. (1996) From outcomes research to disease management: a guide for the perplexed, *Ann Intern Med*, 124: 832–7.

Frich, L.M. (2003) Nursing interventions for patients with chronic conditions, *J Adv Nurs*, 44: 137–53.

Gibson, P.G., Powell, H., Coughlan, J. et al. (2003) Self-management education and regular practitioner review for adults with asthma, *Cochrane Database Syst Rev*, 1: CD001117.

Gillam, S. and Schamroth, A. (2002) The community-oriented primary care experience in the United Kingdom, *Am J Public Health*, 92: 1721–5.

Glasgow, R.E., Orleans, C.T. and Wagner, E.H. (2001) Does the chronic care model serve also as a template for improving prevention? *Milbank Q*, 79: 579–612, iv–v.

Glenngård, A.H. (2005) Sweden: Health systems in transition. *Health Syst Transit*, 7: 1–126.

Griffiths, C., Foster, G., Barnes, N. et al. (2004) Specialist nurse intervention to reduce unscheduled asthma care in a deprived multiethnic area: the east London randomised controlled trial for high risk asthma (ELECTRA), *BMJ*, 328: 144.

Hainsworth, J. and Barlow, J. (2001) Volunteers' experiences of becoming arthritis self-management lay leaders: "It's almost as if I've stopped aging and started to get younger!", *Arthritis Rheum*, 45: 378–83.

Halstead, L.S. (1976) Team care in chronic illness: a critical review of the literature of the past 25 years, *Arch Phys Med Rehabil*, 57: 507–11.

Ham, C., Parker, H., Singh, D. and Wade, E. (2007) *Getting the Basics Right. Final Report on the Care Closer to Home: Making the Shift Programme.* Coventry: Institute for Innovation and Improvement.

Health Council of Canada (2005) *Modernizing the Management of Health Human Resources in Canada: Identifying Areas for Accelerated Change. Report from a National Summit.* Toronto: Health Council of Canada.

Horrocks, S., Anderson, E. and Salisbury, C. (2002) Systematic review of whether nurse practitioners working in primary care can provide equivalent care to doctors, *BMJ*, 324: 819–23.

Hussein, S. and Manthorpe, J. (2005) An international review of the long-term care workforce: policies and shortages, *J Aging Soc Policy*, 17: 75–94.

Institute of Medicine (2001) *Crossing the Quality Chasm : A New Health System for the 21st Century.* Washington, DC: National Academy Press.

Institute of Medicine (2003) *Health Professions Education: a Bridge to Quality.* Washington, DC: National Academy Press.

Institute of Medicine (2004) *Improving Medical Education: Enhancing the Behavioral and Social Science Content of Medical School Curricula.* Washington, DC: National Academy Press.

Jamtvedt, G., Young, J.M. and Kristoffersen, D. (2004) Audit and feedback: effects on professional practice and health care outcomes (Cochrane Review), in *The Cochrane Library*, Issue 2. Chichester, UK: John Wiley.

Kinnersley, P., Anderson, E., Parry, K. et al. (2000) Randomised controlled trial of nurse practitioner versus general practitioner care for patients requesting "same day" consultations in primary care, *BMJ*, 320: 1043–8.

Kobayashi, R.H., Kobayashi, A.D., Lee, N., Fischer, S. and Ochs, H.D. (1990) Home self-administration of intravenous immunoglobulin therapy in children, *Pediatrics*, 85: 705–9.

Kodner, D. (1993) *Case Management: Principles, Practice and Performance*. Brooklyn, NY: Institute for Applied Gerontology.

Kohn, L.T., Corrigan, J.M. and Donaldson, M.S. (2000) *To Err is Human: Building a Safer Health System*. Washington, DC: Institute of Medicine and National Academy Press.

Kruger, D.F., White, K., Galpern, A. et al. (2003) Effect of modem transmission of blood glucose data on telephone consultation time, clinic work flow, and patient satisfaction for patients with gestational diabetes mellitus, *J Am Acad Nurse Pract*, 15: 371–5.

Laine, C. and Davidoff, F. (1996) Patient-centered medicine. A professional evolution, *JAMA*, 275: 152–6.

Lewin, S.A., Skea, Z.C. and Entwistle, V. (2004) Interventions for providers to promote a patient-centred approach in clinical consultations, *Cochrane Database Syst Rev* 2: CD003267.

Lorig, K. and Holman, H.R. (1989) Long-term outcomes of an arthritis self-management study: effects of reinforcement efforts, *Soc Sci Med*, 29: 221–4.

Lorig, K.R., Sobel, D.S. and Stewart, A.L. (1999) Evidence suggesting that a chronic disease self-management program can improve health status while reducing utilization and costs: A randomized trial, *Med Care*, 37: 5–14.

Loveman, E., Royle, P. and Waugh, N. (2003) Specialist nurses in diabetes mellitus, *Cochrane Database Syst Rev*, 2: CD003286.

Lynn, J., Schuster, J.L., The Center to Improve Care of the Dying and the Institute for Healthcare Improvement (2000) *Improving Care for the End of Life: A Sourcebook for Clinicians and Managers*. New York: Oxford University Press.

McDonald, H.P., Garg, A.X. and Haynes, R.B. (2002) Interventions to enhance patient adherence to medication prescriptions: scientific review, *JAMA*, 288: 2868–79.

McDonald, M., McPhee, P.D. and Walker, R.J. (1995) Successful self-care home dialysis in the elderly: a single center's experience, *Perit Dial Int*, 15: 33–6.

McKee, M., Dubois, C.A. and Sibbald, B. (2006) Changing professional boundaries, in C.A. Dubois, M. McKee and E. Nolte (eds) *Human Resources for Health in Europe*, pp.63–78. Maidenhead: Open University Press.

Ministry of Health Planning (2003) *A Framework for a Provincial Chronic Disease Prevention Initiative*. Victoria, BC: Population Health and Wellness.

Montani, S., Bellazzi, R., Quaglini, S. and d'Annunzio, G. (2001) Meta-analysis of the effect of the use of computer-based systems on the metabolic control of patients with diabetes mellitus, *Diabetes Technol Ther* 3: 347–56.

Montori, V.M., Helgemoe, P.K., Guyatt, G.H. et al. (2004) Telecare for patients with type 1 diabetes and inadequate glycemic control: a randomized controlled trial and meta-analysis, *Diabetes Care*, 27: 1088–94.

Moote, C. (1993) Techniques for post-op pain management in the adult, *Can J Anaesth*, 40: R19–28.

Munro, N., Felton, A. and McIntosh, C. (2002) Is multidisciplinary learning effective among those caring for people with diabetes? *Diabet Med* 19: 799–803.

Nancarrow, S. (2004) Dynamic role boundaries in intermediate care services, *J Interprof Care*, 18: 141–51.

Neumeyer-Gromen, A., Lampert, T., Stark, K. and Kallischnigg, G. (2004) Disease management programs for depression: a systematic review and meta-analysis of randomized controlled trials, *Med Care*, 42: 1211–21.

Nodhturft, V., Schneider, J.M., Hebert, P. et al. (2000) Chronic disease self-management: improving health outcomes, *Nurs Clin North Am*, 35: 507–18.

Nolte, E., Knai, C. and McKee, M. (eds) (2008) Managing Chronic conditions: experience in eight countries. Copenhagen: European Observatory on Health Systems and Policies.

Norris, S.L., Glasgow, R.E. and Engelgau, M.M. (2003) Chronic disease management. A definition and systematic approach to component interventions, *Dis Manage Health Outcomes*, 11: 477–88.

Orne, R.M., Garland, D., O'Hara, M., Perfetto, L. and Stielau, J. (1998) Caught in the cross fire of change: nurses' experience with unlicensed assistive personnel, *Appl Nurs Res*, 11: 101–10.

Osman, L.M., Calder, C., Godden, D.J. et al. (2002) A randomised trial of self-management planning for adult patients admitted to hospital with acute asthma, *Thorax*, 57: 869–74.

Ostbye, T., Yarnall, K.S., Krause, K.M. et al. (2005) Is there time for management of patients with chronic diseases in primary care? *Ann Fam Med*, 3: 209–14.

Ouwens, M., Wollersheim, H., Hermens, R., Hulscher, M. and Grol, R. (2005) Integrated care programmes for chronically ill patients: a review of systematic reviews, *Int J Qual Health Care*, 17: 141–6.

Oxman, A.D., Thomson, M.A., Davis, D.A. and Haynes, R.B. (1995) No magic bullets: a systematic review of 102 trials of interventions to improve professional practice, *CMAJ*, 153: 1423–31.

Piette, J.D., McPhee, S.J., Weinberger, M., Mah, C.A. and Kraemer, F.B. (1999) Use of automated telephone disease management calls in an ethnically diverse sample of low-income patients with diabetes, *Diabetes Care*, 22: 1302–9.

Pong, R.W., Saunders, D., Church, J., Wanke, M. and Cappon, P. (1995) *Health Human Resources in Community-based Health Care: A Review of the Literature*. Health Canada, Health Promotion and Programs Branch.

Pratt, L.R. (2006) Long-term conditions 5: meeting the needs of highly complex patients, *Br J Community Nurs*, 11(6): 234–5, 238–40.

Productivity Commission (2005) *Australia's Health Workforce*. Canberra: Productivity Commission.

Pruitt, S.D. and Epping-Jordan, J.E. (2005) Preparing the 21st century global healthcare workforce, *BMJ*, 330(7492): 637–9.

Quill, T.E. and Brody, H. (1996) Physician recommendations and patient autonomy: finding a balance between physician power and patient choice, *Ann Intern Med*, 125(9): 763–9.

Richardson, G., Maynard, A., Cullum, N. and Kindig, D. (1998) Skill mix changes: substitution or service development? *Health Policy*, 45: 119–32.

Robertson, M.K., Umble, K.E. and Cervero, R.M. (2003) Impact studies in continuing education for health professions: update, *J Contin Educ Health Prof*, 23: 146–56.

Schreiber, R., MacDonald, M., Davidson, H. et al. (2003) Advanced nursing practice: opportunities and challenges in British Columbia. Victoria, BC: Canadian Health Services Resource Foundation. http://www.chsrf.ca/final_research/ogc/pdf/schreiber_report.pdf.

Sibbald, B., Shen, J. and McBride, A. (2004) Changing the skill-mix of the health care workforce, *J Health Serv Res Policy*, 9(Suppl 1): 28–38.

Singh, D. (2005a) *Which Staff Improve Care for People with Long-term Conditions? A Rapid Review of the Literature.* Birmingham: University of Birmingham and NHS Modernisation Agency.

Singh, D. (2005b) *Transforming Chronic Care.* Birmingham: University of Birmingham and Surrey and Sussex PCT Alliance.

Smith, S., Bury, G., O'Leary, M. et al. (2004) The North Dublin randomized controlled trial of structured diabetes shared care, *Fam Pract*, 21: 39–45.

Smits, P.B., Verbeek, J.H. and de Buisonje, C.D. (2002) Problem based learning in continuing medical education: a review of controlled evaluation studies, *BMJ*, 324: 153–6.

Sperl-Hillen, J., O'Connor, P.J., Carlson, R.R. et al. (2000) Improving diabetes care in a large health care system: an enhanced primary care approach, *Jt Comm J Qual Improv*, 26: 615–22.

Stevenson, K., Baker, R., Farooqi, A., Sorrie, R. and Khunti, K. (2001) Features of primary health care teams associated with successful quality improvement of diabetes care: a qualitative study, *Fam Pract*, 18: 21–6.

Stott, K. and Walker, A. (1965) *Times, Teamwork and Teambuilding.* New York: Prentice-Hall.

Stromberg, A., Martensson, J., Fridlund, B. and Dahlstrom, U. (2001) Nurse-led heart failure clinics in Sweden, *Eur J Heart Fail*, 3: 139–44.

Stromberg, A., Martensson, J., Fridlund, B. et al. (2003) Nurse-led heart failure clinics improve survival and self-care behaviour in patients with heart failure: results from a prospective, randomised trial, *Eur Heart J*, 24: 1014–23.

Struthers, R., Hodge, F.S., De Cora, L. and Geishirt-Cantrell, B. (2003) The experience of native peer facilitators in the campaign against type 2 diabetes, *J Rural Health*, 19: 174–80.

Stubblefield, C. and Mutha, S. (2002) Provider-patient roles in chronic disease management, *J Allied Health*, 31: 87–92.

Szasz, T.S. and Hollender, M.H. (1956) A contribution to the philosophy of medicine; the basic models of the doctor-patient relationship, *AMA Arch Intern Med*, 97: 585–92.

Von Korff, M., Gruman, J., Schaefer, J., Curry, S.J. and Wagner, E.H. (1997) Collaborative management of chronic illness, *Ann Intern Med*, 127: 1097–102.

Vrijhoef, H.J., Diederiks, J.P. and Spreeuwenberg, C. (2000) Effects on quality of care for patients with NIDDM or COPD when the specialised nurse has a central role: a literature review, *Patient Educ Couns*, 41: 243–50.

Wagner, E.H. (1998) Chronic disease management: what will it take to improve care for chronic illness? *Eff Clin Pract* 1: 2–4.

Wagner, E.H., Austin, B.T., Davis, C. et al. (2001) Improving chronic illness care: translating evidence into action, *Health Aff*, 20: 64–78.

Wakefield, M.K. (2004) *Institute of Medicine Committee on the Future of Rural Health Care. Quality through Collaboration: The Future of Rural Health Care.* Washington DC: National Academy Press.

Wells, K.B., Sherbourne, C., Schoenbaum, M. et al. (2000) Impact of disseminating quality improvement programs for depression in managed primary care: a randomized controlled trial, *JAMA*, 283: 212–20.

Whitmer, A., Seifer, S.D., Finnochio, L., Leslie, J. and O'Neil, E. (1995) Community health workers: integral members of the health care workforce, *Am J Public Health*, 85: 1055–8.

WHO (2005) *Preparing a Workforce for the 21st Century: The Challenge of Chronic Conditions.* Geneva: World Health Organization.

WHO (2002b) *Current and Future Long-term Care Needs, an Analysis Based on the 1990 WHO Study, The Global Burden of Disease.* Geneva: World Health Organization.

WHO (2002c) *Human Resources and National Health Systems. Shaping the Agenda for Action.* Geneva: World Health Organization.

WHO (2002a) *Innovative Care for Chronic Conditions: Building Blocks for Action*. Geneva: World Health Organization.

WHO (2006) *Working Together for Health: the World. Health Report 2006*. Geneva: World Health Organization.

Wunderlich, G. and Kohler, P. (2001) *Improving the Quality of Long-term Care*. Washington, DC: National Academy Press.

Zwar, N., Harris, M., Griffiths, R. et al. (2006) *A Systematic Review of Chronic Disease Management*. Canberra: Australian Primary Health Care Research Institute.

chapter eight

Decision support

Nicholas Glasgow, Isabelle Durand-Zaleski, Elisabeth Chan and Dhigna Rubiano

Introduction

In their seminal 1996 paper *Organizing Care for Patients with Chronic Illness*, Wagner and colleagues (1996) identified comprehensive approaches to care that improved outcomes for patients with chronic illness. They were able to cluster the various common elements in successful approaches in five general areas:

- the use of explicit plans and protocols
- the reorganization of the practice to meet the needs of patients who require more time, a broad array of resources, and closer follow-up
- systematic attention to the information and behavioural-change needs of patients
- ready access to necessary expertise
- supportive information systems.

Here, "decision support" sits within the "expert system" field; it aims to support the decision making of clinicians and is clearly linked to the existing and potential roles electronic communications systems may play in facilitating evidence-based practice (Wagner et al. 1996). More recent iterations of the Chronic Care Model see decision support aiming to "promote clinical care that is consistent with scientific evidence and patient preferences" (Improving Chronic Illness Care 2007) and encompassing strategies that:

- embed evidence-based guidelines into daily clinical practice
- share evidence-based guidelines and information with patients to encourage their participation
- use proven provider education methods
- integrate specialist expertise and primary care.

In his 2003 review of literature on the effectiveness of the components of the Chronic Care Model, Bodenheimer (2003) stated that decision support "involves availability to all clinicians of the best evidence-based knowledge through clinical practice guidelines and physician education".

Those making treatment decisions remain the focus of decision support strategies and tools, although it is acknowledged that these tools may well be used by clinicians in discussions with patients to enhance their patients' understanding of their conditions and their management. Through use of these tools, including evidence-based clinical practice guidelines or protocols and/or clinical pathways, clinical care processes are more likely to be standardized, thereby reducing variation in healthcare, increasing quality outcomes and reducing medical error.

We here explore the strategies and tools that are included in discussions of decision support. We begin with a general overview of decision support and consider the intended "targets" for decision support activities and the increasing importance of e-health in underpinning decision support interventions. We conclude that decision support embraces a broad array of interventions, increasingly reliant on electronic systems for their delivery but having the common purpose of increasing the quality of chronic disease care through the standardization of the delivery of care in accord with best evidence-based practice while containing costs.

Next we consider the connections between wider "e-health" agenda and decision support within the context of chronic disease management. The use of e-health is an essential enabler for the delivery of high-quality chronic disease care, and, therefore, countries must ensure that the necessary e-health building blocks are in place. We discuss computerized clinical decision support systems (CCDSS) in some detail because they are the building blocks for e-health, are supported by an increasing evidence base and provide a means of identifying some challenges that need to be addressed to move forward. In this section, we consider electronic guidelines for clinicians, computerized decision supports directed at enhancing self-management and electronic health records.

Finally we summarize the key challenges for going forward and suggest some priorities for future research.

The scope of decision support for chronic disease management

Decision support strategies and tools

In general, the term decision support denotes any approach that supports healthcare decision making. The Chronic Care Model places the main focus for decision support strategies and tools on clinicians. This focus for decision support has, however, been broadened to include actions directed at other roles within the health system.

Chronic diseases account for approximately 70% of healthcare costs and affect approximately 20% of Western populations; increasing healthcare expenditures are expected as the number of elderly people living with one or more chronic conditions greatly increases. It is clear that not only clinicians but also patients, healthcare organizations and policy makers are all engaged indirectly in decision making and are, therefore, also appropriate targets for decision support systems and tools.

The overall goal of decision support in chronic care remains the same regardless of the target chosen: improving the quality of care given to patients with chronic diseases while containing healthcare costs.

We have reviewed the literature on chronic care and on decision support and have identified the different interests that four groups working in the health system would have in respect of a comprehensive decision support system targeting that group (Table 8.1). As most studies identified (descriptive or experimental) are context specific, this table is intended to give readers a sense of the inherent diversity and to facilitate adaptation to their own context.

One lesson is that the stakeholders may have different expectations and conflicting agendas. Planning the design and implementation of a decision support system for one or several chronic conditions, therefore, requires an initial study of the implications for each stakeholder, building this information into the process of choosing between the different priorities.

Table 8.1 provides a tentative list of the elements to take into account when considering the implementation of a decision support system for chronic conditions. It is not clear from the studies that there is a uniform model for leadership of system implementation. The most common model seems to be initiated by clinicians (Kawamoto et al. 2005) for themselves or colleagues in primary care or academic centres. This could be termed a bottom-up model. Top-down models are also seen, for example where excessive prescribing was identified by the financing administration as part of a package of interventions designed to reduce prescriptions.

Most activity to date has concentrated on decision supports targeting only the clinician. One of the challenges in going forward is to design, implement and evaluate a variety of strategies and tools that can facilitate quality decision making by all those involved in the delivery of chronic disease care.

Conceptualizing decision support

Decision support is broadly conceptualized in the literature. Objectives of decision support systems have been proposed: Imhoff et al. (2001) commenting that clinical decision support "aims at providing healthcare professionals with therapy guidelines directly at the point of care", and Coiera (2003) stating that clinical decision support systems "are by and large intended to support healthcare workers in the normal course of their duties, assisting with tasks that rely on the manipulation of data and knowledge".

Some authors specifically distinguish between the more individualized decision support systems and generic practice guidelines and critical pathways. Trowbridge and Weingarten (2001) noted how decision support systems require the input of patient-specific clinical variables and produce patient-specific recommendations, whereas guidelines and pathways typically provide more general suggestions for care and treatment. Liu et al. (2006) supported this differentiation by defining a clinical decision tool as "an active knowledge resource that uses patient data to generate case-specific advice which supports

Table 8.1 Factors relevant to decision support system design for different health system actors

	Patients	Health professionals	Healthcare organizations	Health policy makers (scope)
Description	Single chronic condition or multiple chronic conditions	Physicians, nurses, pharmacists, allied health professionals, peer instructors	Primary care services, multidisciplinary teams, ambulatory care services, emergency services, acute admissions, managers	Reimbursement; organization of healthcare; continuing (medical) education, career enhancement for health professionals
Characteristics	Well-informed, activated, preference-sensitive decisions	Prepared, proactive	Patient registration and chronic disease registers; continuity of care; linkage of health services to social services	Centralized/decentralized decision and financing
Outcome measures	Behavioural outcomes (subjective); clinical outcomes (objective, e.g. mortality, complications, HbA1c level, blood pressure); patient satisfaction; quality of life; self-efficacy; social support	Behavioural outcomes; process outcomes (quality of care, e.g. number of eye examinations, number of HbA1C blood samples)	Process outcomes: quality of care (e.g. number of emergency room visits, number of specialist consultations); avoidable admission rate	Economic outcomes (cost-effectiveness): direct and indirect costs

HbA1c, glycosylated haemoglobin.

decision making about individual patients by health professionals, the patient themselves or other concerned about them". They identify four distinctive components in clinical decision tools:

- *the target decision maker*: the tool is designed to aid a clinical decision by a health professional and/or patient
- *the target decision*: the decisions concern an individual patient
- *the knowledge component*: the tool uses patient data and knowledge to generate an interpretation that aids clinical decision making
- *the timing*: the tool is used before the health professional or patient takes the relevant decision.

In order to improve understanding of the diversity of decision tools Liu et al. (2006) proposed a typology that enables a conceptualization of the relationships between various clinical decision tools in three broad categories: paper based, electronic based and mechanical (Figure 8.1). Although these categories have some utility in a conceptual sense, they are not in fact mutually exclusive. For example, practice guidelines, care pathways and checklists may all be presented in an electronic format while tables of pre- and post-test probabilities may be presented in card format.

In summary, the notion of decision support can be seen to embrace a broad array of interventions. Some have typically been paper based, such as guidelines and care pathways. Some are delivered through computerized systems, including

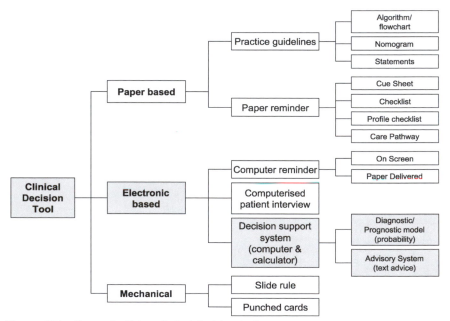

Figure 8.1 Conceptualizing clinical decision tools.

Source: Adapted from Liu J, Wyatt JC, Altman D (2006) Decision tools in healthcare: focus on the problem, not the solution, BMC Medical Informatics and Decision Making 6:4, published through BioMed Central.

prompts and more complex prognostic tools. Some are in the form of educational activities delivered to clinicians or patients through a variety of educational technologies. All are becoming increasingly reliant on electronic systems for their delivery, and all have the common purpose of increasing the quality of chronic disease care through the standardization of the delivery of that care in accordance with best evidence-based practice while containing costs (Table 8.2).

Clinical decision support systems

The Healthcare Information and Management Systems Society defined clinical decision support (Osheroff et al. 2005) as:

> . . . providing clinicians or patients with clinical knowledge and patient-related information, intelligently filtered or presented at appropriate times, to enhance patient care. Clinical knowledge of interest could range from simple facts and relationship to best practices for managing patients with specific disease states, new medical knowledge from clinical research and other types of information.

There are many types of support system. They may be paper based or, increasingly, computer based. A useful categorization of various clinical decision support interventions has been suggested by the Healthcare Information and Management Systems Society (see Table 8.3 below). Decision support mechanisms increase in complexity and in stakeholder involvement.

Paper-based approaches

The simplest forms of support (often paper based) improve physicians' ordering behaviour but do not address issues of continuity of care and patient empowerment. The benefits may be limited to a single episode of care and the tool is a top-down system that does not promote physician or patient education. Context-sensitive support systems are certainly more complex to build and implement, not only because of the technical requirement to incorporate past episodes of care but also because they require cooperation by all stakeholders concerned.

Computerized systems

The evolution of CCDSS since the early 1990s mirrors the evolution of the goals of health policy decision makers: from guideline implementation to patient empowerment.

The boundaries between paper-based systems and electronic based systems are blurred. For example, CCDSS were rapidly identified as the most effective tool for guideline implementation, achieving better professional compliance than continuing medical education, audits or paper reminders (Agence Nationale d'Accrédition et d'Évaluation en Santé 2000). The Australian Department of

Table 8.2 Clinical decision support intervention types

Clinical decision support type	Subtypes	(Stated) benefits
Forms and templates	Prompts for information collection required for advanced DS	Complete document for quality/continuity of care, reimbursement, legal
	Clinician encounter documentation forms	Complete orders
	Patient self-assessment forms prior to encounter	Facilitates other data-driven decision supports
Relevant data presentation	Patient-specific data display for general data review	Optimizes decision-making by ensuring all pertinent data are considered
	Patient-specific data display for context during clinical ordering	
	Situation-specific data display relevant to a setting or a condition	
	Costs and order display	
	Retrospective reporting	
Proactive order suggestions and order sets	Prompts for correct and complete orders and related situation-specific documentation	Makes the right thing the easiest to do
	Condition-specific orders; fully specified or pick lists, fill-in the blank	Ensures that a situation is addressed completely
	Consequent orders: tests (for follow up), interventions (rescue drugs)	Prevents errors of omission
	User-requested access to decision logic/critiquing	Promotes standardization of orders
	Recommendations on preferred diagnostic and treatment interventions	
Support for guidelines, complex protocols, algorithms, clinical pathways	Stepwise processing of multi-step protocol or guideline	Makes the right things the easiest
	Checks ensuring that management protocols are followed in a long-term process	Helps avoid omission errors in care processes stretching over time
	Time-based reminders	
Reference information and guidance	Context-insensitive delivery of reference and guidance materials	Addresses recognized information needs of patients and clinicians
	Context-sensitive delivery of reference and guidance materials	
Reactive alerts (unsolicited by patient or clinical recipient)	Alerts to prevent potential errors	Prevents errors of omission or commission because of unrecognized knowledge needs of physicians or patients
	Alerts to foster preferred or optimal orders and care plans	
	Alerts to promote more cost-effective orders	

Source: Adapted from table 'Clinical decision support intervention types' in HIMSS 2004 guidebook.

Health and Ageing report *Electronic Decision Support for Australia's Health Sector* (National Electronic Decision Support Taskforce 2003) outlined a typology classification of electronic decision support developed from work undertaken by the National Health Information Management Advisory Council and the National Institute of Clinical Studies (Box 8.1). Clearly the technical complexity inherent in each of these types progressively increases.

Careful planning is an important prerequisite when developing any computerized clinical decision support system. The different steps in the development and implementation of these systems are presented in Figure 8.2.

The potential for electronic systems to deliver clinical decision support ranges from the simple presentation of information (such as providing the treatment requirements for diabetic patients drawn from national or international guidelines, without specific reference to the actual patient, doctor or setting) to increasingly complex functionality such as "expert systems" and "machine learning systems" (Coiera 2003). Expert systems contain specific knowledge, typically presented as a set of rules, and are able to combine data from individual patients to propose a decision. Machine learning systems hypothesize relationships within raw data, with some newer technologies even enabling complex characterization of those relationships to be produced. This kind of system is similar to those that Imhoff et al. (2001) referred to as "statistical and artificially intelligent methods".

According to Imhoff et al. (2001), the three methodologies employed to acquire the medical knowledge (the necessary rules and facts) required for a decision support system to operate are:

- traditional expert systems: gathering information from experts in the field
- evidence-based methods: evaluation of available medical knowledge,

Box 8.1   Electronic decision support for Australia's health sector

This has been divided into four types (National Electronic Decision Support Taskforce (2003).

Type 1 provides categorized information that requires further processing and analysis before decisions can be made.

Type 2 presents the clinician with trends of patients' changing clinical status and alerts clinicians to out-of-range assessments and intervention strategies. Clinicians are prompted to review the alerts before arriving at a decision.

Type 3 uses deductive inference engines to operate on a specific knowledge base and automatically generates diagnostic or intervention recommendations based on the changing clinical condition of the patient.

Type 4 uses more complex knowledge management and inference models such as case management reasoning, neural network or statistical discrimination analysis to perform outcome or prognostic predictions. These systems have self-learning capabilities and use advanced mathematical models to deal intelligently and accurately.

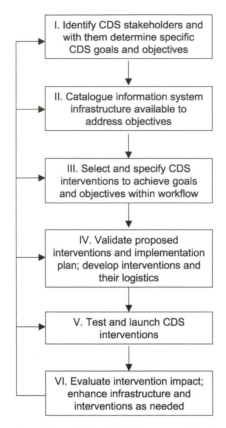

Figure 8.2 Summary of applying clinical decision support to improve outcomes in healthcare organizations.

Source: Adapted from Osheroff et al. (2005).

therapeutic procedures, methods and established behaviour with reference to healthcare decisions
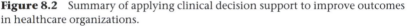
- statistical and artificial intelligence methods: time series analysis combined with methods for knowledge discovery in large databases and applied to a standard clinical information system.

In general, characteristics associated with the development of CCDSS are organizational and technical. The development of CCDSS is favoured by having consistent guidelines and reimbursement systems that do not create conflicting incentives. Optimal CCDSS provide timely information, with data automatically retrieved from the electronic medical record and with their output readily useable in the form of a recommended action, and they are integrated into the clinical workflow (Kawamoto et al. 2005). Criteria that need to be considered in developing CCDSS innovations include:

- patient-specific capabilities

- an interactive interface (e.g. generates feedback and evaluates physician performance)
- occurrence at the point of care: the information needs to be available at the place and time of the physician–patient encounter
- evolutionary system: the system needs to be able to include new features as the requirements of the patients and the physicians evolve, for example through the natural history of the disease or through changes in the ability to use CDSS
- integration into the daily clinical workflow
- integration into the electronic health record
- respect for physician autonomy
- adaptability to patient preference-sensitive subgroups.

Barriers that need to be addressed from the clinician's perspective in order to implement CCDSS into clinical workflow include:

- physician reluctance
- poor computer literacy
- workable guidelines for use in daily practice
- physicians' sense of ownership of guidelines (Kawamoto et al. 2005; Nies et al. 2006).

Chronic disease management and e-health policy initiatives

Managing chronic diseases in the manner envisaged by the Chronic Care Model requires the development, implementation and operation of e-health systems, seen as essential enablers for the delivery of quality chronic disease care.

Implementing e-health policies is expensive. Advances in computer technology occur frequently, and the potential of the latest technology may be grasped before the now "old" technology has been fully exploited. Innovations in e-health often take place within the context of health service reform. Those affected by the proposed changes may be reform weary and, therefore, resistant to change. All of these factors potentially come into play when new interventions in clinical decision support systems are considered.

Examples of e-health platforms

Many developed countries are investing substantial resources in e-health programmes. The increasing burden of chronic disease is one of the key policy drivers for these investments; consequently, many e-health programmes contain elements directly relevant to chronic disease. The e-health platforms in Canada (Canada Health Infoway 2007), Denmark (Medcom 2007), the United Kingdom (NHS Connecting for Health 2007) and Australia (Health Connect 2007), and the recently proposed French plan for the improvement of the quality of life of people with chronic diseases that has as one of its objectives the establishment of an Internet portal for chronic conditions (Ministère de la Santé et des Solidarités 2007), are all examples within which components relevant to chronic disease management can be identified. The stated objectives for these platforms include improving access, increasing patient participation, increasing efficiency of delivery and improving care coordination. These platforms may include guidelines for professionals, information on diseases for patients, patient education programmes and eligibility criteria for benefits. The technical requirements are described below. A further common feature of these systems is a very high level of governance (Ministry of Health or equivalent level), which is consistent with the high stakes in terms of trust and confidentiality.

Examples of e-health building blocks

These programmes identify essential "building blocks" in an e-health system. The following building blocks are considered essential for the delivery of optimal chronic disease care:

- adequate infrastructure, e.g. broadband connectivity, suitable software and hardware
- agreed technical standards, e.g. for sharing of clinical information
- ability to identify individuals (patients and healthcare practitioners) across the healthcare system with reliability and validity
- adequate protections on access to sensitive clinical information
- interoperable electronic health records
- CCDSS.

It is beyond the scope of this chapter to consider all of these in detail. We will however look at CCDSS in detail as these are fundamental to the future of decision support systems.

Computerized clinical decision support in chronic disease management

The use of CCDSS is particularly relevant for chronic disorders. Effective management requires the timely application of evidence-based interventions over time by a healthcare team. In diabetes, for example, decision support systems seek to optimize patient care by ensuring proactive assessments of serum glycosylated haemoglobin (HbA1c) and other relevant clinical measures, foot examinations, eye examinations, dietary advice, exercise advice and medication. The targets of decision support systems include physicians (both hospital and community based) and other members of the multidisciplinary team – nurses, pharmacists, and allied health professionals – as well as those with healthcare management responsibilities.

CCDSS can thus address many aspects of the management of a patient with chronic disease: test ordering, drug dosage adjustment, patient education, coordination, organization of care, assurance of quality of care and facilitating efficiency within the delivery of care. Existing CCDSS combine some of the following:

- alerts and reminders (e.g. test ordering, recall of patients with particular characteristics for clinic visits)
- care plans, organization of care processes
- decision aids (e.g. drug dosing, drug–drug interactions and order entry prompts advising of potential conflicts) and problem solving provided at the time of the consultation based on real-time patient information
- information retrieval
- assessment of practitioner performance.

Several innovative computer-based decision support approaches have been implemented in chronic care settings. We here consider three approaches illustrating innovations designed to (1) support decision making in practice, (2) enhance self-management and (3) reach out to the wider health system (shared electronic health records). For each of these we briefly summarize their role, the evidence base underpinning this role, and potential areas for future development.

Supporting decision making: computerized systems

Practice guidelines for the management of chronic diseases exist in all countries included in the accompanying volume of case studies. Electronic guidelines are available online but on their own are far from sufficient to produce workable CCDSS. During the design process, guidelines must be written in a way that allows their translation into computerized guidelines. The transition from paper-based guidelines to a CCDSS (Aguirre-Junco et al. 2004; Maviglia et al. 2003) requires:

- making choices on which parts of the guideline will and will not be automated
- deciding the knowledge content of the guideline
- implementing the computerized guideline after encoding in a computer-interpretable guideline format
- integrating the automated guideline into the clinical workflow
- tests and validation; evaluation.

Practitioners require recommendations drawn from guidelines to be patient specific. This means that within the CCDSS there must be linkage between the guideline and the patient electronic record. The structure of electronic patient records and guidelines should be compatible (Barretto et al. 2003).

Evidence of effectiveness

CCDSS have been evaluated in the following conditions: hypertension, diabetes, depression, heart failure, asthma and chronic obstructive pulmonary disease, osteoarthritis and end-stage renal disease.

An early systematic review by Hunt et al. (1998) considered the effects of CCDSS on both healthcare practitioner performance and patient outcome. Practitioner performance was assessed as the frequency of compliance with existing guidelines. For chronic conditions such as hypertension, diabetes, heart failure, and for long-term treatments such as anticoagulation for atrial fibrillation or valve replacement, CCDSS uniformly increased compliance with guidelines. The effect on patient outcome was either not measured or moderate. Comparable results were found in subsequent reviews (Garg et al. 2005; Kawamoto et al. 2005). Findings of reported evaluations on the effect of decision supports in clinical practice are summarized in Table 8.3.

Users' opinions are generally positive and favour computerized guidelines over paper-based guidelines. Common problems identified in these studies included poor training or limited computer literacy, reluctance to use the system during patient consultation and limited scope of the problems covered by the CCDSS. However, it must be remembered that many of these studies were undertaken at a time when computers were less deeply entrenched in everyday life than is now the case.

Challenges

The coexistence of more than one chronic condition is very common, particularly for people over the age of 50 years. Two key challenges arise from this: how to construct guidelines that include common comorbidities and how to ensure that, when the guidelines are applied to a particular individual, the CCDSS prompts patient specific information (Van Weel and Schellevis 2006).

Supporting self-management: interactive health communication

One way to make use of electronic connectivity to enhance self-management is through the application of telehealth (Murray et al. 2005): "Interactive Health Communication Applications (IHCAs) are computer-based, usually web-based, information packages for patients that combine health information with at least one of social support, decision support, or behaviour change support." TeleHealth (IHCA) functions include to:

- relay information
- enable informed decision making
- promote health behaviours
- promote peer information exchange and emotional support
- promote self-care
- manage demand on health services.

Because there have been a number of developments in this area, we will discuss it in detail

Evidence of effectiveness

The use of telehealth in chronic diseases has been facilitated by technological developments, greater familiarity with information technology, better information infrastructures and access to the Worldwide Web (Bodenheimer et al. 2002).

Table 8.3 Evidence for the effectiveness of computerized clinical decision support systems

Reference with abbreviated title	Study design	Condition/ treatment	Target	Type of intervention	Patient outcomes		Quality of care	Reduced healthcare costs/use of servicse
					Objective	Subjective		
Garg et al. (2005) Effects of computerized clinical decision support systems	Systematic review	n/a	Physicians	CDSS			+	
O'Connor et al. (2003) Decision aids for people facing health treatment or screening decisions[a]	Systematic review	n/a	Patients	Computer and web-based decision aids		+		–
Eccles et al. (2002) Effect of computerized evidence-based guidelines on management of asthma and angina in adults	RCT	Asthma, angina	GPs	Computerized guidelines	–	–	–	–
Manotti et al. (2001) Effect of computer-aided management on the quality of anticoagulation treatment	RCT	Oral anticoagulant treatment	Physicians in anticoagulant clinic	Computer aided dosing	+		+	+
Rollman et al. (2002) Computerized decision support to improve treatment of major depression in primary care	RCT	Major depression	GPs	CDSS with diagnostic and feedback on treatment	–		–	
McCowan et al. (2001) Lessons from a trial to evaluate computer decision support software to improve the management of asthma	RCT	Asthma	GPs	CDSS	~			~

(Continued Overleaf)

Table 8.3 Continued

Reference with abbreviated title	Study design	Condition/treatment	Target	Type of intervention	Patient outcomes		Quality of care	Reduced healthcare costs/use of servicse
					Objective	Subjective		
Murray et al. (2004) Failure of computerized treatment suggestions to improve health outcomes of outpatients with uncomplicated hypertension	RCT	Hyper-tension	Physicians, pharmacists	Evidence-based treatment suggestions using eHR	–	–	–	
Tierney et al. (2005) Can computer-generated evidence care suggestions enhance evidence-based management of asthma and chronic obstructive pulmonary disease?	RCT	Asthma, COPD	GPs	Computer-based evidence care suggestions	–	–	–	–
Lester et al. (2006) Trial of an informatics-based intervention to increase statin prescription for secondary prevention of coronary disease	RCT	Ischaemic heart disease	GPs	CDSS	+		+	
Plaza et al. (2005) Cost-effectiveness of an intervention based on the Global Initiative for Asthma recommendations using a computerized clinical decision support system	RCT	Asthma	Specialists and GPs	Specialists and CDSS		+		+

CDSS, computerized clinical decision support systems; RCT, randomized controlled trial; n/a, not applicable; eHR, electronic health resource; COPD, chronic obstructive pulmonary disease; GP, general practitioner; +, intervention improves the outcome; ~,intervention does not show any effect on the outcome; –, intervention has a negative effect on the outcome.
[a]This majority of studies included in this review concerned cancer screening and treatment; additionally, 25% of the decision aids reviewed were not computer/ web based. However, the review provided important evidence on the use of decision aids for patients and is, therefore, included here.

Yet despite applications in many chronic conditions, evidence of effectiveness is limited (Table 8.4), although neither is there evidence of negative effects.

Telehealth interventions might also influence the healthcare system beyond chronic care by restructuring relationships among providers, between providers and payers and between providers and patients. For example, many existing reimbursement schedules fail to allow for reimbursement of education and Internet interactions and new health services that are not currently included in existing benefit schedules. An understanding of the need for reform of financing systems and the traditional relationship between healthcare providers is key to success (Park 2006).

Another important outcome for a telehealth programme is its potential ability to improve access to healthcare, not only in terms of geographical access but also for those populations that have traditionally been disadvantaged, such as the elderly, minorities or indigent populations. For example, a recent randomized controlled trial of the use of telemedicine case management found improvements in glycaemic control of elderly patients with diabetes in areas designated as "medically underserved" in the state of New York (Shea et al. 2006).

Supporting health systems: electronic health records

Electronic health records (eHR) serve a number of functions:

- patient care delivery
- patient care management
- patient care support processes
- financial and administrative processes
- patient self-management.

Effective chronic care may ultimately require the widespread availability of electronic health records that can be used as a communication vehicle linking health professionals and patients. When coupled with Internet decision supports, this has been seen as a means to improve the organization of healthcare delivery, in the light of concerns that demands on healthcare practitioners' time have increased (Mechanic 2001).

> Many excellent suggestions exist for how doctors can use the Internet to communicate with patients, to provide information through a practice website, and to link patients with useful, valid, and relevant sources of information. . . . Such communication can facilitate information flow, allow better scheduling of appointments to prevent discontinuity, and avoid gaps in communication. It may also reduce unnecessary appointments, save the patient and doctor time and inconvenience, and contribute to health education and patient responsibility. . . .Combining these technologies with ancillary staff provide the basis for more effective practice designs.

Evidence of effectiveness

Two studies show some improvement in the care process associated with introduction of electronic health records but no effect on subjective or objective

Table 8.4 Evidence of effectiveness of telehealth and interactive health communication applications

Reference with abbreviated title	Study design	Condition/treatment	Target	Type of intervention	Patient outcomes		Quality of care	Reduced healthcare costs/use of services
					Objective	Subjective		
Lewis (1999) Computer-based approaches to patient education	Systematic review	Chronic disease (45% of studies)	Patients	Computer-based patient education		+		
Murray et al. (2005) Interactive health communication applications for people with chronic disease	Systematic review	AIDS/HIV Alzheimer's disease, asthma, diabetes	Patients	IHCA (computer web based)	+	+		
Currell et al. (2000) Telemedicine versus face to face patient care: effects on professional practice and healthcare outcomes	Systematic review	n/a	Health professionals, patients	Telemedicine		~		~
Meigs et al. (2003) Trial of web-based diabetes disease management	RCT	Diabetes type 2	GP	Web-based decision support	+		+	
Shea et al. (2006) Trial comparing telemedicine case management with usual care in older, ethnically diverse, medically underserved patients with diabetes mellitus	RCT	Diabetes	Patients (age 65+)	Telemedicine	+			
Noel et al. (2004) Home telehealth reduces healthcare costs	RCT	Chronic heart failure, lung disease and/or diabetes	Patients (elderly)	Home telehealth integrated into facility's eHR system	+	~	+	+

IHCA, Interactive Health Communication Applications; RCT, randomized controlled trial; +, intervention improves the outcome; ~, intervention does not show any effect on the outcome; –, intervention has a negative effect on the outcomes.

outcomes (O'Connor et al. 2005; Tierney et al. 2005). The key challenges for the development of electronic health records lie in achieving functional interoperability within health systems. Agreeing technical standards are essential. Implementing nationwide (or statewide) electronic medical records has proved problematical. Substantial costs, budget overruns, unforeseen difficulties, negative results and even withdrawal of projects have been reported in the United Kingdom (Hendy et al. 2005), Germany (Tuffs 2004, 2006) and the United States (Burton et al. 2004; Scott et al. 2005).Technical difficulties include flaws in software design, absence of standard formats for physicians' notes and failure to develop interfaces between the different systems, as well as the high costs of programs. However, these problems appear to be common to major information technology procurements in many sectors.

Cultural issues include concerns about liability, privacy and the evidence that disease management programmes using decision support can succeed without a universal electronic medical record (Litaker et al. 2005; Solberg et al. 2005).This means that while government and payers struggle with plans for electronic records, other stakeholders experiment with other aspects of the e-health agenda. However e-health provides a unique opportunity to involve patients in the management of their disease by giving them access to sources of information and to decision aids.

Programmes that support self-management and home-based care for patients with chronic diseases have shown promising results (Warsi et al. 2004; Chodosh et al. 2005; Deakin et al. 2005; Turnock et al. 2005). Although traditionally relying on courses and written material, modern information technology and, in particular, the wide availability of the Internet and cell phones offer new possibilities for reinforcement and monitoring of patient self-management. Patient empowerment through information technology is currently at an experimental stage but may have important implications for the general organization of healthcare by shifting to the patient certain tasks currently performed by healthcare practitioners. The current proportion of patients with chronic disease who might use decision support may not be large, perhaps on average 20% of the population, with a higher proportion among younger patients and patients with higher education (Robinson and Thomson 2001). The pharmaceutical and insurance industries have played a leading role in promoting patient responsibility. Industry-sponsored programmes involving shared decision making and using call centres have allowed patients to take an active part in managing their health (Muir Gray 2002). Physicians may appear to be more reluctant than other stakeholders (Blakeman et al. 2006) and have expressed concerns about the erosion of their professional responsibility (Chapter 7) and the use of this approach by pharmaceutical companies to promote their own products to patients less skilled in critical analysis of evidence of effectiveness.

Quality criteria for assessing patient decision aids have been developed through international consensus and include specific criteria for Internet-based tools. These quality criteria include the delivery of feedback on the personal health information entered (Elwyn et al. 2006).

The development of decision aids for patients poses the same concerns about quality, although on a much larger scale, as does the development of CCDSS for doctors. France has mandated certification of all decision aids for drug prescribing. As patient-orientated computerized decision aids are introduced, it is likely that the same regulation will apply.

Conclusions

Decision support innovations aimed at improving the quality and safety of chronic disease care should target all those involved in the delivery of that care: clinicians (medical, nursing and allied health professionals), patients and their carers, healthcare managers and policy makers. The nature of the particular decision support will vary.

Decision support innovations relevant to chronic disease are inseparably intertwined with e-health agendas. Computers are increasingly the platform for delivery of decision supports.

Within the Chronic Care Model, decision support activities are directly relevant to enhancing self-management through both the electronic presentation of information and telehealth.

Innovations in clinical decision support are occurring in many parts of the health system. Most often these are focused on one particular chronic condition in one specific health service setting. There is evidence of gains in both quality and safety of care through the deployment of decision support systems. Lessons can be learned from these examples, and extrapolations made from the particular to the more general or from a specific context to another context. However, the challenges of reorganizing health systems so that decision supports are present and operational in all parts of the system are very large. There are profound implications for traditional relationships such as those between doctor and patient. Patients can become more activated and empowered. There are also profound implications for those who fund health services. New technologies are expensive and new activities need to be funded. There is no certainty that these new expenditures will be offset by savings elsewhere in the system. Reform weariness on the part of clinicians and managers of health services may result in negative perceptions of proposed new initiatives.

Priorities for future research

From this preliminary overview of the existing evidence on the use of decision supports to help in the management of chronic diseases, we have identified a number of aspects that need further consideration. These should be the subjects of operational research in order that all stakeholders –patients; healthcare providers, payers, healthcare organizations, policy makers and manufacturers – can benefit from adequate tools. The aspects that need consideration can be grouped into three categories:

- research on how to design the tools
- research on implementation
- research on evaluation.

Research on how to design the tools involves the standardization of the steps necessary to translate guidelines into CCDSS. Research on implementation concerns how users of decision supports react to these tools and how best to tailor the tools to their needs. This includes, for example, research on how best to incorporate CCDSS into the clinical workflow of physicians and what adaptations are required to enable patient preference-sensitive interventions. Research on evaluation addresses both the designs of intervention studies (observational, case–control, time series) and the outcomes used. We have seen that outcomes other than traditional clinical endpoints used in trials are appropriate. These include outcomes designed to measure increased cooperation between stakeholders, such as different health professions and patients, and improved access to health and healthcare for underserved populations.

References

Agence Nationale d'Accrédition et d'Évaluation en Santé (2000) *Efficacité des methodes de mise en œuvre des recommandations médicales*. Paris Cedex: ANAES.

Aguirre-Junco, A.R., Colombet, I., Zunino, S. et al. (2004) Computerization of guidelines: a knowledge specification method to convert text to detailed decision tree for electronic implementation, *Medinfo* 11: 115–19.

Barretto, S.A., Warren, J., Goodchild, A. et al. (2003) Linking guidelines to electronic health record design for improved chronic disease management, in *Proceedings of the American Medical Informatics Association*, pp. 66–70.

Blakeman, T., Macdonald, W. and Bower, P. (2006) A qualitative study of GPs' attitudes to self-management of chronic disease, *Br J Gen Pract*, 56: 407–14.

Bodenheimer, T. (2003) Interventions to improve chronic illness care: evaluating their effectiveness, *Dis Manag*, 6: 63–71.

Bodenheimer, T., Lorig, K., Holman, H. and Grumbach, K. (2002) Patient self management of chronic disease in primary care, *JAMA*, 228: 2469–75.

Burton, L.C., Anderson, G.F. and Kues, I.W. (2004) Using electronic health records to help coordinate care, *Milbank Q*, 82: 457–81.

Canada Health Infoway. http://www.infoway-inforoute.ca/en/WhatWeDo/Overview.aspx (accessed October 2007).

Chodosh, J., Morton, S.C., Mojica, W. et al. (2005) Meta-analysis: chronic disease self-management programs for older adults, *Ann Intern Med*, 143: 427–38.

Coiera, E. (2003) Clinical decision support systems, in (eds) *Guide to Health Informatics*, 2nd edn. London: Arnold.

Currell, R., Urquhart, C., Wainwright, P. and Lewis, R. (2000) Telemedicine versus face to face patient care: effects on professional practice and health care outcomes, *Cochrane Database Syst Rev*, 2: CD002098.

Deakin, T., McShane, C.E., Cade, J.E. and Williams, R.D. (2005) Group based training for self-management strategies in people with type 2 diabetes mellitus, *Cochrane Database Syst Rev*, 2: CD003417.

Eccles, M., McColl, E., Steen, N. et al. (2002) Effect of computerised evidence based guidelines on management of asthma and angina in adults in primary care: cluster randomised controlled trial, *BMJ*, 325: 1–7.

Elwyn, G., O'Connor, A. and Stacey, D. (2006) Developing a quality criteria framework for patient decision aids: online international Delphi consensus process, *BMJ*, 336: 417–22.

Garg, A.X., Adhikari, N.K., McDonald, H. et al. (2005) Effects of computerized clinical decision support systems on practitioner performance and patient outcomes: a systematic review, *JAMA*, 293: 1223–38.

Health Connect (2007) http://www.health.gov.au/internet/hconnect/publishing.nsf/ Content/intro (accessed October 2007).

Hendy, J., Reeves, B.C., Fulop, N., Hutchings, A. and Masseria, C. (2005) Challenges to implementing the national programme for information technology (NPfIT): a qualitative study, *BMJ*, 331: 331–6.

Hunt, D.L., Haynes, R.B., Hanna, S.E. and Smith, K. (1998) Effects of computer-based clinical decision support systems on physician performance and patient outcome. A systematic review, *JAMA*, 280: 1339–46.

Imhoff, M., Webb, A. and Goldschmidt, A. (2001) On behalf of the ESICM, *Health Inform Intens Care Med*, 27: 179–86.

Improving Chronic Illness Care (2007) The Chronic Care Model: Decision support. Washington, DC. Association of American Medical Colleges. http:// www.improvingchroniccare.org/index.php?p=Decision_Support&s=24 (accessed October 2007).

Kawamoto, K., Houlihan, C.A., Balas, E.A. and Lobach, D.F. (2005) Improving clinical practice using clinical decison support systems: a systematic review of trials to identify critical features to success, *BMJ*, 330: 765.

Lester, W.T., Grant, R.W., Barnett, G.O. and Chueh, H.C. (2006) Randomized controlled trial of an informatics-based intervention to increase statin prescription for secondary prevention of coronary disease, *J Gen Intern Med*, 21: 22–9.

Lewis, D. (1999) Computer-based approaches to patient education. A review of the literature literature, *J Am Med Infomat Assoc*, 6: 272–82.

Litaker, D., Ritter, C., Ober, S. and Aron, D. (2005) Continuity of care and cardiovascular risk factor management: does care by a single clinician add to informational continuity provided by electronic medical records? *Am J Manag Care*, 11: 689–96.

Liu, J., Wyatt, J.C. and Altman, D.G. (2006) Decision tools in health care: focus on the problem, not the solution, *BMC Med Informat Decision Making*, 6: 4.

Manotti, C., Moia, M., Palareti, G. et al. (2001) Effect of computer-aided management on the quality of treatment in anticoagulated patients: a prospective, randomized, multicenter trial of APROAT (Automated PRogram for Oral Anticoagulant Treatment), *Haematologica*, 86: 1060–70.

Maviglia, S M, Zielstorff, R.D., Paterno, M. et al. (2003) Automating complex guidelines for chronic disease: lessons learned, *J Am Med Informat Assoc*, 10: 154–65.

McCowan, C., Neville, R.G., Ricketts, I.W. et al. (2001) Lessons from a randomized controlled trial designed to evaluate computer decision support software to improve the management of asthma., *Med Inform Internet Med*, 26: 191–201.

Mechanic, D. (2001) How should hamsters run? Some observations about sufficient patient time in primary care, *BMJ*, 323: 266–8.

Medcom (2007) http://www.medcom.dk/wm109991 (accessed October 2007).

Meigs, J.B., Cagliero, E., Dubey, A. et al. (2003) A controlled trial of web-based diabetes disease management, *Diabetes Care*, 26: 750–7.

Ministère de la Santé et des Solidarités (2007) *Plan pour l'Amélioration de la Qualité de vie des Personnes Atteintes de Maladies Chroniques*. Paris: Ministère de la Santé et des Solidarités.

Muir Gray, J.A. (2002) *The Resourceful Patient*. Oxford: eRosetta Press.

Murray, E., Burns, J., See Tai, S., Lai, R. and Nazareth, I. (2005) Interactive health communication applications for people with chronic disease, *Cochrane Database Syst Rev*, 4: CD004274.

Murray, M.D., Harris, L.E., Overhage, J.M. et al. (2004) Failure of computerized treatment suggestions to improve health outcomes of outpatients with uncomplicated hypertension: results of a randomized controlled trial, *Pharmacotherapy*, 24: 324–37.

National Electronic Decision Support Taskforce (2003) *Electronic Decision Support for Australia's Health Sector*. Canberra: Commonwealth of Australia.

NHS Connecting for Health (2007) http://www.connectingforhealth.nhs.uk/ (accessed October 2007).

Nies, J., Colombet, I., Degoutlet, P. and Durieux, P. (2006) Determinants of success of computerized clinical decision support systems integrated in CPOE systems: a systematic review, *AMIA Annu Symp Proc*, 2006: 590–8.

Noel, H.C., Vogel, D.C., Erdos, J.J., Cornwall, D. and Levin, F. (2004) Home telehealth reduces healthcare costs, *Telemed J e-health* 10: 170–83.

O'Connor, A.M., Stacey, D., Entwistle, V. et al. (2003) Decision aids can help people take an active role in making informed decisions about healthcare options. *Cochrane Database Syst Rev*, 1: CD001431.

O'Connor, P.J., Lauren Crain, A., Rush, W.A. et al. (2005) Impact of an electronic medical record on diabetes quality of care, *Ann Fam Med*, 4: 300–6.

Osheroff, J.A., Pifer, E.A., Teich, J.M., Sittig, D.F. and Jenders, R.A. (2005) *Improving Outcomes with Clinical Decision Support: An Implementer's Guide*. Chicago, IL: Healthcare Information and Management Systems Society.

Park, E.J. (2006) Telehealth technology in case/disease management, *Lippincotts Case Manag* 11: 175–82.

Plaza, V., Cobos, A., Ignacio-Garcia, J.M. et al. (2005) Cost-effectiveness of an intervention based on the Global INitiative for Asthma (GINA) recommendations using a computerized clinical decision support system: a physicians randomized trial, *Med Clin (Barcelona)*, 124: 201–6.

Robinson, A. and Thomson, R. (2001) Variability in patient preferences for participating in medical decision making: implication for the use of decision support tools, *Qual Health Care*, 10: 134–8.

Rollman, B.L., Hanusa, B.H., Lowe, H.J. et al. (2002) A randomized trial using computerized decision support to improve treatment of major depression in primary care, *J Gen Intern Med*, 17: 493: 503.

Scott, J.T., Rundall, T.G., Vogt, T.M. and Hsu, J. (2005) Kaiser Permanente's experience of implementing an electronic medical record: a qualitative study, *BMJ*, 331: 1313–16.

Shea, S., Weinstock, R., Starren, J. et al. (2006) A randomized trial comparing telemedicine case management with usual care in older, ethnically diverse, medically underserved patients with diabetes mellitus, *J Am Med Informat Assoc*, 13: 40–51.

Solberg, L.I., Scholle, S.H., Asche, S.E. et al. (2005) Practice systems for chronic care: frequency and dependence on an electronic medical record, *Am J Manag Care*, 11: 789–96.

Tierney, W.M., Overhage, J.M., Murray, M.D. et al. (2005) Can computer-generated evidence-based care suggestions enhance evidence-based management of asthma and chronic obstructive pulmonary disease? A randomized, controlled trial, *Health Serv Res*, 40: 311–15.

Trowbridge, R. and Weingarten, S. (2001) Clinical decision support systems, in K. Shojania, B. Duncan and K.M. McDonald (eds) *Making Health Care Safer: A Critical Analysis of Patient Safety Practices. Evidence Report/Technology Assessment* No. 43. Rockville, MD: Agency for Healthcare Research and Quality.

Tuffs, A. (2004) Germany plans to introduce electronic health card, *BMJ*, 329: 131.

Tuffs, A. (2006) Introduction of Germany's electronic health cards is delayed, *BMJ*, 332: 72.

Turnock, A.C., Walters, E.H., Walters, J.A.E. and Wood-Baker, R. (2005) Action plans for chronic obstructive pulmonary disease, *Cochrane Database Syst Rev*, 4: CD005074.

Van Weel, C. and Schellevis, F.G. (2006) Comorbidity and guidelines: conflicting interests, *Lancet*, 367: 9510.

Wagner, E.H., Austin, B.T. and Von Korff, M. (1996) Organizing care for patients with chronic illness, *Milbank Q*, 74: 511–44.

Warsi, A., Wang, P.S., LaValley, M.P., Avorn, J. and Solomon, D.H. (2004) Self-management education programs in chronic disease. A systematic review and methodological critique of the literature, *Arch Intern Med*, 164: 1641–9.

nine

Paying for chronic
disease care

Reinhard Busse and Nicholas Mays

Introduction

There is no one "best" way to pay for services for people with chronic health problems, but there is little doubt that payment methods have important implications for the nature and quality of services provided. This chapter focuses on the different methods and combinations of methods available for paying for the care of people with chronic conditions, and the incentives generated by these methods. The chapter will cover incentives for payers/purchasers, providers (organizations, teams and individuals) and patients. Financial incentives can serve as primary motivators or reinforcers of behaviour change among providers, patients and other stakeholders. Yet few incentives in current healthcare systems promote effective chronic care, let alone chronic disease management. Instead, the predominant payment schemes represent major barriers. However motivated some healthcare stakeholders may be to implement changes to improve chronic care, few will operate counter to their economic interests (Leatherman et al. 2003). A core element for improving chronic care will, therefore, be to develop and adopt payment approaches that include appropriate financial incentives.

To examine both past and current financing mechanisms, as well as provide policy-relevant options in order to align incentives towards improving care for the chronically ill, the chapter employs an extended triangular model involving the population/payers, the providers and the financial intermediaries (Figure 9.1). The financial intermediaries have, in line with the separation found within most countries, been further subdivided into the "financial pooler", which collects and pools collective resources for health services, and the "payer/ purchaser", which pays for or purchases care for defined parts of the population. The main focus is on how providers are paid to deliver care to people with chronic conditions. However, beyond looking at how such payers/purchasers pay providers (relationship D), the chapter also examines the patient–provider relationship (A) and gives some consideration to financial allocations to payers/purchasers (C), especially in systems where patients have a choice of payer/purchaser.

The chapter examines the main reasons why payers, purchasers, providers and patients may wish to use reimbursement modalities to increase the emphasis given by frontline staff to the management of chronic disease. It covers the main generic (i.e. not specifically developed for chronic care) approaches used to pay providers, including provider organizations, provider groups and individual providers, and summarizes key examples drawn from different countries, including some of the country case studies in the volume accompanying this book. The chapter then gives particular emphasis to describing so called "pay-for-performance" and "quality-based payments" (as defined in Box 9.1) on the grounds that they represent an area of innovation in provider payment that is widely debated in a number of countries, especially the United States and United Kingdom, but potentially relevant to many other high-income settings. Finally, the chapter attempts to summarize the evidence available about the impact of these approaches in terms of effectiveness and cost-effectiveness.

Traditional forms of paying for healthcare and their effects on care for chronic conditions

Before describing and analysing innovative ways of paying for the care of people with chronic illnesses, it is important to briefly review past, and often still current, ways of paying for care and their effects on chronic care.

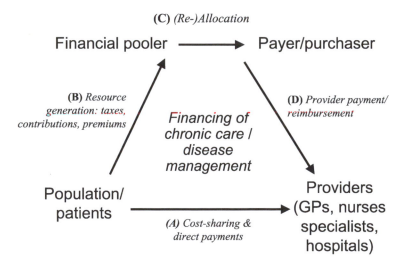

Figure 9.1   Financial flows related to paying for chronic care.

Box 9.1 Definitions of key terms

Chronic disease management. This is defined as a population-based approach to the treatment of chronic illness using evidence-based clinical guidelines, multidisciplinary management and information systems to produce good outcomes at reasonable cost (Couch 1998; see also Chapter 4). Typically, chronic disease management programmes pay physicians and providers for putting in place appropriate structures and processes of care (e.g. better information systems), including paying for changes in the way that physicians and providers provide care.

Pay-for-performance. By contrast, pay-for-performance has tended to focus on paying for the delivery of specific patient-based outcomes of care, not necessarily exclusively in the field of chronic care. Thus it refers to "financial incentives that reward providers for the achievement of a range of payer objectives, including delivery efficiencies, submission of data and measures to payer, and improving quality and patient safety" (McNamara 2006). It can be applied to hospitals, provider organizations, primary care physicians and their practices, specialists, nursing homes, domiciliary care teams and rehabilitation providers, and it can, in theory, be applied to any condition except the most acute. Pay-for-performance can thus be seen as an emerging component of more established approaches to chronic disease management, which typically include a wider range of techniques designed to improve the quality and cost-effectiveness of care.

Quality-based payment. McNamara (2006) defines quality-based payment (or quality-based purchasing) as a narrower concept than pay-for-performance, since it does not generally include an economic component (i.e. incentives for cost savings or efficiency gains); instead it "focuses only on financing schemes that embody explicit financial incentives to reward and penalize providers based on the level of quality of care they deliver". Quality, McNamara continues, "can be pegged to structural benchmarks (e.g. information technology investments), processes of care (e.g. compliance with clinical guidelines), and outcomes, including technical outcomes (lower mortality following surgery) and patients' satisfaction with their care experiences", but not costs.

Provider payment/reimbursement

Traditionally, there have been three ways for paying physicians and other healthcare professionals from pooled resources (i.e. by insurers or governments; resource flow D in Figure 9.1): fee-for-service, capitation and salary. All three have been used to pay providers at different levels in healthcare systems for the management of people with chronic conditions, among other things. However, none of these methods fully aligns financial incentives with the goal of optimal care for patients with chronic conditions. In effect, each creates different perverse incentives for patient care.

Fee-for-service involves paying extra money for each unit of service provided and generally motivates providers to increase the amount of service they provide, assuming that the payment offered exceeds the cost to the provider. The incentive under fee-for-service reimbursement is to provide as many reimbursable services as possible, creating the potential for overuse of such services while failing to provide uncovered services that may be equally or more cost-effective, such as active patient monitoring by phone or computer. The effect on quality is hard to predict. Providers may overprovide services of dubious value on the one hand, yet, on the other hand, they face no incentives to skimp or withhold valuable services. Fee-for-service also minimizes incentives for avoiding patients who are difficult to treat, such as patients with multiple chronic conditions.

Capitation gives physicians (or other healthcare providers) a fixed amount to provide services to patients for a particular time, irrespective of the volume of services consumed by individual patients. Thus it generates the opposite incentives of fee-for-service, namely, to provide as little care as possible to each patient as providers paid by capitation bear the financial risk, creating the potential for underuse of services. Under capitation, physicians have the incentive to sign up more patients and do less for each, as well as to avoid high users of care such as patients with multiple chronic conditions. In theory, some of these incentives are moderated in situations where patients can choose to enrol with other providers. With choice, providers face some incentives to provide high-quality care to retain patients and income, but they must do so within a budget. If the capitation payment is not risk-adjusted (i.e. if providers do not receive higher capitation payments for patients with higher needs), providers will not be interested in caring for the chronically ill as such patients will cost more to provide services to than the capitation sum based on average patients.

Salary gives a provider a guaranteed income for a period of time irrespective of how much work is carried out. As a result, there is no particular incentive on providers to over- or under-provide. However, there is also no specific incentive to provide high-quality care (unless the provider works for an organization in competition with other organizations to retain patient affiliations or maintain workload), and lazy staff may provide little care. While salary may be the most neutral form of clinician reimbursement, much relies on occupational norms, peer pressure and emulation to maintain performance.

The **payment of institutions** (especially acute care hospitals) is one level up in the system, and payment methods include fee-for-service, per diem payments, case fees and budgets. Per diem payments (i.e. a fee per day of inpatient stay) used to be a common way of paying hospitals particularly in social health insurance systems. If per diem prices are uniform across all patients, providers will have incentives to prefer less costly patients or to keep costly patients longer than necessary to recoup their costs through higher total reimbursement. As patients with chronic diseases are increasingly managed primarily in the ambulatory care sector, they are hospitalized only for acute complications, which often makes them high-cost patients who are disadvantaged through this payment mechanism. Case fees, especially those known as "diagnosis related groups" have different incentives. The original system developed in the United States was based on diagnosis only and assumed that all patients in each diagnosis related group generated similar costs for the hospital, thus effectively sharing financial risk with providers, and perhaps perversely encouraging early discharge. The European adaptations, such as in France, Germany or the Netherlands, include, first, so-called "outliers", which justify a higher level of reimbursement for difficult cases, and, second, procedures provided by the hospital for classification (Busse et al. 2006), effectively turning them into a hybrid with fee-for-service. Chronically ill people admitted to hospital should benefit from such developments, but they are at risk of inappropriate overprovision, as under fee-for-service. Institutional budgets have similar incentives to salaries paid to professionals.

In practice, variants of the basic payment methods are often combined into more complex payment systems in order to offset the inherent limitations of each. For example, it is common in the United States to find that salaried staff also receive additional incentive payments or bonuses (e.g. for treating a target number of patients and/or treating them in a timely manner) to mitigate the risk that they will provide poor-quality or too few services. Typically, capitation is coupled with incentives to reward high-quality services whereas salary is linked with output or productivity payments and fee-for-service with inducements to be economical, such as a share of any profit that the provider organization is able to make or by withholding a proportion of the professional's earnings subject to satisfactory performance. Hence, there is a great deal of interest in developing "blended" or "mixed" approaches to payment for chronic disease care as well as for other services. Many pay-for-performance initiatives, as well as paying directly for the delivery of specific measures of quality and/or outcome, use a blend of payment methods. The United Kingdom NHS general practitioner contract first implemented in 2004 can be seen as a pay-for-performance blended payment contract in that it comprises capitation, fee-for-service, infrastructure (capital and information technology) payments plus a substantial element of quality-driven remuneration (see below).

Resource generation and (re)allocation

Often overlooked are the incentives for payers/purchasers related to the management of people with chronic disease. However, these are critical for the whole system to function properly, especially in countries with competing payers/purchasers. Two general situations can be distinguished: the payers receive their financial resources directly from the population (i.e. resource flows B and C in Figure 9.1 are not separated) and the payers receive their financial resources from pooled resources (i.e. through resource flow C in Figure 9.1).

In the first situation, resources allocated to the payers will be either risk related – thereby disadvantaging the chronically ill, who will face high premiums – or not risk related, that is, either income or community rated. While this leads to similar contributions for people with and without chronic illnesses, evidence from several countries shows that expenditure for around 80% of the population insured is *below* average while 20% have above-average expenditure and are bad risks (of whom 5% are very bad risks and are responsible for 50% of expenditure). Financially, insurers will always be better off to try to avoid the (very) bad risks. The insurers are also discouraged from providing high-quality chronic disease management as they risk disproportionately attracting sicker, especially chronically ill, people who want to benefit from paying average contributions.

In the second situation, the attractiveness of patients with chronic conditions will depend on whether the prevalence of morbidity or chronic illness is included in the formula for calculating the allocation to payers, be they sickness funds in social health insurance systems or local health authorities in tax-funded systems. Most formulae have traditionally only included sociodemographic parameters (e.g. age, sex, employment status) and sometimes regional variables (Busse et al. 2006). While in tax-funded systems with no choice of payer, this may disadvantage regions with a higher percentage of chronically ill people, it does not lead to deliberate selection of patients with low risks, or "cream-skimming". Even if active cream-skimming of healthier persons is often not possible (and not allowed) on the part of competing sickness funds in social health insurance systems, the lack of a morbidity variable in the risk-allocation formulae has meant that sickness funds traditionally had no interest in investing in chronic disease management – as successful programmes would have increased their popularity with the chronically ill, thereby leading to financial difficulties. Recently, countries such as the Netherlands, Belgium and Germany have begun to address this issue by including morbidity as a factor in the formulae they use to calculate allocations to sickness funds (Van de Ven et al. 2007).

Cost sharing and direct payments

A final method of payment for chronic care is patient out-of-pocket payment or copayment (resource flow A in Figure 9.1). In most healthcare systems, patient copayments or user charges are the product of historical accident and are rarely designed with chronic care in mind. In general, copayments tend to obstruct good chronic disease care, especially for poorer people, who are normally at greater risk as copayments tend to be attached to the pharmaceuticals essential for good care. In a 2007 meta-analysis of the evidence on cost sharing between 1985 and 2006, Goldman et al. (2007) concluded that increased cost sharing is associated with lower rates of drug treatment, worse adherence by existing users and more frequent discontinuation of therapy. The RAND Health Insurance Experiment, a landmark study performed in the 1980s, demonstrated that cost sharing reduced *appropriate* and necessary office visits and preventive care as well as inappropriate visits, with adverse effects on visual acuity (Lurie et al. 1989), blood pressure control (Keeler et al. 1985) and survival among high-risk patients (Brook et al. 1983).

However, it is possible to see how varying patient copayments in systems where they are widespread could be used to encourage patients either to take part in chronic disease management programmes or to seek out providers who are willing to comply with specific disease management protocols and/or standards (Table 9.2, below, has examples of the use of schemes of this type to promote chronic disease management). The effectiveness of such schemes depends on whether patients interpret the lower out-of-pocket cost or reduced contribution rate as a signal of lower quality and value, or are mainly influenced by the price signals and are thereby attracted to such programmes.

Chronic disease management programmes: rationale, role of incentives and prerequisites

There are three main reasons why chronic disease management programmes have come to prominence with payers and/or purchasers in a number of very different health systems:

First, the clinical profile and needs of patients have altered dramatically over the last 40–50 years. Patients with multiple chronic conditions are now the norm. Unfortunately, the payment modalities in many healthcare systems were developed in an era of largely acute care and are not fitted to contemporary patterns of morbidity.

Second, studies commonly find that some patients do not receive appropriate, high-quality care and are exposed to the risk of medical errors. As a result, payers want to improve quality as a way of containing the rising overall costs of healthcare. A sense of financial "crisis", perceived as threatening sustainability in some healthcare systems, has encouraged the development of better chronic disease care.

Third, it is well known that healthcare professionals, and particularly doctors, respond to financial incentives. Experience has also shown that simply giving comparative performance information to providers and other more traditional educational approaches to improvement have comparatively modest, gradual effects on doctors' performance, but where rapid change is required, it is possible that the rate of improvement could be accelerated by adding financial incentives to the reputation-based incentives produced by making performance information available publicly (either to payers or patients or both).

Professionals tend to stress the importance of intrinsic motivation and worry that professional motivation and flexibility may be damaged by linking financial rewards to the performance of particular activities, whereas managers and payers tend to emphasize the importance of extrinsic motivation in improving quality of services. It is likely that both intrinsic and extrinsic incentives for quality improvement are necessary and need to be carefully balanced. This chapter focuses on the extrinsic aspect of quality improvement for chronic disease care whereas other chapters focus on other ways of motivating improvements in chronic disease management.

The range of reasons for the current vogue for altering payment modalities to encourage better chronic care means that different systems and payers will have different goals in introducing new methods.

The prerequisites described below are based on conceptualization and experience to date rather than rigorous evaluation since such evaluation of different approaches is often lacking (see below). There is still contention as to what are the essential clinical features of good chronic care management or other models (Singh and Ham 2006; see also Chapter 4). However, it is possible to identify many of the wider organizational features of systems that are needed to allow a range of different chronic care approaches a better chance of success.

The evidence presented in Chapter 3 indicates that any net returns to the payer from most chronic disease management programmes tend to occur after the first five years once the up-front investment in programmes has been made. Indeed, the benefits of avoiding severe complications are often only realized after eight to ten years (Eastman et al. 1997). This suggests that *continuity of involvement with patients on the part of funders/insurers* and hence providers (e.g. through patient enrolment), is likely to be one of the most important prerequisites for effective payment systems.

Given that benefits and cost savings tend not to appear for several years, it is noteworthy that in most private medical insurance systems, such as those in the United States, patients only stay with an insurer for an average of about three years. While this has not been the case until recently in social health insurance systems, where choice of sickness fund and competition between insurers is only now being encouraged, such as in Germany or the Netherlands, drop-out rates from disease management programmes (in Germany) or signs of a growing tendency to change funds (in the Netherlands) demonstrate that this may also become relevant in those countries. As a result, most chronic disease management programmes to do not appear to be a good investment for individual insurers.

Yet, as demonstrated in Chapter 3, chronic disease management (e.g. for diabetes) can be a very good investment from a societal point of view because of avoided complications, improved health-related quality of life, long-term cost savings from decreased use of services and less time receiving disability payments, and other benefits such as workplace productivity gains. There is a huge discrepancy between the individual insurer's weak rationale and the strong societal rationale for chronic disease management. Employers stand to gain potentially but are unlikely to invest heavily unless they are confident that they will have a stable workforce.

High-quality chronic disease management programmes also risk disproportionately attracting sicker people, further discouraging insurers and providers to provide such programmes. This suggests that in systems which offer choice of insurer or sickness fund and/or choice of provider, thereby encouraging a fairly rapid turnover of enrolees and patients, there may need to be a separate system of funding for chronic disease management, probably from public sources, to enable a socially efficient level of management to be provided. From this perspective, the prospect held out in the Netherlands of competing private insurers offering chronic disease management packages to their insurees in order to be able subsequently to offer them lower premiums appears naive, or at best unlikely to be sustainable if patients move between insurers in any numbers (Klein-Lankhorst and Spreeuwenberg 2008). An alternative approach in social insurance systems with multiple sickness funds or insurers is to develop a sophisticated risk-equalization formula and process that would operate to reallocate resources between insurers or sickness funds as patients change their affiliations, as well as encouraging insurers to take responsibility for people with chronic conditions (resource flow C in Figure 9.1). This is, however, extremely challenging technically.

Even in collective tax-funded or single-payer social health insurance systems, which, in many ways, are much better placed to facilitate long-term chronic disease care, any significant degree of devolution may encourage the local "insurers" (i.e. planning or purchasing authorities) to take a short-term view and focus on providing more acute care to deal with current demand rather than investing in chronic disease management with its likely longer term benefits. There may well be wider political reasons for so doing (e.g. reducing waiting times for elective surgery rather than investing in chronic disease management programmes) as governments are held to account for their achievements over a relatively short time cycle.

Experience with putting in place chronic disease management programmes indicates that there are a number of other important requirements for effective payment approaches.

- The ability ex ante to identify and stratify patients in terms of severity (i.e. risk adjustment for calibrating performance measures, see below) and requirements for care (i.e. risk adjustment of capitation rates), and to be able to monitor patients' health status over time insofar as performance and outcomes relate to payment.
- The availability of widely accepted, evidence-based or informed guidelines or protocols defining "appropriate" and/or "cost-effective" care for different people, and the ability to implement these guidelines and protocols.
- The development of carefully chosen, risk-adjusted performance measures, where improvements against these measures will produce measurable improvements in the health of enrolled patients. These are generally likely to be process or quality measures, since outcome measures do not contain specific information about what providers should be changing to improve outcomes and often take too much time to achieve (see above). The measures should be as close as possible to the end of the causal chain from processes to outcomes (Chassin 2006).
- Systems are needed that can measure and assess the structure, process quality and outcomes (where relevant) of care ex post.
- Motivation of physicians and staff to empower and support their patients to manage their chronic disease: a collaborative approach to chronic disease management involving active patient self-management as well as encouragement of patient compliance through various forms of care management. This is more usually found in primary healthcare teams and therefore in systems with well-developed primary healthcare.
- An integrated, flexible workforce is required that is willing and able to cross professional boundaries, conventional team structures and job skills in response to financial incentives and payment modalities (Rechel et al. 2006).

The number and range of these prerequisites explains why payment schemes produce both disappointing and variable results.

Specific incentives used to stimulate improved care especially for the chronically ill

Table 9.1 summarizes the main ways in which payers can specifically encourage the provision of appropriate chronic disease care. Financial incentives can apply to the structure, processes and outcomes of care, and should be considered in relation to other, non-financial regulations or incentives.

At present, the bulk of financial incentives in high-income countries other than the United States relate to the structure or process of care. Only the United Kingdom NHS general practitioner contract specifically includes a range of incentive payments focused on the delivery of particular outcomes (see below). In general, there has been a gradual shift of focus from approaches that simply take into account the presence of patients with chronic disease (or who are likely to suffer from chronic illnesses) when funding either purchasers or providers towards payment incentives designed to encourage specific kinds of structural and process response at provider level (e.g. as in the Australian Enhanced Primary Care (EPC) package (Glasgow et al. 2008)).

Case studies in selected high-income countries compiled for the volume accompanying this book provide a range of examples of the main types of payment and regulatory incentive currently in use to encourage chronic care (Durand-Zaleski and Obrecht 2008; Glasgow et al. 2008; Jiwani and Dubois 2008; Karlberg 2008; Klein-Lankhorst and Spreeuwenberg 2008; Schiotz et al. 2008;

Table 9.1 Purpose of financial incentives and regulation for chronic disease care

Focus	Purpose of financial incentives	Purpose of other relevant types of regulation
Structure	To implement DMPs, and recruit and enrol patients in DMPs To put in place "integrated" forms of care (mostly packages that cross institutional/sectoral boundaries)	To implement systems of in-house quality management To detail structural requirements To implement systems of data collection
Process	To keep patients in DMPs for a target period of time To ensure that the care protocols specified in DMPs are followed (e.g. in encounters with a specific provider, over x months) To reach predefined targets on process measures (e.g. proportions of patients treated with a particular drug)	To mandate evidence-based standards (i.e. clinical practice guidelines) To implement/mandate targets on process measures of quality To reach agreement on minimum volume of services
Outcome	To reach predefined targets (e.g. proportion of patients with outcome x) or to reward the top $y\%$ of providers on an indicator	To implement/mandate targets on health outcomes and/or patient satisfaction

DMP, disease management programme.

Siering 2008; Singh and Fahey 2008). The most notable examples of financial incentives in this group of countries are summarized in Table 9.2, organized according to the model for tracing financial flows outlined in Figure 9.1. The policy focus in most high-income countries is on provider incentives, given the importance of healthcare professionals, especially physicians, in determining how patients use health services (between payers/purchasers and providers; flow D in Figure 9.1).

The following sections describe examples of payment initiatives in the countries reviewed for this book and described in the accompanying volume, complemented by a description of the United States experience with Medicare pay-for-performance.

Provider payment incentives

Australian Enhanced Primary Care Practice Incentive Programme and Service Improvement Payments

After a series of experiments in the 1990s in multidisciplinary care planning and coordinated care, the Commonwealth government in Australia introduced the EPC package in 1999, designed to increase the involvement of general practitioners, practice nurses and allied health professionals in structured and coordinated care based on the Chronic Care Model (see Chapter 4) (Glasgow et al. 2008). Pay-for-performance elements (the Practice Incentive Programme and Service Improvement Payments) were subsequently introduced within the EPC, the bulk of which is paid by fee-for-service, the usual method of payment for general practitioner and related services in Australia. The Practice Incentive Programme and the Service Improvement Payments pay general practices according to whether they have met prescribed quality and service criteria for chronic care (Glasgow et al. 2008). Performance-based payments typically account for less than 10% of the income of a practice.

The diabetes Service Improvement Payment pays practices for each patient who has completed an annual cycle of care comprising assessment of glycosylated haemoglobin (HbA1c), blood pressure, lipids, weight, behavioural risk factors and screening for complications, and for the proportion of diabetics in the practice who have completed an annual cycle of care. By 2006, over 90% of eligible practices were taking part in the diabetes Practice Incentive Programme; of these, 70% had received Service Improvement Payments and half of these had achieved their outcome targets. The introduction of these programmes was accompanied, in the early 2000s, by improvements in the quality of care for patients with diabetes, though whether these gains would have occurred in any event is not known.

The United Kingdom NHS general practitioner contract

One of the innovations in the 2004 United Kingdom NHS general practitioner contract is that general practices are rewarded for delivering care exhibiting particular features deemed to be associated with clinical and organizational quality (Roland 2004; Smith and York 2004). The contract addresses quality in two ways.

Table 9.2 Examples of financial incentives for chronic disease care in selected high-income countries

Financial flows (as in Figure 1)	Financial incentives to encourage chronic disease care (patients and services) in different high-income countries			
	Target: patients with chronic conditions	Target: structures	Target: processes	Target: outcomes
Patient to provider (A)	No copayments for services related to their disease (e.g. ALD in FR for 30 mainly chronic diseases until 2004) Lower annual limits on copayments (GER) Certain drugs require lower cost sharing if indication is deemed serious (FR)	ALD exemption only for established and agreed care protocol for each patient (FR since 2004) Cost sharing may be reduced or waived if patients enrol in DMPs (GER) Coverage of additional services (e.g. patient education) for patients in DMP/ALD Patients with chronic conditions/complex needs managed via care plan receive fee rebate for five allied health services per year (e.g. podiatry) (AUS)	ALD exemption only if care protocol is presented to every treating physician on each visit (FR) Lower cost-sharing limit only if patient adheres to therapy (GER, since 2007)	
Patient to financial pooler (B)	Premium reduction of maximum of 10% for insured under group contracts (e.g. chronically ill) (NL)	Insurers are interested in offering premium reductions to DMP participants (NL), but not yet implemented		
Financial pooler to payer/purchaser (C)	Funding (re-) allocation formula between insurers accounts for individual morbidity criteria (i.e. individually risk-rated capitations) (NL, GER from 2009)	Funding (re-) allocation formula (RSCS) takes into account patient enrolment in DMPs: sickness funds receive *more* for patients registered with a DMP and *less* for those not enrolled, thereby encouraging funds to offer DMPs (GER)		

(Continued Overleaf)

Table 9.2 Continued.

Financial flows (as in Figure 1)	Financial incentives to encourage chronic disease care (patients and services) in different high-income countries			
	Target: patients with chronic conditions	Target: structures	Target: processes	Target: outcomes
Payer/purchaser to provider (D)	Piloting of "year of care" payment for complete package of chronic disease management required by individuals with chronic conditions (e.g. based on validated "care pathways" for diabetes) (DK, UK)	Per patient bonus for physicians for acting as gatekeepers for patients with chronic conditions and for setting care protocols (FR) Bonus for DMP recruitment and documentation (GER) 1% of total health budget available for integrated care (GER) Points for achieving structural targets (UK GP contract) Payments to GPs for generic care planning, case conferences, establishing disease registers for patients with chronic disease (AUS, EPC) Additional services (e.g. patient self-management education) only reimbursable if physicians and patients participate in DMP (GER)	Points for reaching process targets (UK GP contract) PIP and SIP payments for meeting prescribed quality and service criteria for chronic conditions over an annual care cycle (e.g. for diabetes) (AUS) Additional services (e.g. patient self-management education) only reimbursable if physicians and patients participate in DMP (GER)	Points for achieving outcome targets (UK GP contract)

ALD, affections de longue dureé; AUS, Australia; DMP, disease management programme; DK, Denmark; EPC, enhanced primary care programme; GP, general practitioner; FR, France; GER, Germany; NL, Netherlands; PIP, practice incentive programme; RSCS, risk structure compensation scheme; SIP, service improvement payments; UK, United Kingdom.

First, it sets out a range of quality-related requirements that have to be fulfilled by providers in order to be contracted to the NHS (e.g. having a practice information leaflet for patients, a system to handle patient complaints, safety policies and a system to enable quality assurance). Second, it includes a system of financial incentives for clinical and organizational quality. Traditionally, NHS funding of general practitioners has been largely on the basis of the number of patients registered with a practice, although there were exceptions such as target-driven payments for cervical cancer screening and child immunizations. Now, quality rewards make a substantial part of the funding (typically 25% of a general practice's income) in addition to capitation and infrastructure payments.

Performance is measured using a Quality and Outcomes Framework (QOF) especially developed for this purpose. The framework focuses on four main components, one of which (clinical standards) is linked directly to the care of people with ten chronic conditions: coronary heart disease, stroke or transient ischaemic attacks, hypertension, diabetes, chronic obstructive pulmonary disease, epilepsy, cancer, mental health problems, hypothyroidism and asthma (Box 9.2).

In 2006–07, other indicators were added covering heart failure, palliative care, dementia, depression, chronic kidney disease, atrial fibrillation, obesity, learning disabilities and smoking, with a greater emphasis on prevention. The other three

Box 9.2   The Quality and Outcomes Framework (QOF) in the United Kingdom NHS general practitioner contract

The Quality and Outcomes Framework (QOF) for achieving clinical quality standards was developed on the basis of the best currently available evidence. To link payments to the achievement of quality standards, a system of points was developed to an original maximum of 1050 (currently 1000). The maximum number of points achievable for each indicator is related to the associated workload. The 80 clinical indicators in 19 areas account for 66% of the total number of points achievable by a practice. Most points are available for ischaemic heart disease (121), hypertension (105) and diabetes (99).

For clinical indicators, indicator points are awarded in a simple linear relationship to achievement between a minimum and maximum achievable. By contrast, points are based on a yes/no determination for organizational or patient experience indicators. For example, for controlling blood pressure in diabetic patients (i.e. achieving a blood pressure of 145/85 mmHg or less) a maximum of 17 points can be achieved. No points are achieved until 25% of patients have controlled blood pressure; the maximum practically achievable has been set at 55%. If a practice achieves this target blood pressure in 55% of its diabetic patients, it will be given the full score for this indicator. If the target is achieved in, say, only 30% of the diabetic patients, the practice will get a score for this indicator of only 2.8 points; i.e. 5(30%−25%) 30^{ths}(55%−25%) of 17.

components of quality are organizational quality standards (in five areas), the experience of patients (consultation length and results of patient surveys) and the provision of additional services (in four areas: cervical screening, child health surveillance, maternity services and contraceptive services). Each component is made operational through a comprehensive list of over 150 indicators that describe performance (selected examples are given in Table 9.3).

The approach is not prescriptive; it leaves it to each practice to decide in which domains of quality and targets to concentrate its efforts. However, the contract includes a small bonus mechanism to reward the breadth of the quality improvement focus, in addition to the incentives described above, which reward the depth of the improvements.

In the first year of the new contract, the median practice achieved 83% of the maximum total number of points (Doran et al. 2006), exceeding the government's predictions. Performance in the second year was even stronger, with the median practice attaining 87% of the maximum number of points. Performance in the third year (2006–07) was stronger still, with 95% of practices scoring the maximum number of points (Information Centre 2007).

In 2006, the QOF was modified, partly in response to a perception that the targets were too easy to achieve. All minimum, and some of the maximum, thresholds attracting points were increased. Thirty indicators were dropped or altered and 18 new clinical areas were introduced (e.g. depression) to give greater weight to areas such as mental health, which was regarded as under-represented in the QOF. The biggest query about the QOF remains whether it genuinely encourages better quality care or simply rewards successful under-taking of specific activities and completeness of recording (see below). Since payments are made in relation to the number of points achieved by a practice, the QOF is not a zero sum game and has resulted in an increase in spending on general practices in the NHS. As a result, the rewards of the better performers have not been at the expense of the poorer performers.

Table 9.3 Examples of indicators, targets and point values for chronic disease management in the United Kingdom NHS general practitioner contract

Type	Indicator	Points	Target range
Structural	The practice establishes a register for patients with stroke or transient ischaemic attack (STROKE1)	4	Yes/no
Process	The percentage of patients with history of myocardial infarction who are currently treated with an angiotensin-converting enzyme inhibitor (CHD11)	7	25–70%
Outcome	The percentage of patients with diabetes in whom the last blood pressure was 145/85 mgHg or less (DM12)	17	25–55%
Outcome	The percentage of patients age 16 years and over on drug treatment for epilepsy who have been convulsion free for last 12 months recorded in last 15 months (EPILEPSY4)	6	25–70%

Source: British Medical Association 2003.

The "year of care" approach

The "year of care" approach is a costed "package" approach to paying for chronic disease care derived from managed care in the United States, but adapted for the circumstances of the United Kingdom NHS and designed to encourage continuity and integration of a full range of care for individuals over a concerted period of time (a year). The NHS defines this approach as, "[t]he ongoing care a person with a chronic condition should expect to receive in a year, including support for self-management, which can then be costed and commissioned. It involves individuals through the care planning process, enabling them to exercise choice in the design of a package to meet their needs" (Centre for Clinical Management Development 2007).

The amount of funding available for the "year of care" is calculated using a risk-adjusted capitation formula based on the likely consumption of a range of necessary health services over a 12-month period for people with specific diagnoses. "Year of care" funding has been developed for people with diabetes and a range of mental health problems and is being piloted and evaluated.

The United States Medicare pay-for-performance demonstration

This Medicare pay-for-performance initiative in the United States comprised a series of demonstration pilots, initially with ten large multispecialty group practices, that started in 2005, though there are plans to extend the demonstration to solo and small group practices with fewer support staff and a narrower range of specialties. Practices are paid by fee-for-service in the normal way, but, in addition, there is a financial incentive for improved chronic care. The practices share 80:20 with the Centers for Medicare and Medicaid Services any savings on the usual cost they are able to make by improving their outcomes and/or reducing their costs of care for patients with costly conditions such as diabetes, congestive heart failure and chronic obstructive pulmonary disease. Half-way through the three-year trials, the practices were reported to be making encouraging progress in identifying Medicare patients with chronic, high-cost conditions and closing the gaps in their care, thereby avoiding costly hospital stays (Klein 2006). The participating groups take the decision to invest their own resources in the systems needed to track and follow up patients on the basis that they can make significant savings. They are being compared with a control group of matched patients in the same geographic area managed by other practices. If the group practice qualifies for the savings bonus, a proportion of it is tied to the group's performance on a range of quality targets to prevent the accumulation of savings simply by reducing the quality of care.

Incentives for payers/purchasers

Risk structure compensation scheme

There are relatively few examples of chronic disease management incentives directed at payers/purchasers. However, in 2002 in Germany, where there is free patient choice among not-for-profit sickness funds, the formula used to reallocate revenue between funds to ensure that each is fairly funded for the likely costs of meeting the healthcare needs of its enrolees was amended to give extra funding for enrolees registered with a chronic disease management programme (initially confined to diabetes, breast cancer, asthma and coronary heart disease and subject to minimum standards) (Busse 2004; Siering 2008). Instead of patients with chronic conditions generating deficits for sickness funds, they are now relatively attractive. Despite contention between the sickness funds and physicians' associations as to what constituted the minimum standards for chronic disease management programmes and the patient care documentation needed, this reform has led to a rapid rise in the provision of disease management programmes by sickness funds and of the number of patients enrolled in them, though critics argue that the scheme does not provide incentives for sickness funds to improve the care of people with chronic conditions as much as to enrol them in schemes and be compensated more highly as a result.

Incentives for patients

Financial incentive schemes targeted directly at patients to promote chronic disease management are also relatively uncommon. For example, hitherto, schemes involving differential copayments have been regarded as politically unacceptable in the United Kingdom NHS. However, there are schemes in both France and Germany where the general use of copayments is more common. In Germany, cost sharing may be reduced or waived entirely for patients enrolled with specific chronic disease management programmes. Patients choosing to become involved in chronic disease management programmes also have access to additional services that other patients are not eligible for, and patients compliant with chronic disease management protocols are eligible for further reductions in their copayments (Siering 2008). In France, patients are exempt from chronic disease management copayments if they present their previously agreed care protocol at every physician visit (Durand-Zaleski and Obrecht 2008). Evaluations of these schemes have yet to be published.

Another theoretical approach to altering what patients pay to promote their involvement in, and access to, chronic care would be to lower patients' insurance contributions (in private and social insurance systems) in return for their participation in validated chronic disease management programmes. This could be combined with lower copayments for specific services (A and B in Figure 9.1).

Evidence about the impact of different payment methods

This section reviews the evidence on the different (financial) incentive systems to encourage better chronic disease management that have been described in the previous section.

There are surprisingly few high-quality studies of different payment methods designed to improve the quality and/or efficiency of care for chronic disease (i.e. pay-for-performance and quality-based purchasing, in particular) despite the strong interest in using financial incentives to improve healthcare quality. The best evidence comes from the United States and so has to be interpreted carefully for use elsewhere. Furthermore, much of the evidence comes from single case studies of schemes rather than rigorous comparative studies. As a result, there is considerable scope for debate as to the relative effectiveness of schemes; how they work; which are the most influential components of programmes; in which circumstances different approaches might work best; the best size, frequency and duration of incentives; whether rewards should be focused on the highest performers, on those who have improved or should relate to an absolute standard; how many performance domains to concentrate on at any one time; how financial incentives interact with other tools for quality improvement (e.g. reputational incentives generated by, for instance, publication of performance information where patients can choose providers); the costs of programmes in relation to their benefits; and the nature of the barriers and enablers of effective approaches.

While earlier reviews consistently concluded that there was a lack of evidence on the effects of different ways of paying providers for chronic care, including pay-for-performance (Eichler et al. 2001; Gosden et al. 2001; Institute of Medicine 2001; Dudley et al. 2004), one of the most recent reviews by Petersen and colleagues (2006) suggested that pay-for-performance has some positive effects, especially when its impact is monitored carefully. However, Frølich and colleagues (2007) remained doubtful, stating: "P4P [pay-for-performance] and PR [public reporting of performance] incentives intended to improve quality are now used worldwide. Despite this, there is relatively little research showing whether such incentives improve quality. We found little empirical evidence upon which to base the design of incentive programs, no comprehensive conceptual models of how incentives should work, and a disconnection between reported research and theory."

Despite some accumulation of information recently, there is little evidence about which performance targets/standards providers should be encouraged to achieve; what sort and scale of financial inducements, and combinations of incentives, are needed for what degree of change; how payments should be structured; and at what level incentives should be targeted (i.e. entire health plans, integrated organizations offering disease management services (e.g. disease-specific "carve outs"), group practices/physician partnerships, individual clinical teams or physicians, patients or some combination of these). It is generally held that incentive schemes should not rely exclusively on patient-level outcome indicators but should include a majority of structure and process measures of quality. This is because chronic disease outcomes are normally dependent on a range of factors, including patient involvement and compliance that are partly outside the control of chronic disease management programmes. Therefore, payments should be for performance largely on the basis of structures and processes rather than patient outcomes since the outcomes achieved are not necessarily always a direct reflection of the quality of services (Beich et al. 2006).

There is clearly growing interest in a range of different ways of changing payment methods to improve the effectiveness and cost-effectiveness of care, including for people with chronic conditions. This has led to more demonstration schemes and increased the scope for empirical work, especially in the

United States, to remedy the relative dearth of evaluative studies. As a result, a number of preliminary evaluations of several different incentive approaches are becoming available.

Quality-based purchasing

The Agency for Healthcare Quality has reviewed the evidence from the United States on the effectiveness and potential of both reputational and payment-driven quality-based purchasing schemes designed to improve the quality of care (Dudley et al. 2004). The review identified eight very varied trials of performance-based payment, each of which used different financial incentives and different measures of performance. The trials were mainly related to prevention and there was only one specifically directed at chronic care. In four studies, the recipient of the incentive was an individual provider, while in the other four the recipient was the provider group or could be either an individual provider or a group. Among the studies targeting individual providers, there were five positive and two negative results; among the studies in which the target was or could be the provider group, there were one positive and two negative results (in general, the term positive was used to mean an effect in the desired direction (i.e. the incentive worked) and negative to mean there was no significant effect of the incentive on the outcome measure). In seven studies, the target of the incentive was a physician. Of the nine dependent variables assessed, five showed a significant relationship to the incentive in the expected direction and four showed no significant change after the incentive was introduced. A single study involved pharmacists and achieved positive results.

There was no consistent relationship between the magnitude of the incentive and response, although the studies were so heterogeneous that this is not surprising. Among the fee-for-service studies, four were positive and one was negative. Among the bonus studies, two were positive and three were negative. There were seven studies of preventive care with nine dependent variables assessed. Among these nine outcomes, five were positive and four were negative. The single study on chronic care was positive. Generally, incentives to achieve performance were found to be more effective when the indicator to be followed required less patient cooperation (e.g. receiving vaccinations or answering questions about smoking) than when significant patient cooperation was needed (e.g. to quit smoking).

The authors concluded that, to date, there are few unequivocal data on which to base a quality-based purchasing strategy, but some evidence that both payment and reputational incentives can work. They suggest that, with appropriate caution, outcome measures can be included among the performance indicators used for quality-based purchasing, and not just structure and process indicators.

Pay-for-performance initiatives in the United States

Even though studies published so far cannot provide definitive evidence, they provide generally positive findings on pay-for-performance at the level of individual hospitals, insurers' programmes or large, integrated healthcare delivery networks. Unfortunately, and not uncommonly, it is still not possible to conclude which aspect of the intervention created the advantage over the comparators and there is no information about the cost-effectiveness of the intervention (Galvin 2006).

Petersen and colleagues (2006) offer perhaps the most up-to-date systematic review of the evidence on explicit financial incentives and improvements in quality measures. They identified 17 studies, 13 assessing process measures of quality, mostly for preventive services. Only two studies compared the type of incentive (bonus versus enhanced fee-for-service). Only five studies were specific to patients with chronic disease. Of these, one used the payment system to encourage skilled nursing home providers to take on elderly patients with chronic disease and improve their health status so that as many as possible could be discharged to their homes (positive effect of bonus payment); a second used the payment system to encourage providers to offer services to young people with substance abuse, psychological problems and criminal histories (to prevent cream-skimming in a system offering additional funding for more effective and efficient services); a third encouraged community mental health centres to provide case management of clients in the community (partial effect of enhanced fee-for-service); a fourth encouraged provider groups to screen diabetic patients for HbA1c (partial effect of bonus per member per month if target rates could be met or exceeded); and the final study encouraged individual physicians to meet quality targets for their diabetic patients based on process and outcome measures (e.g. serum low density lipoprotein and low density lipoprotein cholesterol, retinal examination) (partial effect of bonus paid in relation to achieving or exceeding individual targets and score on composite index of quality).

Five of the six studies of physician-level financial incentives and seven of nine studies of provider group-level financial incentives found partial or positive effects on measures of quality. One of the two studies of incentives at the level of the payment system found a positive effect on access to care, but the other showed signs of patient cream-skimming, indicating that access to care might have deteriorated. The authors found no studies looking at the duration of incentives or the persistence of any effects if incentives were removed. There was only one cost-effectiveness study, which happened to relate to people with chronic conditions. It showed that a combination of incentives could improve patients' access to nursing homes and the outcomes of nursing home care as well as saving US$3000 (€1978) per nursing home stay. However, because of the structure of the payment system, the savings might not accrue to Medicaid, which had paid for the incentives.

Studies to date also raise some important issues, especially about the detailed implementation of pay-for-performance initiatives (Hackbarth 2006).

- Financial incentives for quality are likely to be worth pursuing but require very careful design since there is some evidence of perverse responses to incentives (i.e. excessive focus on incentive-linked versus other tasks or areas of quality, gaming or better reporting without any improvement in quality).
- The objectives of any scheme need to be clearly defined, in particular whether

the goal is to improve the performance at the bottom of the distribution, raise the mean, increase the proportion of providers achieving a standard or reward the best.

- Collecting the data needed for pay-for-performance programmes can be costly and the data may not always accurately capture performance (e.g. risk-adjusted, detailed clinical data are needed to make valid comparisons between providers).
- Providers expend considerable resources trying to earn incentive payments (Chassin 2006); consequently, programmes are costly in terms of providers' time.
- The performance measures used in incentive programmes have to be chosen with great care to ensure that they are associated with health improvements, since providers target their quality-improvement efforts on areas that might earn them additional payments (Chassin 2006); incentives combining process and outcome measures of quality (e.g. provision of smoking cessation advice and quit rates) may mitigate the disadvantages of either approach taken alone (i.e. process measures tend to be more susceptible to gaming and outcome measures may not be sensitive to quality of care since they may be partly outside the control of providers).
- The size of the incentive is probably important though the amount of empirical work on this is negligible, so it is difficult to determine what proportion of provider income should be put at risk in such schemes. In these circumstances, it seems sensible not to offer excessively highly powered incentives.
- Continuous incentives may be more influential than, for instance, an end-of-year bonus.
- Financial incentives alone do not improve care in that incentives must influence frontline staff to alter what they do with, and for, patients, which means that staff must know what to change in terms of the structure of their practices and their processes of care.
- Effects of financial incentives tend to be small at the provider group (or hospital) level but somewhat larger at the level of individual professionals, most likely because individuals cannot obtain the full benefits of their own efforts under schemes operating at higher levels. However, the evidence from studies of the Chronic Care Model (Bodenheimer et al. 2002a, 2002b) tend to show that multidisciplinary teams produce better outcomes, suggesting that incentives at team level might be a feasible compromise between levels. The experience of the US Veterans Health Administration suggests that provider group incentives even without large monetary incentives for physicians can be effective in the presence of rigorous performance monitoring and benchmarking between provider groups (Kerr and Fleming 2007).

Finally, Petersen et al. (2006) offer an interesting theoretical justification for pay-for-performance relating to the information asymmetry that is generally said to lie at the heart of healthcare. They argue that because patient demand may be relatively unresponsive to the technical quality of clinical care, since most patients cannot observe or know the skill expended by clinical staff, financial incentives that reward high quality should contribute to protecting patients' interests, irrespective of their level of awareness of provider quality.

Evaluation of the Quality and Outcomes Framework (QOF) in the United Kingdom

The QOF was introduced in April 2004 when the quality of care for many common chronic diseases in United Kingdom general practices was already steadily improving (Campbell et al. 2005). In the four years since initiation, the QOF has demonstrated two things: generously funded pay-for-performance programmes can be popular with primary care physicians and their staff, and pay-for-performance programmes focus clinical behaviour on the aspects of care that are linked to incentives. Critics have argued that the QOF is poor value-for-money since it merely rewarded practices (handsomely) for what they were already doing in relation to chronic disease management, paid them for more activity not necessarily related to health improvement and simply rewarded the better organized practices excessively for improving their record keeping rather than their care. However, independent evaluation of the quality of care for three common chronic conditions in the QOF (angina, diabetes and asthma) using chart review in a representative sample of practices, rather than QOF returns, indicated strongly that quality (irrespective of value for money) continued to improve after 2004 when the QOF incentives were introduced and at a faster rate for asthma and diabetes than in the earlier period. For example, the percentage of patients with coronary heart disease with a serum cholesterol below 5.0 mmol/l had increased from 18% in 1998 to 61% in 2003, but at the end of the first year of the QOF it had reached 71%. The percentage of patients with diabetes whose HbA1c was less than 7.4 mmol/l increased from 38% in 1998 to 40% in 2003, but 58% after 12 months of the QOF.

There was also a statistically significant difference in improvement between areas of performance linked to incentives by the QOF and those not, suggesting some causal effect of the QOF on quality (Campbell et al. 2007). The authors concluded that pay-for-performance is a useful means to augment other approaches to quality improvement in chronic disease care.

However, general practices in more socioeconomically deprived areas tended to have lower levels of achievement and received less financial reward for the same level of achievement (Guthrie et al. 2006), though the differences between practices in more and less advantaged areas were small (Doran et al. 2006) and there were signs of "catch up" among practices in more-deprived areas over time (Ashworth et al. 2007). In addition, patients in deprived areas were less likely to be registered with a general practice and thereby less likely to be able to benefit from the care improvements reported.

The performance improvements identified are likely to be the result of the better organization of care at general practice level, in particular the provision of more systematic care, which tends to favour larger practices (Wang et al. 2006). This is manifest in a number of ways, such as more effective recall of patients with established risk factors for chronic disease, leading to better follow-up, and greater use of protocol-driven care, including templates for recording consultations, leading to better recording of care and more focused and effective clinical encounters. The QOF is also stimulating an expansion of the role of nurses in primary care. Finally, the quality gains observed would not have been possible without a well-established information technology infrastructure throughout

United Kingdom general practice, allowing practices to understand where they started from before the new contract.

Conclusions

Countries and health systems vary in the degree to which overall system characteristics support or frustrate efforts to enable and support services for people with chronic diseases. In very general terms, systems face the greatest difficulties in adapting their payment arrangements to become more conducive to effective chronic disease care if they have a tradition of patient choice of any provider, and/or of little or no enrolment with particular providers and/or of paying for services episodically using fee-for-service as the predominant method of reimbursement. This is because such systems tend to discourage continuity of care or a provider focus on a population of patients. Many of the most widely discussed approaches to the management of chronic disease are extremely difficult to implement in such fragmented, fee-for-service systems.

Systems with strong primary healthcare are more likely to give greater attention to the management of people with chronic conditions and to obtain better results in this area. For example, the United Kingdom has reasonably good performance on chronic disease outcomes for conditions such as asthma and diabetes compared with similar countries (Nolte et al. 2006). It is also no coincidence that the United Kingdom NHS has recently been able develop some of the most innovative methods internationally of paying for improvements in the quality and outcome of chronic disease care because it has a well-developed primary care system, patient enrolment with primary care physician practices, gatekeeping by general practitioners and experience of paying for ambulatory care through a mixed mode contract that includes elements of capitation, fee-for-service and target payments.

Another commonly experienced barrier to encouraging the appropriate management of people with chronic conditions is the tendency in some systems to pay separately for the care of specific diseases (again, a throwback to a period when it might reasonably be assumed that most patients had a single condition at a time requiring professional attention). Indeed, in most countries, chronic disease management programmes have tended to evolve condition by condition (Anderson and Knickman 2001). Yet, in reality, chronic illness lies along a continuum (i.e. from the asymptomatic person at risk to those with a range of established chronic illnesses) and chronic conditions (and their related risk factors) are increasingly seen as being strongly interrelated.

Yet another, similar, commonly encountered barrier related to system fragmentation, is a tendency in many systems to pay different healthcare professionals separately, thereby perpetuating traditions of independent, solo practice. Much effective care of people with chronic conditions appears to depend on multidisciplinary team work, yet this is frequently frustrated by these payment systems. For example, the Australian EPC initiative has been hampered by the fact that payment for involvement in care planning and case conferences for patients with chronic disease is only available to general practitioners and not to other healthcare professionals whose input is important for effective case management.

In response to such obstacles, policy makers and payers have been increasingly looking for ways of bringing together (bundling) different budgets and sources of funding for different activities and different types of professional to produce more patient-centred methods of payment, rather than paying different professionals separately for individual activities (e.g. the Coordinated Care Trials in Australia and the development of capitated primary health organizations in New Zealand since 2001). They have also begun to develop "blended" or "mixed" approaches to payment for chronic disease care, which attempt to capture the benefits and offset the drawbacks of each separate payment modality. Many pay-for-performance initiatives use a blend of payment methods, including paying directly for the delivery of specific measures of quality and/or outcomes. For example, Goroll et al. (2007) have proposed an alternative to the preponderant encounter-based, fee-for-service payment methods found in the United States in the form of a mix of comprehensive risk-adjusted capitation payments, including an amount for infrastructure and care coordination, and risk-adjusted performance bonuses to mitigate the disadvantages of capitation.

This chapter has focused particularly on recent high-profile pay-for-performance initiatives such as the 2004 general practice contract in the United Kingdom NHS and the current demonstration programmes of the Centers for Medicare and Medicaid Services in the United States. It has shown that financial incentives to encourage providers to undertake desirable activities may be effective in improving performance in chronic care. However, the volume of evaluative research in this field is still comparatively small given the many complexities inherent in designing payment systems, especially ones that include elements of pay-for-performance. For example, there is little or no research where the size of financial incentives has been varied to establish the nature of any "dose–response" relationship or understanding of the costs to providers of complying with the quality goals in programmes. In addition, there is no established conceptual model in the literature as to how financial incentives such as pay-for-performance should work and what factors would facilitate or reduce their impact (Frølich et al. 2007).

In these circumstances, policy development should be cautious. For example, it cannot be assumed that the financial elements in pay-for-performance schemes are always the major motive for professionals to change their practice (Marshall and Harrison 2005). Professionals are motivated by more than remuneration. In particular, physicians and other healthcare professionals respond to reputational incentives, particularly where performance information is published, though remuneration remains a powerful lever for change. There is also extensive psychological evidence that excessive use of externally imposed incentives, particularly financial ones, can "crowd out" the internal motivation to do a good job in areas that are not the subject of extrinsic rewards. This suggests further cautions: that pay-for-performance should not constitute too large a part of the remuneration of the typical provider and that, as far as possible, the indicators of performance used should be supported by the target population of professionals and aligned with their conceptions of what a high-quality service comprises.

References

Anderson, G. and Knickman, J. (2001) Changing the chronic care system to meet people's needs, *Health Aff*, 20: 146–60.

Ashworth, M., Seed, P., Armstrong, D., Durbaba, S. and Jones, R. (2007) The relationship between social deprivation and the quality of primary care: a national survey using indicators from the UK Quality and Outcomes Framework, *Br J Gen Pract*, 57: 441–8.

Beich, J., Scanlon, D., Ulbrecht, J., Ford, E. and Ibrahim, I. (2006) The role of disease management in pay-for-performance programs for improving the care of chronically ill patients, *Med Care Res Rev*, 63(Suppl 1): 96S–116S.

Bodenheimer, T., Wagner, E. and Grumbach, K. (2002a) Improving primary care for patients with chronic illness, *JAMA*, 288: 1775–9.

Bodenheimer, T., Wagner, E. and Grumbach, K. (2002b) Improving primary care for patients with chronic illness: the chronic care model, Part 2, *JAMA*, 288: 1909–14.

British Medical Association (2003) *Investing in General Practice. The New General Medical Services Contract*. London: British Medical Association. http://www.bma.org.uk/ap.nsf/content/investinggp (accessed 19 December 2007).

Brook, R., Ware, J., Rogers, W. et al. (1983) Does free care improve adults' health? Results from a randomized controlled trial, *N Engl J Med*, 309: 1426–34.

Busse, R. (2004) Disease management programmes in Germany's statutory health insurance system, *Health Aff*, 23: 56–67.

Busse, R., Schreyögg, J. and Smith, P. (2006) Hospital case payment systems in Europe, *Health Care Manag Sci*, 9: 211–13.

Campbell, S., Roland, M., Middleton, E. and Reeves, D. (2005) Improvements in the quality of clinical care in English general practice 1998–2003: longitudinal observational study, *BMJ*, 331: 1121–3.

Campbell, S., Reeves, D., Kontopantelis, E. et al. (2007) Quality of primary care in England with the introduction of pay for performance, *N Engl J Med*, 357: 181–90.

Centre for Clinical Management Development (2007) *Definition of Year of Care*. Durham: Durham University. http://www.dur.ac.uk/ccmd/yoc/definition/ (accessed 13 March 2008).

Chassin, M. (2006) Does paying for performance improve the quality of health care? *Med Care Res Rev*, 63(Suppl 1): 122S–5S.

Couch, J. (1998) Disease management: an overview, in J. Couch (ed.) *The Health Professional's Guide to Disease Management: Patient-centered Care for the 21st Century*, pp.1–28. Boston, MA: Jones & Bartlett.

Doran, T., Fullwood, C., Gravelle, H. et al. (2006) Pay-for-performance programs in family practices in the United Kingdom, *N Engl J Med*, 355: 375–84.

Dudley, R., Frolich, A., Robinowitz, D. et al. (2004) *Strategies to Support Quality-based Purchasing: A Review of the Evidence*. Rockville, MD: Agency for Healthcare Research and Quality.

Durand-Zaleski, I. and Obrecht, O. (2008) France, in E. Nolte, C. Knai and M. McKee (eds) *Managing Chronic Conditions: Experience in Eight Countries*. Copenhagen: European Observatory on Health Systems and Policies.

Eastman, R., Javitt, J., Herman, W. et al. (1997) Models of complications of NIDDM. II. Analysis of the health benefits and cost-effectiveness of treating NIDDM with the goal of normoglycaemia, *Diabetes Care*, 20: 685–6.

Eichler, R., Auxila, P. and Pollock, J. (2001) Promoting preventive health care: paying for performance, in Haiti, in P. Brook and S. Smith (eds) *Contracting for Public Services: Output-based Aid and its Applications*. Washington DC: World Bank.

Frølich, A., Talavera, J., Broadhead, P. and Dudley, R. (2007) A behavioural model of clinician responses to incentives to improve quality, *Health Policy*, 80: 179–93.

Galvin, R. (2006) Evaluating the performance of pay for performance, *Med Care Res Rev*, 63(Suppl 1): 126S–30S.

Glasgow, N., Zwar, N., Harris, M., Hasan, I. and Jowsey, T. (2008) Australia, in E. Nolte, C. Knai and M. McKee (eds) *Managing Chronic Conditions: Experience in Eight Countries*. Copenhagen: European Observatory on Health Systems and Policies.

Goldman, D., Joyce, G. and Zheng, Y. (2007) Prescription drug cost sharing: Associations with medication and medical utilization and spending and health, *JAMA*, 298: 61–9.

Goroll, A., Berenson, R., Schoenbaum, S. and Gardner, L. (2007) Fundamental reform of payment for adult primary care: comprehensive payment for comprehensive care, *J Gen Intern Med*, 22: 410–15.

Gosden, T., Forland, F., Kristiansen, I. et al. (2001) Impact of payment method on behaviour of primary care physicians: a systematic review, *J Health Serv Res Policy*, 6: 44–55.

Guthrie, B., McLean, G. and Sutton, M. (2006) Workload and reward in the Quality and Outcomes Framework of the 2004 general practice contract, *Br J Gen Pract*, 56: 836–41.

Hackbarth, G. (2006) Commentary, *Med Care Res Rev*, 63(Suppl 1): 117S–21S.

Information Centre (2007) *National Quality and Outcomes Framework Statistics for England 2006/07*. London: Information Centre. http://www.ic.nhs.uk/webfiles/QOF/2006-07/QOF%202006–07%20Statistical%20Bulletin.pdf (accessed 10 December 2007).

Institute of Medicine (2001) *Crossing the Quality Chasm: A New Health System for the 21st Century*. Washington DC: National Academy Press.

Jiwani, I. and Dubois, C. (2008) Canada, in E. Nolte, C. Knai and M. McKee (eds) *Managing Chronic Conditions: Experience in Eight Countries*. Copenhagen: European Observatory on Health Systems and Policies.

Karlberg, I. (2008) Sweden, in E. Nolte, C. Knai and M. McKee (eds) *Managing Chronic Conditions: Experience in Eight Countries*. Copenhagen: European Observatory on Health Systems and Policies.

Keeler, E., Brook, R., Goldberg, G., Kamberg, C. and Newhouse, J. (1985) How free care reduced hypertension in the health insurance experiment, *JAMA*, 254: 1926–31.

Kerr, E. and Fleming, B. (2007) Making performance indicators work: experiences of US Veterans Health Administration, *BMJ*, 335: 971–3.

Klein, S. (2006) Medicare P4P demo pushes physician care for chronically ill, *Commonwealth Fund Newsletter*, Vol. 20. New York: The Commonwealth Fund. http://www.cmwf.org/publications//publications_show.htm?doc_id=402822.

Klein-Lankhorst, E. and Spreeuwenberg, C. (2008) The Netherlands, in E. Nolte, C. Knai and M. McKee (eds) *Managing Chronic Conditions: Experience in Eight Countries*. Copenhagen: European Observatory on Health Systems and Policies.

Leatherman, S., Berwick, D., Iles, D. et al. (2003) The business case for quality: case studies and an analysis, *Health Aff*, 22: 17–30.

Lurie, N., Kamberg, C., Brook, R., Keeler, E. and Newhouse, J. (1989) How free care improved vision in the health insurance experiment, *Am J Public Health*, 79: 640–2.

Marshall, M. and Harrison, S. (2005) It's about more than money: financial incentives and internal motivation, *Qual Saf Health Care*, 14: 4–5.

McNamara, P. (2006) Foreward: payment matters? The next chapter, *Med Care Res Rev*, 63(Suppl 1): 5S–10S.

Nolte, E., Bain, C. and McKee, M. (2006) Diabetes as a tracer condition in international benchmarking of health systems, *Diabetes Care*, 29: 1007–11.

Petersen, L., Woodard, L., Urech, T., Daw, C. and Sookanan, S. (2006) Does pay-for-performance improve the quality of health care? *Ann Intern Med*, 145: 265–72.

Rechel, B., Dubois, C.-A. and McKee, M. (2006) *The Health Care Workforce in Europe: Learning From Experience*. Copenhagen: World Health Organization Regional Office for Europe on behalf of European Observatory on Health Systems and Policies.

Roland, M. (2004) Linking physicians' pay to the quality of care: a major experiment in the United Kingdom, *N Engl J Med*, 351: 1448–54.

Schiotz, M., Frolich, A. and Krasnik, A. (2008) Denmark, in E. Nolte, C. Knai and M. McKee (eds) *Managing Chronic Conditions: Experience in Eight Countries*. Copenhagen: European Observatory on Health Systems and Policies.

Siering, U. (2008) Germany, in E. Nolte, C. Knai and M. McKee (eds) *Managing Chronic Conditions: Experience in Eight Countries*. Copenhagen: European Observatory on Health Systems and Policies.

Singh, D. and Fahey, D. (2008) England, in E. Nolte, C. Knai and M. McKee (eds) *Managing Chronic Conditions: Experience in Eight Countries*. Copenhagen: European Observatory on Health Systems and Policies.

Singh, D. and Ham, C. (2006) *Improving Care for People with Long-term Conditions. A Review of UK and International Frameworks*. Birmingham: University of Birmingham, NHS Institute for Innovation and Improvement.

Smith, P. and York, N. (2004) Quality incentives: the case of UK general practitioners, *Health Aff*, 23: 112–18.

Van de Ven, W., Beck, K., van de Voorde, C., Wasem, J. and Zmora, I. (2007) Risk adjustment and risk selection in Europe: 6 years later, *Health Policy*, 83: 162–79.

Wang, Y., O'Donnell, C., Mackay, D. and Watt, G. (2006) Practice size and quality attainment under the new GMS contract: a cross-sectional analysis, *Br J Gen Pract*, 56: 830–5.

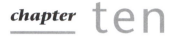
Making it happen

Ellen Nolte and Martin McKee

Introduction

An effective response to the rising burden of chronic diseases will only be possible in a health system that facilitates the development and implementation of structured approaches to management of these conditions. There is now considerable empirical evidence to support the intuitive belief that fragmentation of services makes it difficult to implement the integrated strategies needed (Busse 2004; Epping-Jordan et al. 2004; Segal et al. 2004). However, even when the basic structure of the health system is supportive with, for example, well-developed primary healthcare, there are also barriers to be overcome all along the continuum of care (Calnan et al. 2006).

This concluding chapter explores the challenges that exist and seeks to identify ways of overcoming them. We begin by reviewing the evidence on barriers to coordination and integration. We then examine the various approaches taken by different countries to address them; we describe trends emerging in different healthcare settings, drawing on detailed country case studies published in a companion volume to this book (Nolte et al. 2008). We seek to understand these trends, looking at the drivers of policies, the overall vision underlying them and the understanding and commitment of policy makers, seeking insights into how these shape the resulting strategies. By doing so, we seek to identify facilitators and barriers related to the implementation of successful chronic care policies.

The need for new models of care

This volume demonstrates clearly why the traditional acute episodic model of care is ill-equipped to meet the long-term, fluctuating needs of those with chronic illness and why, as a result, there is a need for new service delivery models that are characterized by collaboration and cooperation among professions and institutions that have traditionally worked separately. The growing recognition of this need (Boerma 2006) is causing many countries to explore new approaches to healthcare delivery that can bridge the boundaries between professions, providers and institutions and so provide appropriate support to patients.

Coordination of care is at the heart of the problem. Patients value coordination of their care, seeing it as an important component of overall quality (Calnan et al. 2006) especially when they have chronic health problems and complex needs (Alazri et al. 2006; Turner et al. 2007). A recent survey of patients' experience in seven countries demonstrated how at least three-quarters of adults considered it important to have somewhere where they are known and where they can obtain assistance in coordinating their care (Schoen et al. 2007). Yet only half of patients with chronic conditions (approximately 60% in Australia and New Zealand) reported having access to a doctor or other source of care that would routinely help coordinate the services they required (a "medical home") (Figure 10.1). Importantly, a relatively high proportion had used multiple providers and care settings, with between 25% (New Zealand) and 55% (Germany) reporting use of multiple specialists in the preceding year, a reflection of suboptimal coordination of care.

Chapter 6 reviewed the now ample evidence that helping patients to self-manage their condition improves clinical and other outcomes (Singh 2005; Zwar et al. 2006), although the precise benefits vary according to the disease processes involved. Yet, the survey of seven countries found that only a small percentage of those with chronic health problems are given written instructions on management of their condition at home, with just over 20% in Germany

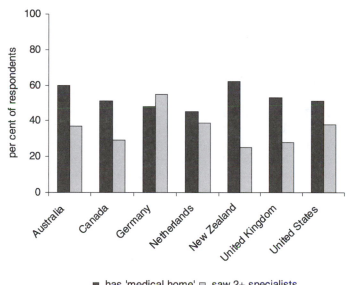

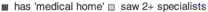

Figure 10.1   Experience of patients with chronic conditions in seven countries.

Source: Adapted from Schoen et al. (2007).

and 33% in Canada, the Netherlands and New Zealand, 40% in Australia and just over 50% in the United States (Schoen et al. 2007). More worryingly, between 15 and 20% of adults with a chronic condition reported frequently having received conflicting information from different providers.

It is noteworthy that failings in care coordination were observed not only in countries traditionally characterized by fragmentation, such as the United States, Australia and Germany, but also in those that are known to have strong primary care such as the Netherlands, New Zealand and the United Kingdom. These countries have a strict gatekeeping system in place, which is often viewed as a mechanism to promote coordination and integration (Starfield et al. 2005; Calnan et al. 2006). Yet, as the findings of Schoen et al. (2007) indicate, this is not necessarily the case and indeed, as Starfield et al. (2005) have pointed out, "[v]ery few health systems, even those that rate high on primary care, achieve high coordination of care". Therefore, problems in achieving coordination and integration of services along the entire care continuum abound in most healthcare settings. The next section explores some of the reasons why.

Overcoming the challenges

Problems of care coordination and integration typically arise at the interfaces between primary and secondary care, health and social care, curative and public health services, and among specialities and professional groups (Boerma 2006), although much of the available evidence relates to the interface between health and social care. To simplify the discussion, we here use notions of integration, coordination, joint or partnership working and related concepts synonymously while recognizing that, in practice, they may not necessarily be identical (Chapter 4).

In an analysis of the United Kingdom experience integrating health and social services in the late 1990s, Hardy et al. (1999) identified a number of major barriers to integration. These include:

- *structural barriers* caused by fragmentation of responsibilities across boundaries between agencies, both within and between sectors
- *procedural barriers* arising from differences in planning and budgetary horizons and cycles and information systems and protocols
- *financial barriers* caused by differences in funding mechanisms and sources and in allocation and flows of financial resources
- *professional barriers* arising from competing ideologies and values, professional self-interest and autonomy, interprofessional competition for domains, threats to job security and potentially conflicting views about service users' interests and roles (Chapter 7)
- *status and legitimacy barriers* as reflected by organizational self-interest and the desire for autonomy.

Similarly, commenting on partnership working in health and social care, Glasby et al. (2006) identified structural divisions, separation of legal and financial frameworks, distinct organizational and professional cultures and differences in terms of governance and accountability as key barriers to bringing together health and social services. Looking more specifically at coordination and integration within the healthcare sector Calnan et al. (2006) identified similar obstacles, in particular structural and financial barriers dividing providers at the primary/secondary care interface as well as professional barriers, such as "professional rivalry" between hospital doctors and general practitioners. More recently, in an analysis of continuity of care in the United Kingdom, Hardy et al. (2006) added frequent organizational change ("organizational turbulence") as a strong impediment towards coordination of care while Plochg et al. (2006) highlighted the potential negative impact of the introduction of a competitive environment on the sustainability of community-based integrated care initiatives.

Financial concerns pose a critical challenge to many initiatives, as there is often a failure to understand that "integration costs before it pays", as Leutz (1999) commented when reviewing attempts in the United States and United Kingdom to integrate health and social services. He argued that successful integration requires sustained investment in staff and support systems (such as training and information systems), funding for start-up costs, and flexibility to respond to needs that emerge during implementation. However, "[f]ailure to anticipate these costs . . . is a typical shortcoming of public initiatives, which are often strapped for cash and may not recognize the new management, training and supervision models that are required".

Leutz (1999) further observed that there is often an expectation that integration initiatives will self-fund from "savings" arising when a new service is substituted for an existing one. This may, however, threaten the position of the existing providers, who may not wish to give up control ("turf guarding"). A recent review of two major research programmes on continuity of care in England and Canada also cautioned that the creation of new coordinating mechanisms will not compensate for lack of resources (Freeman et al. 2007). There may be a temptation to inject one-off extra funding to pay for new services (Leutz 1999), but this will not necessarily ensure long-term sustainability, as illustrated by the example of transmural care in the Netherlands (Box 10.1), an initiative that also highlights the importance of aligning payment schemes with system objectives (Hofmarcher et al. 2007; Chapter 9).

Many initiatives appear to rest on an implicit assumption that integration is "a good thing" (Goodwin et al. 2004; Glasby et al. 2006). Yet the evidence that this is so is scarce; questions remain as to whether such arrangements "really lead to better services and better outcomes", and if so, under what circumstances and how (Glasby et al. 2006). For example, reviewing the evidence on "success", defined as having generated beneficial changes in processes and/or outcomes of partnership working (or, by extension, cooperation) across health and social care in the United Kingdom, Dowling et al. (2004) found that most research focused on process measures, typically relating to the functioning of partnerships. In contrast, evidence about whether or how partnerships improve outcomes, for example by enhancing access to services or improving efficiency, effectiveness or quality of services, was inconsistent or inconclusive. The authors concluded that "research that brings together rigorous and systematic evidence of the outcomes, causality and costs of partnerships has yet to be conducted" (Dowling et al. 2004).

Box 10.1 Transmural care in the Netherlands

Improving the continuity and quality of care for people with long-term conditions by closing the gap between primary and hospital services has been a major objective in Dutch health policy since the 1990s, giving rise to the concept of transmural care (van der Linden et al. 2001). Transmural care has been defined as "care, attuned to the needs of the patient, provided on the basis of cooperation and coordination between general and specialized caregivers with shared overall responsibility and the specification of delegated responsibilities" (van der Linden et al. 2001). This approach has subsequently been developed extensively, with an estimated 500+ initiatives by the end of the 1990s. Most forms of transmural care focus on managing the interface between acute hospital care and alternative settings for those who are not able to return to a fully independent life.

Arrangements are often based on contracts or may be informal. In a few cases, cooperating organizations eventually merged (van der Linden et al. 2001; den Exter et al. 2004). A key challenge has been the provision of sufficient funding in the absence of established financial mechanisms. Many transmural care projects receive grants or subsidies from the local or national government (den Exter et al. 2004). Hospitals may spend up to 3% of their budget on transmural care activities, yet many initiatives have found it difficult to generate additional sources of funding or to restructure their financial mechanisms to cater for the new arrangements (van der Linden et al. 2001).

A recent Cochrane review of shared care arrangements at the interface between primary and speciality care in chronic disease management failed to identify sufficient evidence of significant improvements in patient outcomes, with the possible exception of improved prescribing (Smith et al. 2007). The definition of shared care as "the joint participation of primary care physicians and specialty care physicians in the planned delivery of care" in that review does not exactly match the definition of partnership/joint working described above. However, taken together, these findings highlight the continued difficulty in drawing firm and consistent conclusions about the impact of coordination and integration on outcomes from the available evidence (Chapter 4).

It is also important to note that the often assumed ability of efforts at integration to overcome fragmentation may not be justified. Fabbricotti (2007) found that some forms of integration may, paradoxically, lead to (further) fragmentation. Analysing the formation of integrated delivery systems in the Netherlands, she showed that multidisciplinary teams and case management strategies did increase the alignment of activities by professionals in different organizations but they also decreased opportunities for professionals to coordinate with those monodisciplinary colleagues that remained outside teams. Imbalances of power and resources within the integrated delivery system may cause initiatives to "backfire" as individuals strive to retain their financial and strategic position. Thus, "[p]rocesses of integration and fragmentation take place simultaneously, leading to continually changing and different IDS [integrated delivery systems] structures and alliances between actors" (Fabbricotti 2007).

As these examples show, the available evidence from research provides only limited support for the intuitive belief in the potential of integration to solve many problems. This must be born in mind when looking at the practical experience. The next section explores experiences in a range of countries, focusing, in particular, on how policy makers have sought to establish a policy framework that allows for the development and implementation of coordinated and/or structured approaches to chronic care, thereby, directly or indirectly, overcoming the barriers to integration identified above.

Analysing response in different countries

Reflecting on options to advance the quality of chronic care, Epping-Jordan et al. (2004) noted that "improvement in the care of patients with chronic illness will only occur if the system leaders . . . make it a priority and provide the leadership, incentives and resources necessary to make improvements happen". We here explore whether and how policy makers in different countries have succeeded in this goal.

In many countries, innovative approaches to chronic care are still experimental, with limited evidence of their effectiveness. Few have been adequately documented, although the accompanying volume does provide considerable new information (Nolte et al. 2008). Consequently, the selection of countries reviewed is of necessity pragmatic; they do, however, include a mix of countries with different approaches to funding healthcare that have demonstrated some degree of innovation in chronic care. These are Denmark, England, Germany, the Netherlands, France and Sweden, with the addition of Canada and Australia from outside the European region as these can nevertheless provide useful lessons for Europe. Given the range of approaches adopted in different countries, the analysis inevitably has to be selective, highlighting only key issues; more detailed descriptions can be found in Nolte et al. (2008).

New approaches to chronic care

Health system responses to chronic disease vary widely, reflecting, to a great extent, national approaches to health system governance and responsibilities of different stakeholders in the regulation, funding and delivery of healthcare. The nature and scope of policies on chronic disease are very diverse, with some countries having developed nationally integrated strategies spanning the continuum from health promotion and disease prevention to the management of complex conditions. These include Australia, Denmark and England. Others have implemented a spectrum of parallel policies targeting specific elements along the care continuum (e.g. France, Germany, the Netherlands and some places in Canada and Sweden). The following section briefly summarizes some of the key components of these policies.

Responsibility for health policy in **Australia** is shared by the Commonwealth government and those of the states and territories. Strategies to address chronic disease have focused on quality of care and on reducing resource use (Glasgow et al. 2008). The Commonwealth government's policies include the 2005 *National Chronic Disease Strategy*, which provides an "overarching framework of national direction for improving chronic disease prevention and care across Australia", along with five supporting National Service Improvement Frameworks covering a range of chronic conditions (National Health Priority Action Council 2005). The subsequent 2006 Better Health Initiative, *Better Health for all Australians*, a joint venture from the Australian state and territory governments was designed to reduce the impact of chronic disease through health promotion and early detection and to encourage self-management and improving care coordination (Council of Australian Governments 2006). The Enhanced Primary Care scheme, a system of financial incentives for general practitioners introduced in 1999, encourages coordination of care for patients with chronic conditions with pay-for-performance linked to care quality (Healy et al. 2006; Glasgow et al. 2008; Chapter 9).

The federal division of responsibility in Australia means that implementation of policies depends, to a great extent, on the individual states, whose prime focus tends to be on decreasing the use of hospital resources by reducing admissions, readmissions and length of stay. State responses are numerous and diverse, including, for example, the New South Wales chronic care programme (NSW Department of Health 2004a, 2004b) and the Northern Territory preventable chronic disease strategy (Weeramanthri et al. 2003). Consequently, it has been argued that, despite the existence of a nationally agreed vision in the form of the Better Health Initiative, the momentum for a common national approach has been lost (Glasgow et al. 2008).

Denmark has also developed a national vision of chronic disease control with the government's 2002 *Healthy throughout Life* strategy, which focuses on major preventable diseases and disorders, setting targets to increase life expectancy, improve quality of life and minimize health inequalities (Ministry of the Interior and Health 2003). The strategy was brought into operation in a project by the National Board of Health (2005), followed by a report setting out options for improving the care for those with chronic conditions (National Board of Health 2006). Many of the options proposed are in the form of general recommendations although some are more specific.

Improving care coordination was also an important driver behind the recent structural reform of the Danish health system, which involved reallocation of responsibilities in the healthcare sector between five newly established Danish regions (replacing the previous 14 county councils) and the municipalities (Strandberg-Larsen et al. 2007). As part of the reform, municipal health centres are being developed and evaluated, targeting primarily elderly people and those with chronic health problems (Schiotz et al. 2008). However, the initiative has been criticized as lacking a coherent framework and, importantly, the new centres are limited to provision of non-physician services (Møller Pedersen 2006).

As in Denmark, in England the 2004 White Paper *Choosing Health* set out a broad strategy to improve population health, encompassing health promotion, disease prevention and initiatives designed to improve the care of those with chronic disease (Department of Health 2004a). It built on a series of National Service Frameworks, long-term strategies for improving care in specific areas (e.g. diabetes, cancer, mental health, children, older people, long-term neurological conditions) and the 2004 *National Health Service Improvement Plan* (Department of Health 2004b), which set out a systematic approach to supporting patients with chronic conditions. Strategies included the implementation of case management in all primary care trusts, bodies that are responsible for purchasing care for geographically defined populations on the basis of health need. The 2005 NHS and Social Care Model sets out a comprehensive strategy for improving the care of those with chronic conditions, based on risk stratification to match services to need, case management and establishment of new multidisciplinary teams (Department of Health 2005). The 2006 White Paper *Our Health, Our Care, Our Say* set out the government's vision for community-based care to support elderly people and those with chronic conditions (Department of Health 2006). Key drivers of these policies were the quest for improvement in the quality and accessibility of care for those with chronic disease and the containment or reduction of costs. There is a specific government target to reduce inpatient emergency bed-days by 5% by March 2008, to be achieved, mainly, through the provision of personal care plans for vulnerable people at most risk. The primary care team plays a crucial role in these reforms. Consequently, a new system of paying for primary care has been introduced, which provides financial incentives to encourage general practices to provide high-quality care for selected chronic conditions (Roland 2004), an incentive scheme in which most practices have exceeded expectations (Cole 2005; Chapter 9).

In contrast, no overarching national chronic disease strategies have emerged in France, Germany and the Netherlands, but there has been a spectrum of parallel policies targeting specific elements of the care continuum. This reflects, to some extent, the diverse responsibilities for funding healthcare through (social) health insurance and, in Germany and the Netherlands, the decentralized nature of decision making, involving a range of actors including representatives of the health professions and insurers.

In the **French** healthcare system, concern about a lack of coordination and continuity of care, both in the ambulatory sector and on the interface between ambulatory and hospital care, has prompted a series of changes (Sandier et al. 2004). These include, in 1996, the introduction of mechanisms stimulating experiments with different provider networks at the local level, with initiatives eventually formalized as "health networks" (Réseaux de Santé) in the 2002 *Patients' Rights and Quality of Care Act* (Frossard et al. 2002). This was followed by the 2004 Public Health Law, which defined a series of health targets for (chronic) diseases and risk factors for the period 2005–2009 and foresaw the development of a national public health plan for people with chronic illness, published in 2007 (Ministère de la Santé et des Solidarités 2007), and the 2004 Health Insurance Law, which, among other things, reformed the traditional ALD (*affections de longue durée*) procedure that exempts patients with long-term conditions from co-payments if their care adheres to evidence-based guidelines (Durand-Zaleski and Obrecht 2008). It has been argued that these initiatives lack an integrative vision, with no clearly defined objectives, procedures for implementation, or incentives and sanctions; however, there is an expectation that the 2007 national plan will be an important step towards a more coherent approach to chronic care.

As in France, there is growing concern in **Germany** about the ability to support patients with complex needs in a system that until recently was characterized by a strict separation between the hospital and ambulatory sector, and this has led to a series of initiatives targeting different actors in the healthcare system (Hilfer et al. 2007). In 1993, provisions were introduced to support more integrated models of care, followed by the creation of disease management programmes in 2002 (Busse 2004). In 2004, integrated care obtained further support from the removal of certain legal and financial obstacles by means of the Social Health Insurance Modernization Act. This effectively established integrated care as a distinct sector, enabling health insurance funds to designate financial resources for selective contracting with single providers or network of providers, many of which targeting the interface between acute hospital and rehabilitative care (Busse and Riesberg 2004).

The German disease management programmes have attracted considerable international attention. They are highly structured and regulated and embedded in the social health insurance system. They involve a change in the risk structure compensation scheme that creates strong incentives for sickness funds to enrol patients (Siering 2008). The funding system also creates considerable financial incentives for physicians to participate in the scheme. Existing programmes cover diabetes type 1 and 2, asthma/chronic obstructive pulmonary disease, heart disease and breast cancer. Although disease management programmes are now an integral component of the German healthcare sector, some have questioned their effectiveness and the appropriateness of the financial incentives involved (Gerst and Korzilius 2005).

Similar concerns about continuity and quality of care for people with long-term conditions, especially where their needs straddle the interface between primary and secondary care, has also been a concern in **the Netherlands**. This gave rise to the concept of transmural care in the early 1990s (van der Linden et al. 2001), described in Box 10.1. This has been compared with the "shared care" approaches seen in the United Kingdom (Vondeling 2004). More recently, there has been interest in the development of disease management approaches that support integration of processes along the care pathway for those with chronic conditions (Vrijhoef et al. 2001). Previously, these had attracted some, but limited, interest and, in the early 2000s, approximately 10% of general practitioners in the Netherlands were engaged in some form of disease management (Steuten et al. 2002). It has been argued that an expansion of such programmes was hindered by a lack of a structured framework for implementation and evaluation (Klein-Lankhorst and Spreeuwenberg 2008). However, the 2006 healthcare reform, in which many new market-based elements were introduced, has been interpreted by some as providing potential opportunities to improve care for chronic disease by enabling consumer groups ("collectives") to negotiate group insurance contracts for their members. Thus, a health insurance fund could develop a plan specifically catering for the needs of patients with specific conditions. However, this has so far attracted little interest (Bartholomée and Maarse 2007).

The healthcare systems in Canada and Sweden both devolve considerable responsibilities to the provinces and territories and the counties, respectively. In **Canada**, in 2002, the federal, provincial and territorial ministers of health developed an integrated Pan-Canadian Healthy Living Strategy, focusing on the prevention of chronic disease (Jiwani and Dubois 2008). The strategy reflects the division of responsibilities. Public health is a federal responsibility whereas responsibility for healthcare (within a federal legal framework) lies with the provinces. Consequently, there is considerable diversity in what is happening on the ground, with several provinces developing innovative schemes aimed at care coordination through shared governance of a broad range of health services and increased collaboration among health providers. Examples include Ontario, Quebec, Alberta and British Columbia. In Ontario, there is a Chronic Disease Prevention and Management Framework, which provides a framework for the activities of family health teams, which were created in 2004, and the more recently established (2005) Local Health Integration Networks. The latter are local governance structures mandated to plan, coordinate and fund local health services within specified geographic areas. Many have identified chronic disease prevention and management as a priority (Jiwani and Dubois 2008). In Quebec, initiatives to enhance chronic care have been embedded in an overall strategy to improve health and social care within available resources. This has involved the creation of local services networks (health and social services centres) which bring together all care providers in a region to develop partnerships of relevant groups (such as physicians and community organizations). These are tasked with ensuring provision of a comprehensive basket of services stretching from prevention to end-of-life care.

In **Sweden**, the primary care centre is seen as the foundation for chronic care, guided by regional and local guidelines. Nurses play an increasingly prominent role, taking on advanced care of patients with chronic and complex conditions such as diabetes and asthma, for whom they have limited rights to prescribe (Karlberg 2008). By the late 1990s, two-thirds of hospitals had nurse-led heart failure clinics, based on clinical protocols, with nurses empowered to change medication regimens within the protocols (Stromberg et al. 2001). However, there has been considerable debate in Sweden about the challenges of coordination between providers. This has led to the development of so-called "chains of care" (Andersson and Karlberg 2000), defined as "coordinated activities within healthcare" often involving "several responsible authorities and medical providers" (Ahgren 2003), and comparable to managed clinical networks for specific patient groups that work to common guidelines and agreements (Karlberg 2008). By 2002, most county councils had established at least one chain of care, most focusing on patients with chronic conditions such as diabetes, dementia and rheumatoid disorders. The main driver of these initiatives was the quest to improve quality of care; although success has been mixed, there appears to be a strong motivation among county councils to continue and extend this approach (Ahgren 2003). Since 2005, there has also been a movement to develop local coordinating strategies at county level, under the heading "local healthcare" (*narsjukvard*). This has been defined as "an upgraded family- and community-oriented primary care [system] supported by a flexible hospital system" (Ahgren and Axelsson 2007). Taken together, these developments seek to strengthen links between local providers, especially in relation to elderly people and those with mental disorders such as dementia. Although the chains of care and local healthcare strategies have evolved on essentially parallel tracks, they are being linked in several places (Karlberg 2008). There is an expectation that the newly formed Swedish Association of Local Authorities and Regions may enhance coordination at the local and regional level.

In summary, there are many strategies being implemented in different countries to address chronic disease, with different systems at different stages of the process and with different degrees of comprehensiveness. For example, they vary in the extent to which they span the spectrum from prevention to palliation, or whether they concentrate on only a small part of that spectrum. It is, however, important to note how most of these countries have made chronic care a priority. The next section will explore whether this prioritization has been matched by appropriate investment.

Supporting the development and implementation of new approaches to chronic care

The evidence reviewed in this volume and in the accompanying one highlight several broad areas where attention is needed in the transition from the traditional model of fragmented care to one where the patient's journey is better coordinated. These include:

- the provision of adequate finances, both to bring about the transition, including the development of new structures and skills, and to sustain the new system
- the creation of an appropriately trained and motivated workforce, imbued with an acceptance of the value of joint working
- information technology, with systems designed to support the new approaches to care and built in flexibility to adapt to future changes.

A fourth issue is the creation of systems that enable patients to self-manage effectively (Chapter 6), an issue that can only be addressed successfully if complemented by the three elements listed above.

Financing

Several countries have, directly or indirectly, set aside considerable resources to support the development and implementation of innovative approaches to chronic care. The precise mechanism has varied, depending on the existing lines of accountability and responsibility. Targeted payments have been used where tiers of government have direct control over delivery, while more decentralized systems have tended to use start-up grants to support the development of new approaches, although this distinction is not clear cut.

For example, the Australian federal and state governments committed, in 2006, a total of AU$500 million (€305 million) over five years to the Australian Better Health Initiative. One of its five priority areas supports targeted training for health professionals to assist people with chronic conditions to manage their condition better. A second priority is to improve coordination of services, backed up by provision of incentive funds (Council of Australian Governments 2006). The Australian government has made available a further AU$15 million (€9 million) from 2006–07 to support additional self-management support strategies, following an earlier injection of AU$36.2 million (€22 million) to test different models for self-management of chronic conditions for their suitability to the Australian context (Sharing Health Care Initiative; Jordan and Osborne 2007).

In France, the provider health networks tasked with strengthening the coordination, integration and continuity of healthcare for those with complex needs are supported by the state and by the social health insurance funds, with a total of €650 million invested between 2000 and 2005 (Durand-Zaleski and Obrecht 2008). Funds can be used to finance networks per se (infrastructure and operating costs) or for new services. Investments have included mobile dialysis units; specialized mental health facilities; new cancer centres that combine research, treatment and prevention; and new centres for management of HIV/AIDS (McKee and Healy 2002). By 2006, approximately 450 networks operated in France, mostly targeting patients with chronic conditions, with patients with diabetes forming a large section (although even then covering only around 5% of the diabetic population in France). The budget for the 2007 national plan on the quality of life for the chronically ill has been set at €727 million for the period 2007–11 (Ministère de la Santé et des Solidarités 2007).

Several countries have used start-up grants to support the development of new approaches to care. For example, the federal government in Canada has supported provincial initiatives through the Primary Healthcare Transition Fund (2000–06) (Jiwani and Dubois 2008). This has, for example, assisted the Alberta government to establish a multidisciplinary chronic disease management team in the Calgary Health Region. The Australian government has allocated funds within the National Primary Care Collaborative Programme to improve service delivery, access and integration of care for patients with complex and chronic conditions, with a "second wave" to be supported by a total AU$34.5 million (€21 million) over four years from 2007/08. Activities in the first wave involved approximately 20% of general practices and included the establishment of disease registers, initiation of service and patient management plans and improved access. In Denmark, the municipal health centres have received an initial funding of 170 million Dkr (€22 million) for 28 experimental initiatives, with the expectation that municipalities will assume financial responsibility from 2008 (Møller Pedersen 2006).

Inevitably, there is a danger that, even where evaluations have been positive, innovations will fail to attract long-term support after the start up funding has ended. Success often depends on the new approaches being incorporated into routine care, and while sustained financing will be a necessary requirement it may not be sufficient, especially where the innovation challenges established ways of working (May 2006).

Several countries have introduced financial incentives for providers and/or purchasers/payers to strengthen care coordination or implement structured disease management programmes. Examples include Australia, Denmark, England, France and Germany. As demonstrated in Chapter 9, the success of these schemes has been mixed and it is important to highlight that where fee for service is the main form of payment in primary care, such as in Australia and Germany, the introduction of additional incentives has led to a high administrative burden that, at least in the Australian case, has acted as a main barrier to implementation of more coordinated approaches to care in general practice (Zwar et al. 2005). In Germany, the high administrative burden linked to the disease management programme has been one of the key criticisms expressed by physicians opposing the programme (Siering 2008), with efforts now underway to relieve the situation (Hilfer et al. 2007).

Other approaches to provide incentives for coordination among providers involve changes to funding mechanisms. For example, the recent structural reforms in Denmark that gave municipalities a greater role in health mean that the municipalities now have to contribute 20% to healthcare funding. This was designed to encourage municipalities to invest in health promotion and preventive treatment while developing alternatives to hospital services (Ankjaer-Jensen and Christiansen 2007). However, there is a risk that this could impede coordination and may potentially lead to a duplication of services provided by municipalities and regions. In Germany, integrated care is being financed through a mechanism that redistributes 1% of the income of sickness funds from ambulatory and hospital care to integrated care pilots. This money can only be used for this purpose (Busse and Riesberg 2004) and, in 2006, a total of €571 million was invested in integrated care pilots (Hilfer et al. 2007).

Workforce and capacity

Chapter 7 demonstrated that human resources are central to the development and implementation of new approaches to chronic care. It also showed that, while several countries are attempting to develop new roles and competencies, few countries have a comprehensive policy framework that goes all the way from educational programmes to mechanisms to integrate new roles and competencies into routine practice. For example, in England, the Department of Health has put considerable effort into developing the workforce, including the development of national workforce competency frameworks (Singh and Fahey 2008). One component is the creation of the new title of community matron, intended as a case manager who can support patients with complex health needs. However, this has initially caused friction within the nursing community as the introduction of community matrons took no account of the similar roles already being undertaken in the community (Hudson 2005).

Chapter 7 also drew attention to the necessity of providing appropriate organizational arrangements for chronic care. It is apparent that countries where primary care has traditionally been provided by doctors, typically in single-handed practices with few support staff, face a major challenge in developing and implementing new roles and competencies. In France, for example, there are even legal barriers to redefining roles and delegating tasks to non-medical personnel. Consequently, it required a change in the law on professional responsibilities before hospital dieticians could assume responsibility for diabetic education and counselling, roles previously performed by endocrinologists (Durand-Zaleski and Obrecht 2008). However, even where there are no such restrictions, payment systems often hinder the delegation of tasks from doctors to other health professionals. For example, although the Enhanced Primary Care scheme in Australia was intended to encourage multidisciplinary care, its impact has been limited because payments for participation in many activities are limited to general practitioners (Glasgow et al. 2008). A lack of appropriate incentives has also been identified as creating barriers to greater involvement by general practitioners in integrated approaches to care in Denmark and the Netherlands (Steuten et al. 2002; Schiotz et al. 2008). In France, the payment of providers on a fee-for-service basis does not encourage improved coordination between physicians and nurses (Durand-Zaleski and Obrecht 2008).

These structural barriers to joint working are often reinforced by professional concerns among physicians about delegating tasks in countries where nurses have traditionally played a minimal role in primary care, as in Canada (Bailey et al. 2006), Germany (Rosemann et al. 2006) and Australia (Oldroyd et al. 2003) (see Chapter 7).

Information technology

Complex systems involving multiple professionals, working across interfaces between sectors, can only function if there are effective mechanisms to transfer information (Hofmarcher et al. 2007; Leutz 1999). Many countries are investing considerable resources in the development of electronic health records, including France, Germany and several provinces in Canada. In some cases, this is as part of a wider national strategy, such as the English National Programme for Information Technology (NPfIT) launched in 2002 (House of Commons Health Committee 2007) and the Australian HealthConnect initiative (Glasgow et al. 2008), working towards the development of broad e-health platforms (Chapter 8). However, progress has been slow, and in some instances, such as in Germany, initiatives have met with substantial criticism by providers because of the costs involved (Tuffs 2007). The English initiative has been criticized for delays in implementation, inadequate safeguards against disclosure of personal data (in part reflection of a series of cases in which official data were lost by government agencies), failure to meet the needs of users and threats to patient safety arising from problems with information retrieval (Hendy et al. 2007).

Clinical information systems that link different providers remain relatively underdeveloped in most settings. Where systems have been developed, their (cost-)effectiveness has been questioned. For example, an audit of 12 health networks in France found that an investment of over €30 million in the development and implementation of systems of shared computerized medical records has had very limited results, with only two networks having succeeded in developing a fully operational system (Durand-Zaleski and Obrecht 2008). A recent survey among countries in the Organisation for Economic Co-operation and Development (OECD) on care coordination showed that only a few countries had put policies in place to enhance information collection and transfer (Hofmarcher et al. 2007).

These problems are unsurprising. Challenges already begin with the seemingly simple task of booking appointments in the health system, which commentators often contrast with the relative ease of on-line booking of airline tickets on the Internet. Yet this is not a valid comparison in the area of chronic disease. Airline websites make it easy to book single journeys, analogous to an acute episode of care. They are much less useful for the traveller seeking to follow a complex journey through many different cities (analogous to a patient with a chronic disease), and even if the passenger succeeds in getting a ticket there is no guarantee that he or she will make all the connections, and even less that their luggage will follow them to their ultimate destination. The demands on information systems designed to support chronic disease management are an order of magnitude more complicated than many of those used to support simple commercial transactions. The difficulties are compounded with increasingly mobile populations, a growing number of whom may be receiving care in different countries. With the possible exception of some localized small-scale projects, existing clinical information systems do not seem to be up to the challenge.

Evaluation

This volume demonstrates clearly how all countries are facing similar challenges in responding to chronic disease yet none have fully satisfactory solutions. There is a critical need to facilitate sharing of experiences, so that countries can learn from each other. This book and the companion volume seek to support this process. Yet reviews such as these can only reflect the available evidence of what works and what does not. It will be apparent to the reader that the expenditure of many millions of euros on innovative approaches to chronic disease management has not been matched by a corresponding effort to evaluate them.

There are, however, a few exceptions. In Australia, all programmes implemented by the federal government are formally evaluated for appropriateness, effectiveness and efficiency, usually by contractors independent of government (Glasgow et al. 2008). These evaluations are designed to inform the government whether or not programmes should be continued (although they do not determine what the decision will be; Box 10.2). In Germany, the legislation enabling the creation of disease management programmes included a statutory requirement that sickness funds would evaluate them to ensure that the programmes complied with the criteria for funding and their goals were being achieved (Siering 2008). Evaluation has to be undertaken by independent contractors, working to methodological specifications established by the Federal Insurance Office, which accredits disease management programmes. However, these evaluations are limited in scope (Hilfer et al. 2007) and, recognizing their shortcomings, one large sickness fund has commissioned a scientific evaluation that will compare prospectively disease management programmes with usual care (Joos et al. 2005).

Initiatives to improve care of those with chronic diseases have also been evaluated in Denmark. The Chronic Disease Self-Management Programme, initially developed in the United States (Chapter 6) to use lay trainers to help patients to develop the necessary skills to coordinate the various elements of their care, was piloted in two sites to ascertain whether it would translate to the Danish context (Schiotz et al. 2008) (the programme was also tested for appropriateness in

Box 10.2   Evaluating the Australian Asthma 3+ Visit Plan

The Asthma 3+ Visit Plan formed part of the Australian asthma management plan. It incorporated financial incentives for general practitioners, with payments claimable if the patient had had at least three asthma-related consultations over four weeks to four months. Consultations had to cover diagnosis and assessment of severity, review of asthma-related medication, provision of a written asthma action plan and education of the patient. It was evaluated at local and national level by researchers independent of government, using multiple methods including eliciting views from general practitioners (survey) and service users (interviews), analysis of Medicare data and focus groups comprising both service users and providers. An additional component focused on its use among Aboriginals and Aboriginal and Torres Strait Islanders. The evaluation revealed several important issues, including difficulties in getting people with asthma to return for all three visits and the challenges that general practitioners confronted when attempting to integrate the relative inflexible structure of the plan into routine practice. In response, the government launched an Asthma Cycle of Care initiative (from 1 November 2006), reducing the number of visits to two and increasing the time permitted to complete the cycle to one year while maintaining the content of the Asthma 3+ Visit Plan. Yet, despite these modifications, there has been little change in the take-up of this approach, indicating the importance of other barriers to changing practice. (Adapted from Glasgow et al. 2008.)

Australia (Australian Government Department of Health and Ageing 2005) and England (Kennedy et al. 2007)). The evaluation was positive, achieving similar results to those in the United States, and the Danish government now works towards rolling the programme out nationally, with the regions to establish a network to ensure the quality of the programme (National Board of Health 2006).

Although the English National Health Service has a large research and development programme, including a Service Delivery and Organization programme, the scale and speed of new initiatives has made it difficult to keep pace with them (Singh and Fahey 2008). In some instances, pilot initiatives have been rolled out before evidence from evaluations was available, illustrated by the example of case management, introduced in nine pilot projects in 2003 but rapidly adopted as national strategy (Department of Health 2004b) (Chapter 4). A subsequent evaluation of the pilots did not find evidence that they had reduced emergency admissions, one of the key goals (Gravelle et al. 2007).

In France there has been less evaluation, although health networks are subject to regular external audit every three years (Durand-Zaleski and Obrecht 2008). The regional health authorities paying for the networks are entitled to discontinue funding if the audits produce adverse findings (Box 10.3). Other care systems are not being evaluated on a systematic basis, which is also the case in

Box 10.3   Auditing health networks in France

In its 2006 report on health networks, the ministerial audit group responsible for health and social affairs noted that the agencies funding the
networks (the state and social health insurance funds) had failed to act on
the networks' internal audits or to request in-depth evaluations where
there was cause for concern. It found no tangible evidence of improved
coordination of the work of office-based and hospital-based physicians
and other health professionals. New management tools, such as electronic
medical records and decision support systems, were mostly viewed as not
sustainable. The cost of networks was considered high (€500 million)
in relation to the results obtained. Yet, despite these findings, there is an
expectation that the networks will ultimately lead to improvements.
(From Durand-Zaleski and Obrecht 2008.)

Germany where, except for the statutory requirement of evaluation disease
management programmes, there is no systematic approach to evaluate other
forms of care targeted at those with chronic illness.

Moving forward

This chapter has identified three key elements that ought to be in place for an
effective response to chronic disease. These are sustained financing, skilled and
motivated health professionals, and supportive information systems. Yet, on
their own, these are not sufficient. Given the limited successes so far, this final
section must be somewhat speculative. Nonetheless, it is possible to draw some
tentative conclusions about what is needed.

First, there is a need to recognize that there is a problem that requires action.
The complexity of chronic diseases and the potential responses to them mean
that solutions will not emerge spontaneously. Those with oversight of the
health system, whether they are health ministries, regional authorities, sickness
funds or provider networks, often working together, must take charge to ensure
that the necessary actions are taken to reconfigure organizational structures,
remove barriers to change and invest in training and information technology.
They must also ensure that the responses are comprehensive, consistent and
contextually appropriate. This volume has provided several examples of ideas
that, in themselves, might have been expected to bring benefits but achieved
less than they might have because they failed to take account of the context in
which they were being implemented or they were not coordinated with other
initiatives.

Second, there is a need to ensure that payment systems encourage rather than
discourage coordination. In some countries, a quest for apparent "efficiency" or
reduction in waiting lists has stimulated the introduction of payment based on
activity. Examples include the use of diagnosis-related groups in Germany and
the so-called "payment by results" policy in England, both of which encourage

the repeated admission of patients to hospital, precisely the opposite of what is desirable for the optimal management of chronic disease.

Third, there is a great need to learn from the many experiences across Europe. In particular, there is a need to understand not only what works but also what works in what circumstances. In other words, what are the structural, organizational and cultural prerequisites for success. It cannot be assumed that something that works in one setting, where there may already be consensus of the value of multidisciplinary working, will work in another.

There are also some questions that those in charge might ask themselves. One relates to the balance, in a particular country, between centrally defined requirements and local autonomy. Given the system of accountability linking the centre and periphery, what is the best way to bring about change? The answer will depend on the national context. The creation of a strict national regulatory framework in Germany has been viewed as beneficial in ensuring that disease management programmes meet an appropriate standard but it has also been criticized for inhibiting further improvements in response to local circumstances (Siering 2008). In contrast, and somewhat unusually given the otherwise highly centralized nature of the system, the lack of "regulation" in England has been seen as contributing to the considerable local variation that exists (Singh and Fahey 2008). A related issue is the balance between top-down versus bottom-up approaches. Ham (2003) has highlighted how competing pressures on organizations arising from policies initiated by healthcare reformers on one hand and established ways of delivery, on the other, are likely to result in a gap between policy intent and actual implementation. A critical role is to be played by professionals, who exert a large degree of control in healthcare organizations such as primary care practices and hospitals. Failure to engage them in the reform process is likely to hamper sustainable change. Indeed, as work on "chains of care" in Sweden has demonstrated, approaches that engaged professionals, or were indeed initiated by professionals themselves, succeeded in developing improved interorganizational and interprofessional coordinated structures while those initiated top-down by councils did not (Ahgren and Axelsson 2007). However, a supportive policy environment was also found to be critical for success.

Another question is whether it will actually be possible to implement change in the existing system or will it require fundamental reform, especially where there are major structural barriers to collaboration (Plochg and Klazinga 2002). Glasgow et al. (2008) noted, "[t]he Australian government together with the State and Territory governments have made a substantial financial commitment to realising improved chronic disease and mental health outcomes . . . The reforms planned are incremental rather than radical and the fundamental division of responsibilities in healthcare between the federal and state governments looks likely to remain. The jury is out on whether these reforms will be able to be carried through and will be sufficient to respond to the challenge of chronic disease." The German disease management programmes involve a financing system that is a departure from the existing payment mechanisms in the social insurance system. However, does this call these existing mechanisms into question?

A related question is whether restructuring undertaken for other reasons will make the response to chronic disease easier or more difficult. In Denmark, recent administrative reforms are seen as providing an opportunity to improve coordination, although several commentators noted that it could potentially increase resource use (Ankjaer-Jensen and Christiansen 2007; Strandberg-Larsen et al. 2007). Similarly, recent reforms in the Netherlands, introducing greater competition, have been seen by some as offering the possibility of implementing more integrated approaches while others suggest that they may make it more difficult (Custers et al. 2007). In England, the relentless pace of reorganization of the National Health Service is viewed as having impeded initiatives to coordinate care (Hardy et al. 2006).

Conclusions

The increased burden of complex chronic diseases, coupled with the growing clinical and organizational opportunities to manage them, poses the greatest challenge to health policy makers over the coming decades. It is no longer possible to muddle through, hoping that appropriate responses will somehow emerge. Instead, it is necessary to understand the nature of changing health needs, to design an effective response, to implement it and, recognizing the fact that nothing stands still, to monitor and reassess. Success is not impossible, but the difficulties should not be underestimated. A first step is to recognize that something must be done. A second, which we hope will be facilitated by the evidence provided in this book, is to realize that something actually can be done, and that they can do it.

References

Ahgren, B. (2003) Chain of Care development in Sweden: results of a national study, *Int J Integr Care*, 3: e01.

Ahgren, B. and Axelsson, R. (2007) Determinants of integrated health care development: chains of care in Sweden, *Int J Health Plann Manage*, 22: 145–57.

Alazri, M., Neal, R., Heywood, P. and Leese, B. (2006) Patients' experiences of continuity in the care of type 2 diabetes: a focus group study in primary care *Br J Gen Pract*, 56: 488–95.

Andersson, G. and Karlberg, I. (2000) Integrated care for the elderly. The background and effects of the reform of Swedish care of the elderly, *Int J Integr Care*, 1: 1–12.

Ankjaer-Jensen, A. and Christiansen, T. (2007) Municipal co-payment for health care services. *Health Policy Monitor*, October. http://www.hpm.org/survey/dk/a10/3 (accessed 11 February 2008).

Australian Government Department of Health and Ageing (2005) *National Evaluation of the Sharing Health Care Initiative. Final Technical Report.* Canberra: Australian Government Department of Health and Ageing.

Bailey, P., Jones, L. and Way, D. (2006) Family physician/nurse practitioner: stories of collaboration, *J Adv Nursing*, 53: 381–91.

Bartholomée, Y. and Maarse, H. (2007) Empowering the chronically ill? Patient collectives in the new Dutch health insurance system, *Health Policy* 84: 162–9.

Boerma, W. (2006) Coordination and integration in European primary care, in R. Saltman,

A. Rico and W. Boerma (eds) *Primary Care in the Driver's Seat? Organizational Reform in European Primary Care*, pp.3–21. Maidenhead, UK: Open University Press.

Busse, R. (2004) Disease management programmes in Germany's statutory health insurance system, *Health Aff*, 23: 56–67.

Busse, R. and Riesberg, A. (2004) *Health Care Systems in Transition: Germany*. Copenhagen: WHO Regional Office for Europe on behalf of the European Observatory on Health Systems and Policies.

Calnan, M., Hutten, J. and Tiljak, H. (2006) The challenge of coordination: the role of primary care professionals in promoting care across the interface, in R. Saltman, A. Rico and W. Boerma (eds) *Primary Care in the Driver's Seat? Organizational Reform in European Primary Care*, pp.85–104. Maidenhead: Open University Press.

Cole, A. (2005) UK GP activity exceeds expectations, *BMJ*, 331: 536.

Council of Australian Governments (2006) *Better Health for all Australians. Action Plan*. Canberra: Council of Australian Governments.

Custers, T., Arah, O.A. and Klazinga, N.S. (2007) Is there a business case for quality in the Netherlands? A critical analysis of the recent reforms of the health care system, *Health Policy*, 82: 226–39.

den Exter, A., Hermans, H., Dosljak, M. and Busse, R. (2004) *Health Care Systems in Transition: The Netherlands*. Copenhagen: WHO Regional Office for Europe on behalf of the European Observatory on Health Systems and Policies.

Department of Health (2004a) *Choosing Health. Making Healthy Choices Easier*. London: Department of Health.

Department of Health (2004b) *NHS Improvement Plan. Putting People at the Heart of Public Services*. London: Department of Health.

Department of Health (2005) *Supporting People with Long Term Conditions. An NHS and Social Care Model to Support Local Innovation and Integration*. London: Department of Health.

Department of Health (2006) *Our Health, Our Care, Our Say: A New Direction for Community Services*. London: Department of Health.

Dowling, B., Powell, M. and Glendinning, C. (2004) Conceptualising successful partnerships, *Health Soc Care Commun*, 12: 309–17.

Durand-Zaleski, I. and Obrecht, O. (2008) France, in E. Nolte, C. Knai and M. McKee (eds) *Managing Chronic Conditions: Experience in Eight Countries*. Copenhagen: European Observatory on Health Systems and Policies.

Epping-Jordan, J., Pruitt, S., Bengoa, R. and Wagner, E. (2004) Improving the quality of care for chronic conditions, *Qual Saf Health Care*, 13: 299–305.

Fabbricotti, I. (2007) *Taking Care of Integrated Care: Integration and Fragmentation in the Development of Integrated Care Arrangements*. Rotterdam: Erasmus University.

Freeman, G., Woloshynowych, M., Baker, R. et al. (2007) *Continuity of Care 2006: What Have We Learned since 2000 and What are Policy Imperatives Now?* London: National Co-ordinating Centre for NHS Service Delivery and Organisation R&D.

Frossard, M., Benin, N., Guisset, M. and Villez, A. (2002) *Providing Integrated Health and Social Care for Older Persons in France: An Old Idea with a Great Future*. Paris: Union Nationale Interfédédérale des Oeuvres et Organismes Privés Sanitaires et Sociaux.

Gerst, T. and Korzilius, H. (2005) Disease-Management-Programme: Viel Geld im Spiel, *Dtsch Ärztebl*, 102: A2904–9.

Glasby, J., Dickinson, H. and Peck, E. (2006) Guest editorial: partnership working in health and social care, *Health Soc Care Commun*, 14: 373–4.

Glasgow, N., Zwar, N., Harris, M., Hasan, I. and Jowsey, T. (2008) Australia, in E. Nolte, C. Knai and M. McKee (eds) *Managing Chronic Conditions: Experience in Eight Countries*. Copenhagen: European Observatory on Health Systems and Policies.

Goodwin, N., Perri, 6, Peck, E., Freeman, T. and Posaner, R. (2004) *Managing Across Diverse*

Networks of Care: Lessons from Other Sectors. London: National Co-ordinating Centre for NHS Service Delivery and Organisation R&D.

Gravelle, H., Dusheiko, M., Sheaff, R. et al. (2007) Impact of case management (Evercare) on frail elderly patients: controlled before and after analysis of quantitative outcome data, *BMJ*, 334: 31–4.

Ham, C. (2003) Improving the performance of health services: the role of clinical leadership, *Lancet*, 361: 1978–80.

Hardy, B., Mur-Veemanu, I., Steenbergen, M. and Wistow, G. (1999) Inter-agency services in England and the Netherlands, *Health Policy*, 48: 87–105.

Hardy, B., Hudson, B., Keen, J., Young, R. and Robinson, M. (2006) *Partnership and Complexity in Continuity of Care: A Study of Vertical and Horizontal Integration Across Organisational and Professional Boundaries*. London: National Co-ordinating Centre for NHS Service Delivery and Organisation R&D.

Healy, J., Sharman, E. and Lokuge, B. (2006) Australia: health system review. *Health Syst Transit*, 8:1–158.

Hendy, J., Fulop, N., Reeves, B.C., Hutchings, A. and Collin, S. (2007) Implementing the NHS information technology programme: qualitative study of progress in acute trusts, *BMJ*, 334: 1360.

Hilfer, S., Riesberg, A. and Egger, B. (2007) Adapting social security health care systems to trends in chronic disease: Germany, in *Proceedings of the ISSA Technical Commission on Medical Care and Sickness Insurance*. Moscow: World Health Organization and the International Social Security Association.

Hofmarcher, M., Oxley, H. and Rusticelli, E. (2007) *Improved Health System Performance Through Better Care Coordination*. Paris: OECD.

House of Commons Health Committee (2007) *The Electronic Patient Record*. London: The Stationary Office.

Hudson, B. (2005) Sea change or quick fix? Policy on long-term conditions in England, *Health Soc Care Commun*, 13: 378–85.

Jiwani, I. and Dubois, C. (2008) Canada, in E. Nolte, C. Knai and M. McKee (eds) *Managing Chronic Conditions: Experience in Eight Countries*. Copenhagen: European Observatory on Health Systems and Policies.

Joos, S., Rosemann, T., Heiderhoff, M. et al. (2005) ELSID-Diabetes study-evaluation of a large scale implementation of disease management programmes for patients with type 2 diabetes. Rationale, design and conduct: a study protocol, *BMC Public Health*, 5: 99.

Jordan, J.E. and Osborne, R.H. (2007) Chronic disease self-management education programs: challenges ahead, *MJA*, 186: 84–7.

Karlberg, I. (2008) Sweden, in E. Nolte, C. Knai and M. McKee (eds) *Managing Chronic Conditions: Experience in Eight Countries*. Copenhagen: European Observatory on Health Systems and Policies.

Kennedy, A., Reeves, D., Bower, P. et al. (2007) The effectiveness and cost effectiveness of a national lay-led self care support programme for patients with long-term conditions: a pragmatic randomised controlled trial, *J Epidemiol Commun Health*, 61: 254–61.

Klein-Lankhorst, E. and Spreeuwenberg, C. (2008) The Netherlands, in E. Nolte, C. Knai and M. McKee (eds) *Managing Chronic Conditions: Experience in Eight Countries*. Copenhagen: European Observatory on Health Systems and Policies.

Leutz, W. (1999) Five laws for integrating medical and social services: lessons from the United States and the United Kingdom, *Milbank Q*, 77: 77–110.

May, C. (2006) A rational model for assessing and evaluating complex interventions in health care, *BMC Health Serv Res*, 6: 86.

McKee, M. and Healy, J. (2002) Réorganisation des systèmes hospitaliers: leçons tirées de l'Europe de l'Ouest, *Rev Med Assur Mal*, 33: 31–6.

Ministère de la Santé et des Solidarités (2007) *Plan pour l'amélioration de la Qualité de Vie des Personnes atteintes de maladies chroniques*. Paris: Ministère de la Santé et des Solidarités.

Ministry of the Interior and Health (2003) *Healthy throughout Life: The Targets and Strategies for Public Health Policy of the Government of Denmark, 2002–2010*. Copenhagen: Ministry of the Interior and Health.

Møller Pedersen, K. (2006) Experiments with municipal health centres, *Health Policy Monitor* 2006. http://hpm.org/survey/dk/a8/1 (accessed 18 February 2008).

National Board of Health (2005) *National Board of Health Project on Major Noncommunicable Diseases*. Copenhagen: Danish National Board of Health.

National Board of Health (2006) *Chronic Conditions: Patients, Healthcare and Community*. Copenhagen: Danish National Board of Health.

National Health Priority Action Council (2005) *National Chronic Disease Strategy*. Canberra: Australian Government Department of Health and Ageing.

Nolte, E., Knai, C. and McKee, M. (eds) (2008) *Managing Chronic Conditions: Experience in Eight Countries*. Copenhagen, European Observatory on Health Systems and Policies.

NSW Department of Health (2004a) *NSW Chronic Care Program 2000–2003. Strengthening Capacity for Chronic Care in the NSW Health System*. Sydney: NSW Department of Health.

NSW Department of Health (2004b) *NSW Chronic Care Program. Phase Two 2003–2006*. Sydney: NSW Department of Health.

Oldroyd, J., Proudfoot, J., Infante, F. et al. (2003) Providing healthcare for people with chronic illness: the views of Australian GPs, *Med J Aust*, 179: 30–3.

Plochg, T. and Klazinga, N. (2002) Community-based integrated care: myth or must? *Int J Qual Health Care*, 14: 91–101.

Plochg, T., Delnoij, D., Hoogedoorn, N. and Klazinga, N. (2006) Collaborating while competing? The sustainability of community-based integrated care initiatives through a health partnership, *BMC Health Serv Res*, 6: 37.

Roland, M. (2004) Linking physicians' pay to the quality of care: a major experiment in the United Kingdom, *N Engl J Med*, 351: 1448–54.

Rosemann, T., Joest, K., Körner, T. et al. (2006) How can the practice nurse be more involved in the care of the chronically ill? The perspectives of GPs, patients and practice nurses, *BMC Fam Pract*, 7: 14.

Sandier, S., Paris, V. and Polton, D. (2004) France: health care systems in transition. *Health Syst Transit*, 6:1–156.

Schiotz, M., Frolich, A. and Krasnik, A. (2008) Denmark, in E. Nolte, C. Knai and M. McKee (eds) *Managing Chronic Conditions: Experience in Eight Countries*. Copenhagen: European Observatory on Health Systems and Policies.

Schoen, C., Osborn, R., Doty, M. et al. (2007) Toward higher-performance health systems: adults' health care experiences in seven countries, 2007, *Health Aff*, 26: w717–34.

Segal, L., Dunt, D. and Day, S. (2004) Introducing coordinated care (2): evaluation of design features and implementation processes implications for a preferred health system reform model, *Health Policy*, 69: 215–28.

Siering, U. (2008) Germany, in E. Nolte, C. Knai and M. McKee (eds) *Managing Chronic Conditions: Experience in Eight Countries*. Copenhagen: European Observatory on Health Systems and Policies.

Singh, D. (2005) *Transforming Chronic Care. Evidence about Improving Care for People with Long-term Conditions*. Birmingham: University of Birmingham, Surrey and Sussex PCT Alliance.

Singh, D. and Fahey, D. (2008) England, in E. Nolte, C. Knai and M. McKee (eds) *Managing Chronic Conditions: Experience in Eight Countries*. Copenhagen: European Observatory on Health Systems and Policies.

Smith, S., Allwright, S. and O'Dowd, T. (2007) Effectiveness of shared care across the interface between primary and specialty care in chronic disease management, *CochraneDatabase Syst Rev*, CD004910.

Starfield, B., Shi, L. and Macinko, J. (2005) Contribution of primary care to health systems and health, *Milbank Q*, 83: 457–502.

Steuten, L.M. G., Vrijhief, H.J.M., Spreeuwenberg, C. and Van Merode, G.G. (2002) Participation of general practitioners in disease management: experiences from the Netherlands, *Int J Integr Care* 2: e24.

Strandberg-Larsen, M., Nielsen, M., Vallgårda, S. et al. (2007) Denmark: Health system review, *Health Syst Transit*, 9: 1–64.

Stromberg, A., Martensson, J., Fridlund, B. and Dahlstrom, U. (2001) Nurse-led heart failure clinics in Sweden, *Eur J Heart Fail*, 3: 139–44.

Tuffs, A. (2007) German doctors threaten to boycott patient record project, *BMJ*, 334: 63.

Turner, D., Tarrant, C., Windridge, K. et al. (2007) Do patients value continuity of care in general practice? An investigation using stated preference discrete choice experiments, *J Health Serv Res Policy*, 12: 132–7.

van der Linden, B., Spreeuwenberg, C. and Schrijvers, A. (2001) Integration of care in the Netherlands: the development of transmural care since 1994, *Health Policy*, 55: 111–20.

Vondeling, H. (2004) Economic evaluation of integrated care: an introduction, *Int J Integr Care*, 4: e20.

Vrijhoef, H., Spreeuwenberg, C., Eijkelberg, I., Wolffenbuttel, B. and van Merode, G. (2001) Adoption of disease management model for diabetes in region of Maastricht, *BMJ*, 323: 983–5.

Weeramanthri, T., Hendy, S., Connors, C. et al. (2003) The Northern Territory preventable chronic disease strategy: promoting an integrated and life course approach to chronic disease in Australia, *Aust Health Rev*, 26: 31–42.

Zwar, N., Comino, E., Hasan, I. and Harris, M. (2005) General practitioner views on barriers and facilitators to implementation of the Asthma 3+ Visit Plan, *Med J Aust*, 183: 64–7.

Zwar, N., Harris, M., Griffiths, R. et al. (2006) *A Systematic Review of Chronic Disease Management*. Sydney: Australian Primary Health Care Institute.

Index

absenteeism, 129, 158
accountability, 35, 83, 109, 147, 224, 239
acquired immunodeficiency syndrome
    (AIDS), 1, 16, 42, 105, 233
action planning, 134
active living, 107, 111
acute care, 7, 152, 198, 226
acute medical model, 145, 222
adherence, 103
administrative burden, 162, 234
administrative workers, 153
advanced practice nurses, 74, 82
adverse reactions, 3
adverse selection costs, 53
advertising bans, 96, 97, 103
advice, 103, 138, 150
advocacy, 111
affections de longue durée (ALD), 229
ageing, 17–18, 106, 143
Agency for Healthcare Quality, 213
alcohol
    abuse, 92, 94, 103–4, 110, 124
    consumption, 102, 106, 121, 153
    policy, 97
Alcoholics Anonymous, 103
ALD, see affections de longue durée
alternative care, 5, 70
alternative contact methods, 137
ambulatory care, 160, 217
ambulatory peritoneal dialysis, 153

anal carcinoma, 105
angina, 120
antibiotics, 105, 106
anticoagulation, 184
antihypertensive drugs, 102, 103, 110
anxiety, 45, 130
appointments, 235–6
architects, 108
arthritis, 16, 32, 124, 128–31, 153
Arthritis Self-Management Program (ASMP),
    128, 130
ASE model, *see* attitude/social influence/self-
    efficacy model
ASMP, *see* Arthritis Self-Management Program
assessment, 75, 145, 183
assistants, 158
asthma
    as chronic disease, 1
    DALYs, 28
    epidemiological data, 8
    in children, 16, 25, 27, 125
    management, 68, 237
    morbidity, 27
    mortality, 16, 25, 27–9
    nurses, 84, 155
    participation of patients, 5
    prevalence, 25, 27
    projected trends, 27–8
    self-management support programmes, 128
    use of CCDSS for, 183

Asthma Cycle of Care Initiative, 237
atrial fibrillation, 184
attitude/social influence/self-efficacy (ASE)
    model, 122, 123
audits, 36, 79, 147, 165, 177, 238
Australia
    advice from doctors in, 138
    ASMP in, 128
    Asthma 3+ Visit Plan, 237
    Better Health Initiative, 232–3
    Coordinated Care Trials, 218
    coordination of care in, 223
    diabetes self-management education, 129
    disease management programmes, 233
    e-health platforms in, 181
    electronic decision support, 179
    Enhanced Primary Care package, 204, 205,
        217, 228, 235
    evaluation of programmes, 56, 236, 237
    health policy, 228
    influence of CCM in, 75, 76
    innovation in chronic care, 227
    payment models, 163
    quality of care in, 2
    self-care in, 117
    self-management support in, 137
    shortage of human resources, 154
autonomy, 125, 127, 181, 224

bariatric surgery, 100, 102
barriers
    to change, 10, 238
    to collaboration, 222, 239
    to computerized clinical decision support
        systems, 181
    to cooperation, 43
    to coordination, 222
    to integration, 222, 224, 227
    to multidisciplinary team work, 163
    to optimal payment systems, 10
    to self-management, 121, 135
bed days, 82
behaviour change, 4, 102, 120
behavioural control, 123
behavioural counselling, 110
behavioural management, 128
behavioural risk factors, 205
behavioural theories, 125
Belgium
    sickness fund calculations, 200
    unipolar depressive disorders, 30
    use of HPV vaccination, 105
benchmarking, 197, 215
Bentham, Jeremy, 121
bereavement, 45
best practices, 2
Better Health Initiative (Australia), 228, 232–3
biofeedback, 130
birth rates, 154
blended payments, 163, 199, 218
blood glucose, 19, 110, 129, 136

blood pressure, 19, 56, 94, 98, 102, 103, 110,
    129, 136, 200, 205, 208
body mass index, 30, 48, 100, 101
bone loss, 104
bonuses, 199, 213
bottlenecks, 162
bottom-up models, 174, 239
breast cancer, 98, 104, 109
breast feeding, 101
breathlessness, 22
brief negotiation, 121
buddying, 135
budgetary horizons, 224
budgets, 108, 198
built environment, 100
bupropion, 97, 110
burden of disease framework, 93, 94
business case, 58, 60

call centres, 137, 189
Canada
    advice from doctors in, 138
    ASMP, 128
    CDSMP, 128
    comorbidity in, 32, 33
    disease management in, 56
    e-health platforms in, 181
    electronic health records in, 235
    fears of deskilling in, 158
    healthcare system, 231
    influence of CCM in, 75
    innovation in chronic care, 227
    interdisciplinary teamwork initiatives, 159
    payment models, 163
    primary care networks in, 155
    self-management support programmes, 129
    shortage of human resources, 154
    use of incentives, 150
    written self-care instructions, 224
cancer
    alcohol abuse and, 103
    mortality from, 36, 95, 97
    obesity and, 98
    prevention, 105
    registries, 34
    role of individual behaviour, 153
    role of viruses, 104
    screening, 109
    sedentary lifestyle and, 104
    support programmes for, 128
    tobacco and, 94–7
    use of hospices for, 5
cancer centres, 233
capitation, 136, 197, 198, 199, 203, 208, 217,
    218
cardiac disease, *see* heart disease
cardiovascular damage, 101
cardiovascular disease, 100, 101, 109, 153; *see
    also* heart disease
    costs, 46
    diabetes and, 22

impact, 50, 116
mortality, 36, 95, 96
obesity and, 98
prevention, 95, 109
risk factors, 102
tobacco as cause, 94
care; *see also* health care *and* social care
coordination, 218
involvement of professionals in, 5
management, 74
models, 65, 151, 222–4
multidisciplinary, 70, 145, 205
planning, 78, 155, 157, 163, 183, 217
preventive, 150, 213
primary, 73, 74, 83–5, 122, 149, 150, 155,
    161, 172, 216, 217, 224–6, 234
processes, 162, 183
protocol driven, 6
rehabilitative, 230
secondary, 84, 149, 150, 155, 224, 225
shared, 226, 230
transmural, 225, 226, 230
variations in preferences for, 4
carers, 127, 130, 144, 152
carved-out programmes, 68
case conferences, 163, 217
case fees, 198, 199
case-level coordination, 146
case management, 9, 65, 70, 72, 74, 77, 81–3,
    145, 150, 157, 179, 214, 218, 226, 229,
    234
Caucasus, 34
causality, 47, 48, 50
CCDSS, *see* computerized clinical decision
    support systems
CCM, *see* Chronic Care Model
CDSMP, *see* Chronic Disease Self-management
    Program
cell phones, 189
central Asian republics, 19, 28
cerebrovascular disease, 16, 18–21, 42; *see also*
    stroke
cervical cancer, 105, 109
cervical screening, 209
cessation services, 97
chains of care, 231, 239
change management, 158
checklists, 176
Chechnya, 34
chemoprevention, 109
chemotherapy, 110
CHESS, *see* Comprehensive Health
    Enhancement Support System
CHF, *see* congestive heart failure
child health surveillance, 209
children
    asthma, 16, 25, 27, 125
    hepatitis B vaccine for, 105
    increasing incidence of chronic disease, 18
    lack of self-management support
        programmes for, 128

management of illness in, 43
mental disorders, 28
obesity, 18, 19, 98, 99, 107, 111
physical activity in, 104
sedentary lifestyles, 107
cholesterol, 94, 98, 103, 106
chronic bronchitis, 22; *see also* chronic
    obstructive pulmonary disease
chronic care, 9, 64–91, 143–71, 202, 227,
    232–8
Chronic Care Model (CCM), 6, 7, 10, 64,
    75–81, 83, 85, 116, 119, 120, 144, 160,
    172, 173, 181, 190, 205, 215
chronic disease
    burden, 1, 8, 44–53
    cause of disability, 15
    complexity, 10
    computerized clinical decision support,
        182–3
    costs, 3, 8, 44, 53–5, 195–221
    data collection, 35
    definition, 1, 7, 42
    determinants, 93
    distal influences, 106–7
    impact, 92
    integration of care, 64–91
    management, 7–10, 43–70, 77–9, 81–5, 109,
        119, 143, 148–50, 181–2, 189, 196, 200–4,
        226, 231, 233
    measurement, 36
    mortality from, 15, 36, 49
    prevalence, 15, 64
    prevention, 9, 35, 43–64, 92–115, 231
    psychological effects, 117
    risk factors, 1, 9, 36, 46, 92–107
Chronic Disease Management Programme,
    119
Chronic Disease Prevention and Management
    Framework, 231
Chronic Disease Self-management Program
    (CDSMP), 126, 127, 128, 129, 130, 133,
    236
chronic obstructive pulmonary disease
    (COPD), 16, 22, 25, 126
    as chronic disease, 42
    definition, 35
    effectiveness of computerized decision
        support systems, 183–4
    epidemiological data, 8
    knowledge about medication as factor, 134
    mortality from, 22, 25, 26
    nurse-led clinics, 84
    rehabilitation for, 157
    smoking as causative factor, 25
clean indoor air legislation, 111
clinical information systems, 6, 79, 80, 83,
    150, 163, 235
cognitive-behavioural interventions, 120, 125
collaborative approach, 6, 120, 203
collaborative care, 65, 120
collaborative training, 160

colon cancer, 104
communicable disease, 1, 16, 43
communication, 126, 128, 133, 146, 158
communication systems, 107, 111
community-based care, 97, 154, 161, 229
community health services, 44
community interventions, 137
community matrons, 82, 83, 150, 234
community perspective, 75
community resources, 79
community service models, 7
comorbidity, 3, 32–3, 69, 131, 132, 133, 151,
    184; *see also* multimorbidity
competing demands, 132
complaints, 208
complementary insurance, 54
complex continuing care, 159
complex needs, 131–3
compliance, 157, 177, 203
Comprehensive Health Enhancement
    Support System (CHESS), 127
comprehensiveness, 83
compression of morbidity, 17–18
computer literacy, 181, 184
computer-based decision support tools, 132
computer-based support systems, 177, 179–81
computerized clinical decision support
    systems (CCDSS), 173, 177, 179–86
computerized guidelines, 183, 184
community linkages, 83
condom use, 124
congestive heart failure (CHF), 2, 16, 17, 68,
    77, 79
consultations, 136, 209
consumer groups, 230
contingency theory, 66
continuing medical education, 177
continuing professional development, 161
continuity of care, 9, 83, 152, 225
continuous incentives, 215
contraceptive services, 209
cooperation, 43, 90, 222, 225, 226
coordination, 8–10, 65, 70, 83, 90, 146, 182,
    205, 223, 224, 226, 228, 229, 231, 232,
    235
copayment, 200, 211
COPD, *see* chronic obstructive pulmonary
    disease
coping strategies, 133
coronary artery disease, 47, 80, 104
coronary heart disease, 47, 80
corruption, 97
cost-benefit comparison, 63
cost controllers, 67
cost-effectiveness, 52, 63, 65, 109
costs
    adverse selection, 53
    concepts, 44
    containment, 158
    direct, 44–6
    economic, 44

employer, 53, 54
external, 52
indirect, 8, 45, 46, 158
internal, 51
macroeconomic, 44, 49
measurement, 63
medications, 8
microeconomic, 44, 47–8
of beneficial behaviours, 121
of cardiovascular disease, 46
of care for older people, 81
of CCM interventions, 77
of chronic disease, 3, 8, 44, 53–5
of diagnosis, 44
of e-health initiative in Germany, 235
of hospitalization, 63
of illness, 44–7
of new technology, 10
of obesity interventions, 100, 102
of prevention, 44
of risky behaviours, 121
of treatment, 44
operating, 53
private, 51
reductions, 77, 156
relevant/irrelevant, 44, 51–2
savings, 55, 57, 67
set-up, 53
true economic, 50–1
welfare, 44, 50–1
cost sharing, 200–1
counselling, 103, 109, 133, 134, 147, 148
counterfactuals, 47
cream skimming, 200, 214
crime, 104, 107
critical pathways, 174
cultural integration, 71
cultural issues, 4, 135, 189
current wheezing, 25
cycles, 224
Czech Republic, 21, 100

DALYs, *see* disability-adjusted life years
data
    analysis, 36
    audit trails, 36
    collection, 36
    epidemiological, 8
    lack of, 15
    mortality, 16, 50
    utilization, 19
deaths; *see also* mortality
    attributable to risk factors, 94
    problems in certifying, 34
decision aids, 183, 189, 190
decisional balance theory, 121
decision making, 123, 158, 184, 189
decision support, 10, 77, 79, 80, 83, 172–94
    intervention types, 178
    research, 190–1
    strategies, 173–4

systems, 10, 163, 174–84, 190, 238
tools, 133, 143, 173–6
DECODE study, 22
deductive inference engines, 179
delegation, 147, 158, 235
deliberative model, 148
delivery
  models, 72–7
  systems, 6, 10, 77, 79, 80, 83, 144
demedicalization, 66
dementia, 16, 19, 30, 35, 127
demographic changes, 92, 93, 106
Denmark
  administrative reforms, 240
  ASMP in, 128
  barriers to integrated approaches, 235
  COPD in, 25
  disease management programmes, 233
  evaluation of programmes, 236
  greater role of municipalities in health, 234
  health policy, 228
  innovation in chronic care, 227
  municipal health centres, 233
  reform of health system, 228
  self-care in, 117
dependency ratio, 106, 154
depression, 1, 8, 16, 19, 28, 30, 32, 36, 42, 47,
    78, 80, 104, 123, 128, 130–3, 183
deprofessionalization, 157
dermatological conditions, 98
deskilling, 158
diabetes
  as chronic disease, 1
  as growing burden, 36
  blood pressure control, 208
  cardiovascular disease and, 22
  care programmes, 77, 128
  centres, 129
  coexistence with CHF, 17
  DALYs lost through, 21
  decision support systems for, 182–4
  depression and, 32
  disease management programmes and, 56
  epidemiological data, 8
  evidence-based interventions, 120
  expenditure on, 3, 47
  impact, 116
  impact of CCM, 80
  in France, 233
  management, 57, 68, 77, 80, 81
  mortality, 16, 22, 24,
  networks, 129
  nurse-led clinics, 84
  nurses, 84, 155
  obesity and, 98–101
  participation of patients, 5
  patients' access to education, 134
  physicians, 84
  prevalence, 16, 21, 22, 23, 34–5
  provider education, 78
  quality of care, 2, 80

role of individual behaviour, 153
screening, 109, 214
sedentary lifestyle and, 104
self-management education, 129
self-management support programmes, 119
stroke and, 19
tobacco use, 94
diagnosis, 7, 22, 44, 149, 158
diagnosis related groups, 199
diastolic blood pressure, 102
diet, 92, 94, 101, 102, 110, 121, 124, 153
dietary advice, 182
dietary energy, 100
dieticians, 84, 129, 155, 234
differentiation, 66
direct costs, 44–6
direct payments, 200–1
direct provision, 146
disability, 15, 16, 18, 19, 21, 30, 41, 49, 93,
    131, 132, 135
disability-adjusted life years (DALYs), 16, 18,
    19, 21, 28
disadvantaged groups, 9, 133
discharge, 57
Disease Control Priorities Project, 95, 108
disease prevention, *see* prevention
disease registers, 233
disease-specific carveouts, 212
disfigurement, 124
disincentives to interprofessional practice,
    162
distal influences, 106–7
district nurses, 146
diversification, 157
documentation, 36
drinking history, 110
drugs
  abuse, 124
  adverse reactions, 3
  combinations of, 3
  dosage adjustment, 182
  trials, 3
drunk-driving laws, 103
Dutch National Panel of the Chronically Ill
    and Disabled, 132
dyspepsia, 105, 106

early detection/diagnosis, 149, 150
econometric approach, 63
economic costs, 44
economic efficiency, 158
economic evaluation, 53
economic growth, 49, 50
economics, 43–64
education, 48, 77–8, 103, 111, 120, 134–6,
    147, 155–7, 160, 165, 172, 176
educational materials, 79
educational programmes, 67
educational sessions, 79
educational technology, 176
efficiency, 51

e-health, 173, 181–2, 189, 190, 235
elderly people, *see* older people
electronic clinical decision tools, 176
electronic guidelines, 183
electronic health records, 163, 182, 187, 189,
    190, 235
electronic medical records, 137, 238
electronic systems, 10, 173
eligibility criteria, 72
emergency admissions, 82, 83
emergency bed-days, 229
emergency departments, 77
emergency room, 57
emergency services, 81
emergency visits, 148
emotional impact, 120
emotional management, 128
emotional support, 148
emphysema, 22; *see also* chronic obstructive
    pulmonary disease
employer costs, 53, 54
employer perspectives, 53
empowerment, 1, 4, 9, 120, 136, 177, 189,
    190, 203
endocrinologists, 84, 234
end-of-year bonus, 215
endoscopy, 106
England
    case management in, 82–3
    influence of CCM in, 75
    integrated organizations in, 146
    lack of regulation in, 239
Enhanced Primary Care (EPC) (Australia), 204,
    205, 217, 228, 235
environment, 4, 92, 93, 100, 107
EPC, *see* Enhanced Primary Care
epidemiological approach, 63
epidemiological evidence, 8
episodic model, 2, 64
Epstein-Barr virus, 105
errors, 151, 201
ethnicity, 135
ethnic minorities, 133, 187
European Health Survey System, 35
Eurostat, 35
evaluation, 53, 56, 181, 236–8
Evercare model, 74, 76, 81, 82
evidence
    balance with intuition, 6
    epidemiological, 8
    for cost-effectiveness, 52
    for impact of CCM, 80, 85
evidence-based guidelines, 79, 172, 173, 196,
    229
evidence-based interventions, 120, 182
evidence-based practice, 2, 9, 97, 143, 151
evolutionary systems, 181
exercise, 102, 110, 121, 128, 130, 153, 182
    on prescription, 137
Expanded Chronic Care framework, 149
Expert Patient Programme, 119, 128, 129, 136

expert systems, 172, 179
external costs, 52
externalities, 52
eye examinations, 155, 182

factor VIII, 153
falls, 104
family members, 127, 130, 153
Family Partnership Intervention, 127
family therapy, 103, 110
fasting blood glucose, 110
fatigue, 126
fat intake reduction and exercise
    (REVESDIAB), 129
fat tax, 99
FCTC, *see* Framework Convention on Tobacco
    Control
fear of encroachment, 157
Federal Insurance Office (Germany), 236
feedback, 78, 79, 135, 147, 163, 165, 181, 189
fee-for-service payments, 162, 197, 198, 199,
    205, 210, 213, 214, 217, 218
fertility, 15, 106
financial barriers, 224
financial flows, 196
financial frameworks, 224
financial incentives, 123, 136, 204–15, 218,
    233, 234, 237
financial management, 71
financial needs, 70
financing, 67, 195, 232–4, 238
Finland, 25, 30, 95, 96, 100
fixed-dose therapies, 103
folic acid, 103
food history, 110
food policy, 97, 111
food prohibitions, 100
food service workers, 153
foot care, 129
foot examinations, 2, 155, 182
foot therapists, 84
formal caregivers, 152, 154
fragmentation, 69, 217, 222, 224, 226, 227,
    232
Framework Convention on Tobacco Control
    (FCTC), 97
frameworks, 72–7, 93, 165
Framingham study, 19
France
    asthma in, 25
    auditing health networks in, 238
    case fees in, 199
    comorbidity in, 33
    concerns regarding coordination and
        continuity, 229
    DALYs due to stroke, 19, 21
    diabetes networks, 129
    discouragement of self-management
        support in, 136
    disease management programmes, 233
    electronic health records in, 235

evaluation of programmes, 237–8
innovations in chronic care, 227, 229–30
Internet portal for chronic conditions, 181
legal barriers to role redefinition, 234
legal definition of professional roles, 155
unipolar depressive disorders in, 30
use of copayments in, 211
functional ability, 124
functional independence, 4
functional integration, 71
functional status, 129
funder/insurers, 196, 202
funding, 10, 72, 143, 146, 150, 225, 227, 229

gall bladder disease, 98
gastric cancer, 105
gastritis, 105
gatekeeping, 83, 84, 217, 224
general practitioner contract, 199
generic competences, 10, 158–61
Germany
    asthma in, 25
    case fees in, 199
    comorbidity in, 33
    coordination of care, 223
    decentralization in, 229
    diagnosis-related groups, 238
    disease management programmes, 233
    electronic health records in, 235
    evaluation of programmes, 236, 238
    innovations in chronic care, 227, 230
    integrated care in, 234
    management incentives for payers/
        purchasers, 210–11
    national regulatory framework, 239
    prevalence of diabetes in, 22
    sickness fund calculations, 200
    use of copayments in, 211
    written self-care instructions, 223
Global Burden of Disease Study, 16, 28, 41, 43
globalization, 92, 93, 98, 99, 106–7
glucose control, 133
glycosylated haemoglobin, 205
goal setting, 120, 134, 135
grants, 226
Greece, 22, 28, 30
group education, 147
Group Health Centre, Ontario, 56
group interventions, 137
group visits, 136
guidelines, 2, 3, 78, 79, 103, 136, 165, 172–8,
    181, 183, 184, 191, 229
guilt-provoking language, 127

haemophilia, 153
Health and Protection Directorate-General, 35
health behaviour, 120
Health Canada, 159
healthcare; *see also* care
    access to, 5, 148
    advances in, 2, 32

approaches, 9
continuity of, 9, 83, 152, 225
delivering, 85, 227
financing, 10, 67
growing complexity, 5, 7, 8
interface with social care, 65, 224
key issues, 2
models, 6, 5, 151, 222–4
services, 151
skills, 148
system, 9, 111, 112, 116
utilization, 3, 77
Healthcare Information and Management
    Systems Society, 177–81
health centres, 146, 228
HealthConnect, 235
health education, 111
Health First, 137
HealthIn-site, 137
health insurance schemes, 53
health networks (France), 229, 238
health plans, 53, 212
health promotion, 108, 152, 159, 229
health services, 108–11
health statistics, 36
health status, 120
Healthy Throughout Life strategy (Denmark),
    228
heart disease, 1, 95, 101–3; *see also*
    cardiovascular disease
heart failure, 2, 3, 17, 42, 68, 84, 119, 120,
    183, 184
heart failure clinics, 84, 156
Helicobacter pylori, 105, 109
hepatic cancer, 105
hepatic cirrhosis, 103
hepatitis, 104, 105
hepatitis B, 109
hepatitis B vaccine, 105
hepatitis C virus, 105
herpes simplex, 105
HIV, *see* human immunodeficiency virus
holistic perspective, 143
home care, 127, 153, 189
home monitoring devices, 137
home visits, 77
hospices, 5
hospital admissions, 77, 82, 83, 129, 148, 150
hospital discharge rates, 19, 21
hospitalization, 63, 81, 82, 116, 120
hospitalization rates, 56
hospitals, 5
housekeeping staff, 153
housing, 149
human-capital approach, 45
HPV *see* human papilloma virus
human immunodeficiency virus (HIV), 1, 16,
    42, 105, 233
human papilloma virus (HPV), 104, 105, 109
human resource continuum, 152–4
human resources, 10, 71, 143–71, 234–5

Hungary, 21, 95
hypercholesterolaemia, 92, 94, 101
hyperlipidaemia, 78
hypertension, 17, 78, 84, 92, 94, 101, 102, 106, 120, 129, 183, 184

ICHA, *see* Interactive Health Communication Applications
IECPCP, *see* Interprofessional Education for Collaborative Patient-centred Practice Initiative
illness representations, 123, 135
immigration, 106
immunization, 105, 109
inactivity, 132
inappropriate prescribing, 3
incentives, 121, 123, 136, 163, 195, 198, 199, 201–15, 218, 230, 233–5, 237
incidence approach, 63
income, 49, 132, 133, 135
index conditions, 32
indicators, 16, 36, 209
indigent populations, 187
indirect costs, 8, 45, 46, 158
individual care plans, 82
individual education, 147
individualized care planning, 150
individualized treatment plans, 4
individual prevention programmes, 108
infectious diseases, 34, 92, 94, 104–6
infertility, 98
informal carers, 130, 144, 152, 153, 154, 161
information dissemination, 111
information infrastructures, 184
information management, 71
information shocks, 95
information systems, 6, 10, 162, 163, 172, 196, 224, 225, 238
information technology, 6, 11, 43, 159, 163, 184, 197, 216, 232, 235–6, 238
infrastructure payments, 199, 208
in-house disease management, 68
Innovative Care for Chronic Conditions, 76, 149
inpatient care, 44, 161
insulin, 98, 110, 129
insurance, 9, 49, 53, 54, 58, 68, 133, 135, 189, 200, 202, 230
intangible costs, 45–7
integration, 9, 10, 64–91, 111, 143–7, 164, 204, 212, 224, 225–7, 234, 235, 240
Interactive Health Communication Applications (ICHAs), 184, 188
interagency coordination, 146
interdisciplinary working, 146, 147, 159
intermediate care, 147
internal costs, 51
internalities, 52
internal motivation, 218
International Obesity Task Force, 98
Internet, 4, 6, 127, 137, 181, 187, 189

interprofessional coordination, 146
Interprofessional Education for Collaborative Patient-centred Practice Initiative (IECPCP), 159
intra-personal externalities, 52
intrinsic motivation, 201
intuition, 6
investment, 48, 225, 233
Ireland, 21, 28
ISARE project, 36
ischaemic heart disease, 95, 101, 102
Israel, 19, 22, 30
Italy, 21, 32, 33

job design, 10, 163
job diversification, 10
job expansion, 10
job security, 224
joint working group practices, 71
junk food businesses, 108

Kaiser Foundation Health Plan, 90–1
Kaiser Foundation Hospitals, 91
Kaiser Permanente, 57, 73, 74, 90, 121
Kaiser triangle, 76
Kazakhstan, 19, 34
knowledge, 133, 135
Kyrgyzstan, 19, 25, 34

labelling restrictions, 97
laboratory testing, 110
labour productivity, 48–9, 55, 57
labour supply, 48, 49
language, 133, 134, 135
Latvia, 25
lay caregivers, 152
lay workers, 153
leadership, 10, 108, 129, 227
legal frameworks, 224
legislation, 157
legitimacy barriers, 224
length of stay, 56
levels of care, 74
liability, 189
liaison nurses, 157
licensing, 103
life cycle approach, 63
life expectancy, 49, 228
lifespan, 154
lifestyle, 1, 101, 108, 110, 111, 120, 123, 128, 149
linkage, 72, 90, 145
lipids, 98, 110, 133, 205
Lithuania, 21
Live Better Everyday programme, 128
liver cancers, 105
liver flukes, 105
Live well with COPD, 148
local government, 104
local healthcare (*narsjukvard*) (Sweden), 231
local health integration networks, 231

local services networks, 231
longevity, 1, 18
longitudinality, 83
long-term beds, 21
long-term treatment, 2
low-income communities, 153
lung cancer, 93–6
Luxembourg, 105

machine learning systems, 179
macroeconomic costs/consequences, 44, 49
macro-level principles, 76
maintenance, 123
malaria, 50
malnutrition, 50
managed care, 9, 65, 67
management, 146
management style, 164
maternity services, 209
measurement instruments, 36
measures of utilization, 78
mechanical clinical decision tools, 176
Medicaid, 68, 214, 218
Medicare, 68, 74, 136, 210, 218
medication, 8, 45, 121, 126, 128, 133, 134,
    151, 157, 182
mental disorders, 1, 8, 28
mental health centres, 214
mental health facilities, 233
mental health navigators, 155
mental illness, 16, 41, 47, 132, 133
mergers contracting, 71
meso-level principles, 76
meta-analyses, 77, 78, 79, 129, 200
meta-guidelines, 133
methodology, 33, 35, 49, 56, 130–1
microeconomic costs/consequences, 44, 47–8
micro-level principles, 76
micromanagement techniques, 73
migration, 5
Mill, John Stuart, 121
mixed payment models, 218
mobile dialysis units, 233
modelling, 124
models of care, 65, 151, 222–4
Moldova, 34
MONICA Project, 34
monitoring, 82, 103, 135, 136, 145, 164
morbidity
    attributable to chronic disease, 34
    compression of, 17–18
    from asthma, 27
    from ischemic heart disease, 101
    in allocations to sickness funds, 200
    indirect costs of, 45
    in Global Burden of Disease study, 43
    markers, 34
    monetary value of, 47
    patterns, 8
    prevention, 93
mortality

data, 16, 50
effects of case management, 82
from asthma, 16, 25, 27–9
from cancer, 36, 95, 97
from cardiovascular diseases, 36, 95, 96
from cerebrovascular disease/stroke, 16, 19,
    20
from chronic disease, 15, 36, 49
from COPD, 22, 25, 26
from diabetes, 16, 22, 24
from heart disease/failure, 17, 95, 101
impact on economic growth, 50
in Global Burden of Disease study, 43
monetary value of, 47
predictor of economic growth, 49
risk, 51, 106
smoking-attributable, 96
statistics, 33–4
motivation, 10, 79, 121, 125, 134–5, 151, 195,
    201, 203, 218, 232, 238
motivators, 195
MRFIT, *see* Multiple Risk Factor Intervention
    Trial
multicollinearity, 63
multicomponent approaches, 130
multidisciplinary care, 70, 145, 205
multidisciplinary management, 196
multidisciplinary teams, 77, 79, 148, 162, 182,
    215, 217, 226, 229, 239
multimorbidity, 2–4, 32–3, 35, 116, 131, 132,
    133, 157, 198; *see also* comorbidity
multinational cooperation, 107
multiple conditions, *see* multimorbidity *and*
    comorbidity
multiple medication, 3–4
Multiple Risk Factor Intervention Trial
    (MRFIT), 106
multiple risk factor reduction approach, 112
multiple sclerosis, as chronic disease, 42
multiprofessionalism, 146
multi-skilled workers, 157
multispeciality teams, 77
municipal health centres (Denmark), 233
municipalities (Denmark), 234
muscular strength, 104
musculoskeletal disorders, 1, 98
myocardial infarction, 123

National Chronic Disease Strategy (Australia),
    228
National Health Information Management
    Advisory Council (Australia), 179
National Institute of Clinical Studies, 179
National Integrated Diabetes Program, 56
National Library of Medicine, 42
nationally integrated strategies, 227
National Primary Care Collaborative
    Programme (Australia), 233
National Programme for Information
    Technology (NPfIT), 235
National Service Frameworks, 229

National Service Improvement Frameworks (Australia), 228
national workforce competency frameworks, 234
NCDs, *see* non-communicable diseases
needs, 70–7, 156
  complex, 131–3, 157
  financial, 70
  for behavioural change, 172
  future, 5
  psychosocial, 70
  support, 131–5
Netherlands
  ASMP in, 128
  asthma in, 27
  barriers to integrated approaches, 235
  case fees in, 199
  comorbidity in, 33
  competing private insurers in, 202
  DALYs due to stroke in, 21
  decentralization in, 229
  diabetes management programme, 57
  GP contracts in, 136
  innovation in chronic care, 227
  integrated delivery systems in, 226
  primary care, 84
  reforms in, 240
  regulation of professional qualifications, 155
  sickness fund calculations, 200
  study on inactivity, 133
  transmural care in, 225, 226, 230
networks, 71
neural network, 179
neuropsychiatric diseases, 28, 30, 32
newsletters, 129
New South Wales, 76
New Zealand
  advice from doctors in, 138
  capitated primary health organizations, 218
  coordination of care in, 223
  disability from stroke in, 21
  quality of care in, 2
  written self-care instructions, 224
NHS and Social Care Model, 76, 229
nicotine therapies, 97, 110
non-communicable diseases (NCDs), 16
non-directive counselling, 110
non-institutional services, 73
Nordrheinische Gemeinsame Einrichtung Disease Management Programme, 85
North Karelia Project, 95
Norway
  comorbidity in, 33
  COPD in, 25
  unipolar depressive disorders in, 32
  use of HPV vaccination in, 105
nurse aides, 158
nurse anaesthetists, 155
nurse-led clinics, 77, 84, 129, 155, 156

nurse practitioners, 155, 158
nurses' education, 147

obesity
  as risk factor, 92, 101, 107
  chemotherapy for, 110
  control, 100
  cost of intervention, 100, 102
  expenditure, 47
  in children, 18, 19, 98, 99, 107, 111
  integrated interventions, 111–12
  mortality, 94, 106
  prevalence, 98
  relationship with blood pressure, 98
  relationship with cancer, 98
  relationship with cardiovascular disease, 98
  relationship with dementia, 30
  relationship with diabetes, 98–101
  relationship with respiratory disease, 98
  stigma, 49
  surgery for, 110
observational learning, 124
occupational therapists, 155
off-site programmes, 68
older people
  access to healthcare, 187
  case management for, 82
  community-based care for, 229
  complex needs, 131
  costs of care, 81
  disability in, 30
  in Denmark, 228
  increasing number of chronically ill, 173
  in Sweden, 232
  mental health problems, 133
  multiple health problems, 2
  self-management interventions, 125, 129
  support for, 84
  weight-bearing exercises for, 204
Omega-3 fatty acids, 110
on-site programmes, 68
operating costs, 53
optimization of therapy, 75
oral hypoglycaemic drugs, 110
organizational change, 159, 225
organizational competencies, 151
organizational culture, 162, 164
organizational philosophy/values, 164
organizational quality standards, 209
organizational structures, 10
organizational theory, 66
organizational turbulence, 225
Orlistat, 102
osteoarthritis, 104, 129, 183
osteoporosis, 98
osteoporotic fractures, 104
outcomes, 124, 156, 162, 172, 173, 175, 180, 197, 203, 212, 225, 81
outliers, 199
out-of-pocket payment, 200, 201
output payments, 199

outreach work, 155
overweight, 94, 98–101, 110; *see also* obesity

pain, 45, 121, 124, 126, 129, 130, 131
pain killers, 117
palliative care, 153
Pan-Canadian Healthy Living Strategy, 231
Papanicolau tests, 105
paper-based clinical decision tools, 176, 177
paper-based guidelines, 183–4
paper reminders, 177
partnering model, 148
partnerships, 159, 225
passive smoking, 94
paternalistic model, 147, 148
path dependency, 85
pathways, 176
patient activation, 120, 135, 190
patient-centred care, 9, 65, 158
patient education, 130, 182
patient-oriented approach, 81
patient–provider relationship, 136
patients
    behaviour, 4, 9
    chronic disease management and, 53
    collaboration with professionals, 6
    compliance, 203
    disadvantaged, 9, 33
    education, 77, 78, 79, 120, 134
    empowerment, 1, 4, 9, 136, 177, 189, 190,
        203
    guides, 129
    incentives for, 211
    monitoring, 136
    motivational counselling, 79
    needs, 70, 156
    perspectives, 53
    preferences, 4
    satisfaction, 156, 157
    self-management support, 79
    support for, 64, 131–5
patient surveys, 209
payer/purchaser, 195, 196
payment by activity, 59
payment by results, 59, 238
payment for performance, 136, 196, 197, 205,
    211, 213–16, 218, 228
payment methods, 10, 162, 163, 211–17, 235
PCNs, *see* primary care networks, 155
peak respiratory flow, 136
peer modelling, 124
peer support, 124, 135, 153
peer-to-peer mentorship, 137
penile cancer, 105
pensions, 49
per diem payments, 198
performance-based payment; *see* payment for
    performance
performance information, 218
performance measures, 203
performance monitoring, 215

performance targets, 212
Permanente Medical Group, 91
personal data, 235
person-centred approaches, 66, 145, 148, 149,
    164
perspectives, 53, 75
pharmaceutical companies, 67
pharmaceutical industry, 108, 189
pharmacists, 155
physical activity, 101, 102, 104, 106, 107, 110,
    112
physical environment, 149
physical functioning, 9
physical inactivity, 63, 94
physical work, 104
Physician's Service Agreement, 136
pilot initiatives, 237
Pittsburgh, 80
Planet health, 102
planners, 154
planning, 100, 145, 146, 172, 224
plaque formation, 103
Poland, 21, 100
policing, 103
policy
    alcohol, 97, 103–4, 161
    food, 97
    public, 44, 51–2
policy makers, 9, 43, 64, 138, 154, 175
pollution, 107
polypills, 103, 110
pooler, 195
pooling, 73
population-based approaches, 9, 33, 68, 145,
    149, 159, 164
population goals, 101
population health promotion, 149
population management (care) model, 73
Portugal, 22
post-hospital discharge follow-up, 157
poverty, 92, 106; *see also* disadvantaged
    groups
practice-based commissioners, 59, 146
practice environment, 162–4
practice guidelines, 183
Practice Incentive Programme, 205
practice information leaflets, 208
practitioners
    education sessions for, 165
    fear of encroachment, 157
    role, 148
precontemplation, 123, 134
premiums, 54
prerequisites, 201–3
prescribing, 3, 226
prevalence approach, 63
prevalence rates
    as markers of morbidity, 34
    asthma, 25, 27
    diabetes, 16, 21, 22, 23, 34–5
    difficulty in estimating, 34, 35

obesity, 98
of chronic disease, 15
stroke, 19, 21
prevention
activities, 159
balancing with treatment, 5
costs, 44
evidence based, 9
of cancer, 105
of cardiovascular disease, 103, 109
of chronic disease, 9, 35, 43–64, 92–115,
149, 229
primary, 93, 100, 102
responsibility for, 9
secondary, 93, 102
strategies, 121
tertiary, 93
preventive care, 150, 213
preventive practice standards, 111
primary care, 73, 74, 83–5, 122, 149, 150, 155,
161, 172, 216, 217, 224–6, 234
primary care centres (Sweden), 174, 231
primary care networks (PCNs), 155
primary care nurses, 156
primary care trusts, 58, 146, 229
primary data collection, 36
primary healthcare, *see* primary care
Primary Healthcare Transition Fund (Canada),
163, 233
primary prevention, 93, 100, 102
priorities, 80
priority indicators, 36
privacy, 189
private costs, 51
private home care, 153
private insurance systems, 202
private-public partnership, 108
private sector, 9, 112
proactive order, 6, 178
proactive teams, 135
problem solving, 120, 127, 131
procedural barriers, 224
process quality, 203
productivity, 8, 44, 48–9, 55, 57, 87, 199
professional barriers, 224, 225
professional boundaries, 64, 155
professional cultures, 224
professional education, 160
professional integration, 71
professional interest groups, 155
professional rivalry, 225
professional roles, 157
professionals
collaboration with patients, 6
communication with, 126
in self-management support, 120
involvement in care, 5
professional values, 147
programmatic interventions, 120
promotion bans, 96
protocol-driven care, 6

protocols, 78, 84, 163, 172, 173, 178, 201,
203, 204, 207, 211, 224, 231
provider payment incentives, 205, 208–10
provider payment/reimbursement, 197
providers, 9, 64, 85, 154, 195, 202, 231
psychobehavioural methods, 130
psychological effects, 117
psychological functioning, 9
psychological support, 148
psychosocial needs, 70
psychosocial support, 82, 130, 152
psychotherapy, 125
public information, 95, 99, 100, 111
public policy, 51–2
public reporting of performance, 212
pulmonary rehabilitation, 157
purchase, 146
pyramid of care, 74

QOF, *see* Quality and Outcomes Framework
quality-adjusted life years, 102
Quality and Outcomes Framework (QOF),
208, 216–17
quality assurance, 208
quality-based payment, 196, 197
quality-based purchasing, 197, 211, 212, 213
quality improvement, 57, 71, 145, 149–51,
164, 201
Quality Improvement and Outcomes
Framework, 163
quality management, 159
quality measures, 214
quality of care, 2, 80, 82, 157, 158, 182, 231
quality of life, 56, 123, 127, 130, 131, 152, 228
quality of service, 201, 212
quality-related requirements, 208
quality rewards, 208
quasi-externalities, 52
Quebec, 32, 148

race, 107
RAND Health Insurance Experiment, 200
randomized controlled trials, 56
rational choice theory, 121–3
rationality, 51, 52
reactive alerts, 178
readiness to change, 135
readmissions, 56
reconfiguring roles, 154–8
recording, 216
recreational facilities, 107
reference information, 178
referrals, 82, 103, 110, 146, 155
reflexive attitude, 145
regression analysis, 63
regulation, 204, 227
regulatory boundaries, 155
rehabilitation, 44, 45, 152, 159
rehabilitative care, 230
reimbursement schedules, 187
reinforcers, 195

relapse, 123
relevant/irrelevant costs, 44, 51–2
reminders, 78, 147, 183
remission, 124
renal disease, 101, 102, 183
renal failure, 16, 42
reputational incentives, 211, 212, 213, 218
research
    decision support, 190–1
    into partnership working, 225
    on self-management support programmes,
        137
resources, 82, 133–4, 153, 162, 163, 164,
    199–200, 228
respiratory disease, 22–8, 98
respiratory rehabilitation programme, 126
retirement, 48, 49
reverse causality, 50
rheumatoid arthritis, 129–30
risk-adjusted capitation formula, 210
risk-adjusted performance bonuses, 218
risk adjustment, 203
risk assessment tools, 150
risk associations, 93
risk-equalization formula, 202
risk-equalization mechanisms, 54
risk factors, 1, 9, 36, 46, 92–107, 111, 205,
    216
risk minimization, 7
risk stratification, 74, 229
risk structure compensation scheme, 210–11,
    230
road safety, 107
robotics, 164
roles, 10, 120, 128, 135, 147, 154–8
Romania, 28
Russian Federation, 19, 28

safety, 107, 151, 159, 197, 198, 208, 235
salary, 197, 198
savings, 48
schistosomes, 105
schizophrenia, 1, 28, 47
school lunches, 111
school programmes, 100
schools, 111
screening, 72, 103, 109, 133, 149, 214
seamless care, 65
secondary care, 84, 149, 150, 155, 224, 225
secondary prevention, 93, 102
second-generation disease management, 69
second-hand smoke, 111
sedentary lifestyle, 92, 94, 101, 104, 107
segregation, 90
self-care, 57, 116–43, 156,
    providers, 152, 153, 161
self-caregivers, 144, 154
self-determination theory, 122, 125
self-efficacy, 120, 123, 124, 128, 131, 133
self-help manuals, 97
self-interest, 224

self-management support, 6, 9, 75, 77, 79, 80,
    83, 116–42, 150, 158, 184–7, 189, 190
self-monitoring, 80
self-perception theory, 121
self-regulation, 122, 123, 128, 131
self-reports, 22, 130
senior nurses, 82, 83
serology, 105
serum glycosylated haemoglobin, 56, 182
serum lipids, 56
service delivery, 64, 74, 76, 163, 222
Service Delivery and Organization
    programme (England), 237
Service Improvement Payments, 205
service navigation, 157
service users' perspectives, 147–8
set-up costs, 53
shared care, 226, 230
shared learning approaches, 165
Sharing Healthcare Initiative, 57
sickness funds, 210, 211
single-payer social health insurance schemes,
    203
skills, 10, 125, 131, 135, 145, 147, 148, 151,
    155, 157, 158, 161, 162
Slovakia, 21
Slovenia, 21, 30
smokers, 109, 111
smoker's cough, 22
smoking, 25, 93–6, 101, 106, 110, 112, 121,
    124, 153, 213
smuggling, 97
social care, 45, 65, 67, 69, 148, 153, 224, 225
social cognitive theory, 122, 124
social deprivation, 116
social disadvantage, 111
social functioning, 9
social health insurance funds (France), 233
Social Health Modernization Act (Germany),
    230
social inequalities, 106
social influences, 124
social insurance, 58, 84, 202
social integration, 71
social justice, 106
social learning theory, 122, 124, 128
socially disadvantaged people, 104
social models, 7
social network, 125, 135
social norms, 124
social services, 150
social support, 124, 128, 133, 156
social welfare, 50
socioeconomic factors, 4, 16
socioeconomic status, 93, 107, 149
software design, 189
Spain
    asthma in, 27
    COPD in, 25
    lung cancer mortality, 95
    unipolar depressive disorders in, 30

specialist nurses, 74, 82, 129, 155, 156
speciality care, 226
specialization, 156
sports, 104
staff competences, 158
stages of change theory, 123
stakeholders, 2, 174, 180, 189
standardized education, 78
standards, 107, 212
Stanford Patient Education Research Center, 130
Starfield, Barbara, 83
start-up costs, 225
start-up grants, 232, 233
statins, 103
statistical discrimination analysis, 179
status barriers, 224
stomach cancer, 105
stomach ulcer, 105
strategic alliances, 71
strategic planning, 71
street walkability, 107
stress, 106, 122–5
stress-coping model, 124–5
stress-coping theory, 122
stroke; *see also* cerebrovascular disease
    as cause of disability, 19, 21
    association with depression, 19
    association with diabetes, 19
    epidemiological data, 8
    hypertension and, 101, 102
    impact, 116
    increased risk of dementia after, 19
    mortality from, 19, 20
    prevalence, 19, 21
    regional variations, 19–21
    sedentary lifestyle and, 104
    self-management support programmes for, 127
structural barriers, 224, 239
stumbling, 104
subjective norms, 123
subsidies, 100, 226
substitution effect, 48
substitutive insurance, 54
suicide, 28
supplementary insurance, 54
support groups, 125
support needs, 131–5
support workers, 153, 158
Sweden
    asthma in, 27
    chains of care, 239
    chronic care services, 146
    coordination between providers in, 231
    diabetes self-management support, 129
    innovation in chronic care, 227
    nurse-led clinics, 84
    redefinition of nurses' role in, 156
    use of HPV vaccination in, 105

Swedish Association of Local Authorities and Regions, 232
Switzerland, 19, 21, 105
symptom management, 121, 128, 130
system change, 83, 159
systems approach, 66, 75, 109
systolic blood pressure, 102

target-driven payments, 208, 217
targets, 173, 209, 228, 229
task-oriented approach, 145
taxation, 58, 99, 100, 103, 200, 203
taxonomies, 32, 70–2
teaching methods, 130
teams, 146, 162
teamwork, 10, 160
technology, 143, 157, 162–4
telecare, 137
telecommunications devices, 164
teleHealth, 184, 187, 190
telemedicine, 157
telephone-based nursing, 133
terminal phase, 127
tertiary prevention, 93
test ordering, 182
text messaging, 137
theory of planned behaviour, 122, 123
theory of reasoned action, 122
therapeutic advances, 18
therapeutic alliance, 109
therpeutic support communities, 103
time-consistent preferences, 51, 52
T-lymphotrophic virus, 105
tobacco
    as risk factor, 107
    control programmes, 94–6
    expenditure, 47
    industry, 108
    interventions, 95–7
    socioeconomic status and, 106
    use, 92
top-down models, 174, 239
Toronto Rehabilitation, 159
Torres Strait Islanders, 237
Tower of Babel story, 65
trade policy, 107, 111
traffic safety, 104
training, 10, 77, 147, 155, 158–61, 164, 184, 225, 232, 238
Transdnistria, 34
trans-fatty acids, 99, 100, 111
transitions, 72, 145, 159
transmural care, 65, 225, 226, 230
transparency, 35
transport emissions, 107
transport systems, 111
trans-theoretical model, 122, 123–4, 134
treatment, 2, 4, 5, 18, 19, 44, 70
triangle of care, 74, 195
true economic costs, 50–1

turf guarding, 225
Turkey, 21

ulcer-causing factors, 106
unipolar depressive disorders, 16, 28, 30–2
United Kingdom
  ASMP, 128
  asthma, 27, 28
  chronic disease management programmes,
    109
  COPD, 25
  DALYs due to stroke, 21
  e-health platforms, 181
  electronic medical records, 189
  Expert Patient Programme, 129
  future needs for healthcare, 5
  GP contracts, 136, 199, 205, 208–9
  health strategy, 228–9
  lack of advice from doctors in, 138
  lung cancer in, 97
  partnership working in, 225
  payments in, 196, 204
  prevalence of stroke in, 21
  primary care, 84
  Quality and Outcome Framework, 208,
    216–17
  quality of care, 2
  shared care, 230
  specialist nurses, 155
  use of HPV vaccination, 105
  year of care approach, 210
United States
  ASMP, 128
  CDSMP, 129
  comorbidity, 33
  development of case fees, 199
  disease management initiatives, 68
  electronic medical records, 189
  evidence on disease management, 81
  lack of advice from doctors, 138
  lung cancer, 94

payment in, 10, 196, 213–15
prevalence of diabetes, 21
prevalence of stroke, 21
research, 44
shortage of human resources, 154
use of hepatitis B vaccine, 105
written self-care instructions, 224
UnitedHealth Group, 74
urban design, 107
urban planning, 107, 108
user–provider relationships, 158
utilization data, 19
utilization management, 57

vaccination, 43, 109, 213
value for money, 52
valve replacement, 184
vascular disease, 103
vertical delegation, 147
Veterans Health Administration, 83, 215
visual acuity, 200
voluntary services, 154
vouchers, 121
Wagner, Edward, 75
waiting times, 43, 203, 238
walking programmes, 137
Warfarin, 3
weight, 104, 110, 121, 124, 129, 137,
  205
welfare costs, 44, 50–1
whole-systems approach, 66, 136, 151
willingness-to-pay method, 45, 50
workforce, 6, 10, 143–71, 234–5
workplaces, 111
work practices, 10
worksite-based health risk reduction, 107
World Bank, 95
World Health Organization, 1, 20, 34
written care instructions, 222, 223

year of care approach, 210